Pharmaceutical Engineering

Pharmaceutical Engineering

D. Yashwant Dugyala

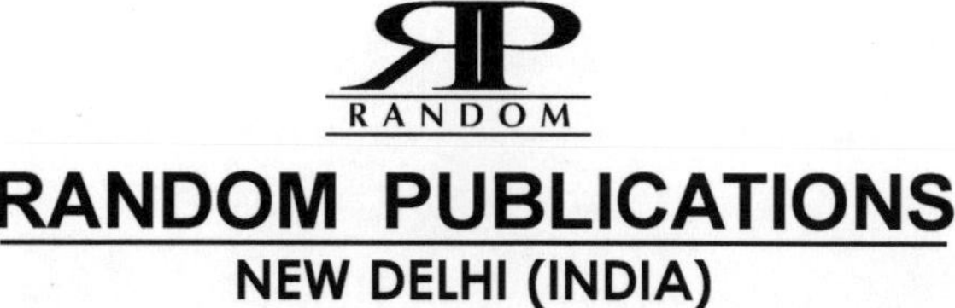

Pharmaceutical Engineering

ISBN 978-93-5111-576-2

Published in 2015 in India by

RANDOM PUBLICATIONS

Reprint : 2015

4376-A/4B, Gali Murari Lal, Ansari Road

New Delhi-110 002

Phone : +9111-43580356, 011-23289044, 011-43142548

e-mail: sales@randompublications.com,

info@randompublications.com, randomexports@gmail.com

Type Setting by : Friends Media, Delhi-110089

Digitally Printed at: Replika Press Pvt. Ltd.

Preface

Pharmaceutical Engineering is a branch of pharmaceutical science and technology that involves development and manufacturing of products, processes, and components in the pharmaceuticals industry. While developing pharmaceutical products involves many interrelated disciplines, the specific subfield of "pharmaceutical engineering" has only emerged recently as a distinct engineering discipline. This now brings the problem-solving principles and quantitative training of engineering to complement the other scientific fields already involved in drug development. Pharmaceutical engineers are involved in the conception, design, construction, and operation of research facilities and manufacturing plants, where they also are involved in the conception, design, scale-up, manufacturing, and labeling and packaging processes in the conversion of chemical and biological materials into valuable pharmaceuticals and pharmaceutical therapies. They have to implement FDA regulations, validation assurance (VA), quality control, and maintain Good Manufacturing Practices (GMP) compliant facilities. In addition to the safety of the end product, they have to maintain a level of personal and environmental safety.

I would like to thank my team for standing beside me throughout my career and writing this book. My special thanks go to "Random Publications" who have published the book.

– D. Yashwant Dugyala

Contents

1

Introduction

Pharmaceutical Engineering is a branch of pharmaceutical science and technology that involves development and manufacturing of products, processes, and components in the pharmaceuticals industry. While developing pharmaceutical products involves many interrelated disciplines, the specific subfield of "pharmaceutical engineering" has only emerged recently as a distinct engineering discipline. This now brings the problem-solving principles and quantitative training of *engineering* to complement the other scientific fields already involved in drug development.

ACADEMIC PROGRAMMES

There are still relatively few academic programmes with this explicit focus. The first one began at the University of Michigan, as a joint project between their College of Engineering and School of Pharmacy. Because such programmes are not yet common, many pharmaceutical engineers have had their formal engineering training in chemical or biomedical engineering.

Most Pharmaceutical Engineering programmes are graduate-level, and as with Biomedical Engineering there is generally an expectation that engineers and scientists working in pharmaceutical engineering should have some relevant graduate-level education. Many have a masters or PhD degree in chemical or biomedical engineering, or a related science. In Italy there is a university degree course (5 years) in Chemistry and Pharmaceutical Technologies(Chimica e Tecnologie Farmaceutiche), different from pharmacy, that ability as a pharmacist and different roles in the industry as an engineer (for the Italian legislation is not really an engineer though performs the same tasks).

PROFESSIONAL LICENSURE/CERTIFICATION

In most jurisdictions, engineering licensure (*e.g.* Licensed "Professional Engineer" or P.E.) is not discipline-specific, so any licensed engineer with competency in pharmaceutical engineering may qualify as licensed. However, in the U.S., most pharmaceutical engineers fall under the "industrial exemption," which does not require a (P.E.) license for those engineers whose work is completely internal and for a private employer. There are ongoing debates about whether to narrow or eliminate this exemption from engineering licensure, and the Executive Director of the National Society of Professional Engineers (NSPE) recently advocated requiring licensure for engineers in the pharmaceutical industry (among a few others).

Most U.S. jurisdictions require two examinations as part of their licensing criteria, the second of which allows electing a particular discipline of emphasis (while not affecting the license itself, as noted above), so pharmaceutical engineers are likely to select the testing option of either chemical engineering or biomedical engineering (which are generally considered the closest available options).

There is also a private (non-governmental) certification offered by the professional organization International Society for Pharmaceutical Engineering (ISPE), known as *Certified Pharmaceutical Industry Professional (CPIP)*. This tends to focus more on (later-stage) manufacturing and commercialization issues, etc., rather than early-stage things like drug design, discovery assays, and preclinical development.

COMMON SPECIALTIES

- *Pharmaceutical Development Sciences*: Broadly, assays or techniques for discovering, modifying, or designing drug substances or excipients; in particular, *rational drug design* - as a relatively recent alternative to traditional trial-and-error drug discovery processes - relies upon principles of engineering more than many other pharmaceutical sciences such as formulation or medicinal chemistry.
- *Bio-/Pharmaceutical Manufacturing Science*: Optimal processes for producing drug substances and products with quality and efficiency
- *Clinical Science:* Applying engineering principles towards conduct of studies to assess safety and efficacy, for the medical community and regulators
- *Regulatory Science:* Scientific bases for regulatory decision-making (typically by the FDA, in the U.S.), with an emphasis on risk-benefit analysis
- *Pharmaceutical Devices*: Designing instruments, tools, or implants which facilitate the making, handling, or use of drugs (*e.g.* drug delivery chips)

These specialties overlap with other engineering areas as well as non-engineering scientific and medical fields, although in all specialties Pharmaceutical Engineers tend to have a distinct focus on product and process design and quantitative analysis.

And in addition to these technical areas, some pharmaceutical engineers pursue careers as business or legal professionals. Their scientific and engineering background is often suitable for careers in management, patent law, or even entrepreneurship - for example.

PHARMACOLOGY

Pharmacology is the branch of medicine and biology concerned with the study of drug action, where a drug can be broadly defined as any man-made, natural, or endogenous (within the body) molecule which exerts a biochemical and/or physiological effect on the cell, tissue, organ, or organism. More specifically, it is the study of the interactions that occur between a living organism and chemicals that affect normal or abnormal biochemical function. If substances have medicinal properties, they are considered pharmaceuticals.

The field encompasses drug composition and properties, synthesis and drug design, molecular and cellular mechanisms, organ/systems mechanisms, signal transduction/cellular communication, molecular diagnostics, interactions, toxicology, chemical biology, therapy, and medical applications and antipathogenic capabilities.

The two main areas of pharmacology are pharmacodynamics and pharmacokinetics. The former studies the effects of the drug on biological systems, and the latter the effects of biological systems on the drug. In broad terms, pharmacodynamics discusses the chemicals with biological receptors, and pharmacokinetics discusses the absorption, distribution, metabolism, and excretion (ADME) of chemicals from the biological systems. Pharmacology is not synonymous with pharmacy and the two terms are frequently confused.

Pharmacology, a biomedical science, deals with the research, discovery, and characterization of chemicals which show biological effects and the elucidation of cellular and organismal function in relation to these chemicals. In contrast, pharmacy, a health services profession, is concerned with application of the principles learned from pharmacology in its clinical settings; whether it be in a dispensing or clinical care role.

In either field, the primary contrast between the two are their distinctions between direct-patient care, for pharmacy practice, and the science-oriented research field, driven by pharmacology.

The origins of clinical pharmacology date back to the Middle Ages in Avicenna's *The Canon of Medicine*, Peter of Spain's *Commentary on Isaac*, and John of St Amand's *Commentary on the Antedotary of Nicholas*. Clinical pharmacology owes much of its foundation to the work of William Withering. Pharmacology as a scientific discipline did not further advance until the mid-19th century amid the great biomedical resurgence of that period.

Before the second half of the nineteenth century, the remarkable potency and specificity of the actions of drugs such as morphine, quinine and digitalis were explained vaguely and with reference to extraordinary chemical powers and affinities to certain organs or tissues. The first pharmacology department was set up by Rudolf Buchheim in 1847, in recognition of the need to understand how therapeutic drugs and poisons produced their effects.

Early pharmacologists focused on natural substances, mainly plant extracts. Pharmacology developed in the 19th century as a biomedical science that applied the principles of scientific experimentation to therapeutic contexts. Today Pharmacologists harness the power of genetics, molecular biology, chemistry, and other advanced tools to transform information about molecular mechanisms and targets into therapies directed against disease, defects or pathogens, and create methods for preventative care, diagnostics, and ultimately personalized medicine.

DIVISIONS

The discipline of pharmacology can be divided into many sub disciplines each with a specific focus.

- *Clinical pharmacology*: Clinical pharmacology is the basic science of pharmacology with an added focus on the application of pharmacological principles and methods in the medical clinic and towards patient care and outcomes.
- *Neuropharmacology*: Neuropharmacology is the study of the effects of medication on central and peripheral nervous system functioning.
- *Psychopharmacology*: Psychopharmacology is the study of the effects of medication on the psyche, observing changed behaviours of the body and mind, and how molecular events are manifest in a measurable behavioural form.
- *Pharmacogenetics*: Pharmacogenetics is clinical testing of genetic variation that gives rise to differing response to drugs.
- *Pharmacogenomics*: Pharmacogenomics is the application of genomic technologies to drug discovery and further characterization of older drugs. Identification of the genetic basis for polymorphic expression of a gene is done through intronic or exomic single-nucleotide polymorphisms (SNPs) which abolishes the need for different mechanisms for explaining the variability in drug metabolism. SNPs based variations in membrane receptors lead to multidrug resistance (MDR) and the drug–drug interactions. Even drug induced toxicity and many adverse effects can be explained by GWA studies. The multitude of SNPs help in understanding gene pharmacokinetic (PK) or pharmacodynamic (PD) pathways.
- *Pharmacoepidemiology*: Pharmacoepidemiology is the study of the effects of drugs in large numbers of people.
- *Toxicology*: Toxicology is the study of the adverse effects, molecular targets, and characterization of drugs or any chemical substance in excess (including those beneficial in lower doses).

- *Theoretical pharmacology*: Theoretical pharmacology is the study of metrics in pharmacology.
- *Posology*: Posology is the study of how medicines are dosed. It also depends upon various factors including age, climate, weight, and sex.
- *Pharmacognosy*: Pharmacognosy is a branch of pharmacology dealing especially with the composition, use, and development of medicinal substances of biological origin and especially medicinal substances obtained from plants.
- *Behavioural pharmacology*: Behavioural pharmacology, also referred to as psychopharmacology, is an interdisciplinary field which studies behavioural effects of psychoactivedrugs. It incorporates approaches and techniques from neuropharmacology, animal behaviour and behavioural neuroscience, and is interested in the behavioural and neurobiological mechanisms of action of psychoactive drugs. Another goal of behavioural pharmacology is to develop animal behavioural models to screen chemical compounds with therapeutic potentials. People in this field (called behavioural pharmacologists) typically use small animals (*e.g.* rodents) to study psychotherapeutic drugs such as antipsychotics, antidepressants and anxiolytics, and drugs of abuse such as nicotine, cocaine, methamphetamine, etc.
- *Environmental pharmacology*: Environmental pharmacology is a new discipline. Focus is being given to understand gene–environment interaction, drug-environment interaction and toxin-environment interaction. There is a close collaboration between environmental science and medicine in addressing these issues, as health care itself can be a cause of environmental damage or remediation. Human health and ecology are intimately related. Demand for more pharmaceutical products may place the public at risk through the destruction of species. The entry of chemicals and drugs into the aquatic ecosystem is a more serious concern today. In addition, the production of some illegal drugs pollutes drinking water supply by releasing carcinogens. This field is intimately linked with Public Health fields.

SCIENTIFIC BACKGROUND

The study of chemicals requires intimate knowledge of the biological system affected. With the knowledge of cell biology and biochemistry increasing, the field of pharmacology has also changed substantially.

It has become possible, through molecular analysis of receptors, to design chemicals that act on specific cellular signaling or metabolic pathways by affecting sites directly on cell-surface receptors (which modulate and mediate cellular signaling pathways controlling cellular function).

A chemical has, from the pharmacological point-of-view, various properties. Pharmacokinetics describes the effect of the body on the chemical (*e.g.* half-life and volume of distribution), and pharmacodynamics describes the chemical's effect on the body (desired or toxic).

When describing the pharmacokinetic properties of the chemical that is the active ingredient or active pharmaceutical ingredient (API), pharmacologists are often interested in *L-ADME*:

- *Liberation:* How is the API disintegrated (for solid oral forms (breaking down into smaller particles)), dispersed, or dissolved from the medication?
- *Absorption*: How is the API absorbed (through the skin, the intestine, the oral mucosa)?
- *Distribution*: How does the API spread through the organism?
- *Metabolism:* Is the API converted chemically inside the body, and into which substances. Are these active (as well)? Could they be toxic?
- *Excretion*: How is the API excreted (through the bile, urine, breath, skin)?

Medication is said to have a narrow or wide *therapeutic index* or *therapeutic window*. This describes the ratio of desired effect to toxic effect. A compound with a narrow therapeutic index (close to one) exerts its desired effect at a dose close to its toxic dose. A compound with a wide therapeutic index (greater than five) exerts its desired effect at a dose substantially below its toxic dose. Those with a narrow margin are more difficult to dose and administer, and may require therapeutic drug monitoring (examples are warfarin, some antiepileptics, aminoglycoside antibiotics). Most anti-cancer drugs have a narrow therapeutic margin: toxic side-effects are almost always encountered at doses used to kill tumors.

MEDICINE DEVELOPMENT AND SAFETY TESTING

Development of medication is a vital concern to medicine, but also has strong economical and political implications. To protect the consumer and prevent abuse, many governments regulate the manufacture, sale, and administration of medication. In the United States, the main body that regulates pharmaceuticals is the Food and Drug Administration and they enforce standards set by the United States Pharmacopoeia.

In the European Union, the main body that regulates pharmaceuticals is the EMEA and they enforce standards set by the European Pharmacopoeia.

The metabolic stability and the reactivity of a library of candidate drug compounds have to be assessed for drug metabolism and toxicological studies. Many methods have been proposed for quantitative predictions in drug metabolism; one example of a recent computational method is Sporcalc.

If the chemical structure of a medicinal compound is altered slightly, this could slightly or dramatically alter the medicinal properties of the compound depending on the level of alteration as it relates to the structural composition of the substrate or receptor site on which it exerts its medicinal effect, a concept referred to as the structural activity relationship (SAR). This means that when a useful activity has been identified, chemists will make many similar compounds called analogues, in an attempt to maximize the desired medicinal effect(s) of the compound. This development phase can take anywhere from a few years to a decade or more and is very expensive.

These new analogues need to be developed. It needs to be determined how safe the medicine is for human consumption, its stability in the human body and the best form for delivery to the desired organ system, like tablet or aerosol. After extensive testing, which can take up to 6 years, the new medicine is ready for marketing and selling. As a result of the long time required to develop analogues and test a new medicine and the fact that of every 5000 potential new medicines typically only one will ever reach the open market, this is an expensive way of doing things, often costing over 1 billion dollars. To recoup this outlay pharmaceutical companies may do a number of things:

- Carefully research the demand for their potential new product before spending an outlay of company funds.
- Obtain a patent on the new medicine preventing other companies from producing that medicine for a certain allocation of time.

DRUG LEGISLATION AND SAFETY

In the United States, the Food and Drug Administration (FDA) is responsible for creating guidelines for the approval and use of drugs. The FDA requires that all approved drugs fulfill two requirements:

- The drug must be found to be effective against the disease for which it is seeking approval (where 'effective' means only that the drug performed better than placebo or competitors in at least two trials).
- The drug must meet safety criteria by being subject to animal and controlled human testing.

Gaining FDA approval usually takes several years to attain. Testing done on animals must be extensive and must include several species to help in the evaluation of both the effectiveness and toxicity of the drug. The dosage of any drug approved for use is intended to fall within a range in which the drug produces a therapeutic effect or desired outcome.

The safety and effectiveness of prescription drugs in the U.S. is regulated by the federal Prescription Drug Marketing Act of 1987. The Medicines and Health care products Regulatory Agency (MHRA) has a similar role in the UK.

EDUCATION

Students of pharmacology are trained as Biomedical Scientists, studying the effects of drugs on living organisms. This can lead to new drug discoveries, as well as a better understanding of the way in which the human body works.

Students of pharmacology must have detailed working knowledge of aspects of physiology, pathology and chemistry. During a typical degree they will cover areas such as (but not limited to) Biochemistry, Biology, Physiology, Genetics, Medical Microbiology and Neuroscience.

Whereas a pharmacy student will eventually work in a pharmacy dispensing medications, a pharmacologist will typically work within a laboratory setting. Careers for a pharmacologist include academic positions (medical and non-medical), governmental positions, private industrial positions, science writing, scientific patents and law, consultation, biotech and pharmaceutical employment, the alcohol industry, food industry, forensics/law enforcement, and public health or environmental/ecological sciences.

PHARMACODYNAMICS

Pharmacodynamics is the study of the biochemical and physiological effects of drugs on the body or on microorganisms or parasites within or on the body and the mechanisms of drug action and the relationship between drug concentration and effect. One dominant example is drug-receptor interactions as modeled by

$$L + R \rightleftharpoons L \cdot R$$

where L=ligand(drug), R=receptor (attachment site), reaction dynamics that can be studied mathematically through tools such as free energy maps. Pharmacodynamics is often summarized as the study of what a drug does to the body, whereas pharmacokinetics is the study of what the body does to a drug.

Pharmacodynamics is sometimes abbreviated as "PD", while pharmacokinetics can be referred to as "PK". See PK/PD models.

EFFECTS ON THE BODY

The majority of drugs either:

- Mimic or inhibit normal physiological/biochemical processes or inhibit pathological processes in animals or
- Inhibit vital processes of endo- or ectoparasites and microbial organisms. There are 7 main drug actions:
  - Stimulating action through direct receptor agonism and downstream effects
  - Depressing action through direct receptor agonism and downstream effects (ex.: inverse agonist)
  - Blocking/antagonising action (as with silent antagonists), the drug binds the receptor but does not activate it
  - Stabilising action, the drug seems to act neither as a stimulant or as a depressant (ex.: some drugs possess receptor activity that allows them to stabilize general receptor activation, like

buprenorphine in opioid dependent individuals or aripiprazole in schizophrenia, all depending on the dose and the recipient)
- Exchanging/replacing substances or accumulating them to form a reserve (ex.: glycogen storage)
- Direct beneficial chemical reaction as in free radical scavenging.
- Direct harmful chemical reaction which might result in damage or destruction of the cells, through induced toxic or lethal damage (cytotoxicity or irritation)

Desired Activity

The desired activity of a drug is mainly due to successful targeting of one of the following:

- Cellular membrane disruption.
- Chemical reaction with downstream effects.
- Interaction with enzyme proteins.
- Interaction with structural proteins.
- Interaction with carrier proteins.
- Interaction with ion channels.
- Ligand binding to receptors:
  - Hormone receptors,
  - Neuromodulator receptors,
  - Neurotransmitter receptors.

General anesthetics were once thought to work by disordering the neural membranes, thereby altering the Na influx. Antacids and chelating agents combine chemically in the body. Enzyme-substrate binding is a way to alter the production or metabolism of key endogenous chemicals, for example aspirin irreversibly inhibits the enzyme prostaglandin synthetase (cyclooxygenase) thereby preventing inflammatory response.

Colchicine, a drug for gout, interferes with the function of the structural protein tubulin, while Digitalis, a drug still used in heart failure, inhibits the activity of the carrier molecule, Na-K-ATPase pump.

The widest class of drugs act as ligands which bind to receptors which determine cellular effects. Upon drug binding, receptors can elicit their normal action (agonist), blocked action (antagonist), or even action opposite to normal (inverse agonist).

In principle, a pharmacologist would aim for a target plasma concentration of the drug for a desired level of response. In reality, there are many factors affecting this goal.

Pharmacokinetic factors determine peak concentrations, and concentrations cannot be maintained with absolute consistency because of metabolic breakdown and excretory clearance. Genetic factors may exist which would alter metabolism or drug action itself, and a patient's immediate status may also affect indicated dosage.

Undesirable Effects

Undesirable effects of a drug include:

- Increased probability of cell mutation (carcinogenic activity)
- A multitude of simultaneous assorted actions which may be deleterious
- Interaction (additive, multiplicative, or metabolic)
- Induced physiological damage, or abnormal chronic conditions

Therapeutic Window

The therapeutic window is the amount of a medication between the amount that gives an effect (effective dose) and the amount that gives more adverse effects than desired effects. For instance, medication with a small pharmaceutical window must be administered with care and control, *e.g.* by frequently measuring blood concentration of the drug, since it easily loses effects or gives adverse effects.

Duration of Action

The *duration of action* of a drug is the length of time that particular drug is effective. Duration of action is a function of several parameters including plasma half-life, the time to equilibrate between plasma and target compartments, and the off rate of the drug from its biological target.

RECEPTOR BINDING

The binding of ligands (drug) to receptors is governed by the *law of mass action* which relates the large-scale status to the rate of numerous molecular processes. The rates of formation and un-formation can be used to determine the equilibrium concentration of bound receptors. The *equilibrium dissociation constant* is defined by:

$$L + R \leftrightarrow L \cdot R$$

$$K_d = \frac{[L][R]}{[L \cdot R]}$$

where L=ligand, R=receptor, square brackets [] denote concentration. The fraction of bound receptors is:

$$\text{Fraction Bound} = K_d = \frac{[L \cdot R]}{R + [L \cdot R]} = \frac{1}{1 + \frac{K_d}{[L]}}$$

This expression is one way to consider the effect of a drug, in which the response is related to the fraction of bound receptors. The fraction of bound receptors is known as occupancy. The relationship between occupancy and pharmacological response is usually non-linear. This explains the so-called *receptor reserve* phenomenon *i.e.* the concentration producing 50per cent occupancy is typically higher than the concentration producing 50per cent of maximum response. The receptor reserve phenomenon is the model that states there are excess receptors on the cell surface than what is necessary for full effect.

Often the response is determined as a function of $log[L]$ to consider many orders of magnitude of concentration. However, there is no biological or physical theory which relates effects to the log of concentration. It is just convenient for graphing purposes. It is useful to note that 50per cent of the receptors are bound when $[L] = K_d$.

The graph shown represents the conc-response for two hypothetical receptor agonists, plotted in a semi-log fashion. The curve towards the left represents a higher potency (potency arrow does not indicate direction of increase) since lower concentrations are needed for a given response. The effect increases as a function of concentration.

MULTICELLULAR PHARMACODYNAMICS

The concept of pharmacodynamics has been expanded to include Multicellular Pharmacodynamics (MCPD). MCPD is the study of the static and dynamic properties and relationships between a set of drugs and a dynamic and diverse multicellular four-dimensional organization. It is the study of the workings of a drug on a minimal multicellular system (mMCS), both *in vivo* and *in silico*. Networked Multicellular Pharmacodynamics (Net-MCPD) further extends the concept of MCPD to model regulatory genomic networks together with signal transduction pathways, as part of a complex of interacting components in the cell.

TOXICODYNAMICS

Pharmacokinetics and pharmacodynamics are termed toxicokinetics and toxicodynamics in the field of ecotoxicology. Here, the focus is on toxic effects on a wide range of organisms. The corresponding models are called toxicokinetic-toxicodynamic models (more details can be found at Ecotoxmodels.org).

TOXICOLOGY

Toxicology is a branch of biology, chemistry, and medicine (more specifically pharmacology) concerned with the study of the adverse effects of chemicals on living organisms. It also studies the harmful effects of chemical, biological and physical agents in biological systems that establishes the extent of damage in living organisms. The relationship between dose and its effects on the exposed organism is of high significance in toxicology. Factors that influence chemical toxicity include the dosage (and whether it is acute or chronic); the route of exposure, the species, age, sex and environment.

Dioscorides, a Greek physician in the court of the Roman emperor Nero, made the first attempt to classify plants according to their toxic and therapeutic effect. Ibn Wahshiya wrote the *Book on Poisons* in the 9th or 10th century.

Mathieu Orfila is considered the modern father of toxicology, having given the subject its first formal treatment in 1813 in his *Traité des poisons*, also called *Toxicologie générale*.

In 1850, Jean Stas gave the evidence that the Belgian Count Hippolyte Visart de Bocarmé killed his brother-in-law by poisoning him with nicotine.

Theophrastus Phillipus Auroleus Bombastus von Hohenheim (1493–1541) (also referred to as Paracelsus, from his belief that his studies were above or beyond the work of Celsus – a Roman physician from the first century) is also considered "the father" of toxicology. He is credited with the classic toxicology maxim, *"Alle Dinge sind Gift und nichts ist ohne Gift; allein die Dosis macht, dass ein Ding kein Gift ist."* which translates as, "All things are poison and nothing is without poison; only the dose makes a thing not a poison." This is often condensed to: "The dose makes the poison" or in Latin "Sola dosis facit venenum".

BASIC TRADITIONAL TOXICOLOGY

The relationship between dose and its effects on the exposed organism is of high significance in toxicology. The chief criterion regarding the toxicity of a chemical is the dose, *i.e.* the amount of exposure to the substance. All substances are toxic under the right conditions. The term LD_{50} refers to the dose of a toxic substance that kills 50 percent of a test population (typically rats or other surrogates when the test concerns human toxicity).

The conventional relationship (more exposure equals higher risk) has been challenged in the study of endocrine disruptors. Toxicity is species-specific, lending cross-species analysis problematic. Newer methods are available to bypass animal-testing.

A nontechnical popularization of traditional toxicology is available in the book *The Dose Makes the Poison*. Factors that influence chemical toxicity:

- Dosage,
  - Both large single exposures (acute) and continuous small exposures (chronic) are studied.
- Route of exposure,
  - Ingestion, inhalation or skin absorption.
- Other factors.
  - Species,
  - Age,
  - Sex,

- Health,
- Environment,
- Individual characteristics.

Foods safe for humans are not necessarily safe for pets. A young healthy pregnant woman in a supportive environment has a different set of chemical sensitivities than an aged homeless male drug addict. Chemicals safe to drink may not be safe to inject. Eating a peanut is life-threatening for some.

The classic experimental tool of toxicology is animal testing. Alternative tests have been and are being developed. One example of a test that has been developed is Corrositex, a toxicology test that is much more accurate than animal testing. Separate test protocols are used for acute and chronic toxicity, irritation, sensitization (allergies), reproductive toxicity and carcinogenesis (cancer).

Few antidotes to poisons exist. Treatment usually consists of removing the poison, repairing damage and providing life support. The testing of one chemical for its cancer-causing properties took 5 years, cost more than $6.5 million in 1980 and utilized 24,000 mice.

DOSE RESPONSE COMPLEXITIES

Most chemicals display a classic dose response curve – at a low dose (below a threshold), no effect is observed. Some show a phenomenon known as sufficient challenge – a small exposure produces animals that "grow more rapidly, have better general appearance and coat quality, have fewer tumors, and live longer than the control animals". A few chemicals have no well-defined safe level of exposure. These are treated with special care. Some chemicals are subject to bioaccumulation as they are stored in rather than being excreted from the body; these also receive special consideration.

PHARMACOGENOMICS

Pharmacogenomics (a portmanteau of pharmacology and genomics) is the study of the role of genetics in drug response. It deals with the influence of acquired and inherited genetic variation on drug response in patients by correlating gene expression or single-nucleotide polymorphisms with drug absorption, distribution, metabolism and elimination, as well as drug receptor target effects. The term pharmacogenomics is often used interchangeably with pharmacogenetics. Although both terms relate to drug response based on genetic influences, pharmacogenetics focuses on single drug-gene interactions, while pharmacogenomics encompasses a more genome-wide association approach, incorporating genomics and epigenetics while dealing with the effects of multiple genes on drug response.

Pharmacogenomics aims to develop rational means to optimize drug therapy, with respect to the patients' genotype, to ensure maximum efficacy with minimal adverse effects. Through the utilization of pharmacogenomics, it is hoped that drug treatments can deviate from what is dubbed as the "one-dose-fits-all" approach. It attempts to eliminate the trial-and-error method of prescribing, allowing physicians to take into consideration their patient's genes, the functionality of these genes, and how this may affect the efficacy of the patient's current and/or future treatments (and where applicable, provide an explanation for the failure of past treatments). Such approaches promise the advent of "personalized medicine"; in which drugs and drug combinations are optimized for each individual's unique genetic makeup. Whether used to explain a patient's response or lack thereof to a treatment, or act as a predictive tool, it hopes to achieve better treatment outcomes, greater efficacy, minimization of the occurrence of drug toxicities and adverse drug reactions (ADRs). For patients who have lack of therapeutic response to a treatment, alternative therapies can be prescribed that would best suit their requirements. In order to provide pharmacogenomic-based recommendations for a given drug, two possible types of input can be used: genotyping or exome or whole genome sequencing. Sequencing provides many more data points, including detection of mutations that prematurely terminate the synthesized protein (early stop codon).

Pharmacogenomics was first recognized by Pythagoras around 510 BC when he made a connection between the dangers of fava bean ingestion with hemolytic anemia and oxidative stress. Interestingly, this identification was later validated and attributed to deficiency of G6PD in the 1950s and called favism. Although the first official publication dates back to 1961, circa 1950s marked the unofficial beginnings of this science.

Reports of prolonged paralysis and fatal reactions linked to genetic variants in patients who lacked butyryl-cholinesterase ('pseudocholinesterase') following administration of succinylcholine injection during anesthesia were first reported in 1956.

The term pharmacogenetic was first coined in 1959 by Friedrich Vogel of Heidelberg, Germany (although some papers suggest it was 1957). In the late 1960s, twin studies supported the inference of genetic involvement in drug metabolism, with identical twins sharing remarkable similarities to drug response compared to fraternity twins. The term pharmacogenomics first began appearing around the 1990s.

DRUG-METABOLISING ENZYMES

There are several known genes which are largely responsible for variances in drug metabolism and response. The focus of this article will remain on the genes that are more widely accepted and utilized clinically for brevity.

- Cytochrome P450s
- VKORC1
- TPMT

Cytochrome P450

The most prevalent drug-metabolising enzymes (DME) are the Cytochrome P450 (CYP) enzymes. The term Cytochrome P450 was coined by Omura and Sato in 1962 to describe the membrane-bound, heme-containing protein characterized by 450 nm spectral peak when complexed with carbon monoxide. The human CYP family consists of 57 genes, with 18 families and 44 subfamilies. CYP proteins are conveniently arranged into these families and subfamilies on the basis of similarities identified between the amino acid sequences. Enzymes that share 35-40per cent identity are assigned to the same family by an Arabic numeral, and those that share 55-70per cent make up a particular subfamily with a designated letter. For example, CYP2D6 refers to family 2, subfamily D, and gene number 6.

From a clinical perspective, the most commonly tested CYPs include: CYP2D6, CYP2C19, CYP2C9, CYP3A4 and CYP3A5. These genes account for the metabolism of approximately 80-90per cent of currently available prescription drugs. The table below provides a summary for some of the medications that take these pathways.

Table. Drug Metabolism of Major CYPs.

Enzyme	Fraction of drug metabolism (per cent)	Example Drugs
CYP2C9	10	Tolbutamide, ibuprofen, mefenamic acid, tetrahydrocannabinol, losartan, diclofenac
CYP2C19	5	S-mephenytoin, amitriptyline, diazepam, omeprazole, proguanil, hexobarbital, propranolol, imipramine
CYP2D6	20-30	Debrisoquine, metoprolol, sparteine, propranolol, encainide, codeine, dextromethorphan, clozapine, desipramine, haloperidol, amitriptyline, imipramine
CYP3A4	40-45	Erythromycin, ethinyl estradiol, nifedipine, triazolam, cyclosporine, amitriptyline, imipramine
CYP3A5	<1	Erythromycin, ethinyl estradiol, nifedipine, triazolam, cyclosporine, amitriptyline, aldosterone

CYP2D6

Also known as debrisoquine hydroxylase (named after the drug that led to its discovery), CYP2D6 is the most well-known and extensively studied CYP gene. It is a gene of great interest also due to its highly polymorphic nature, and involvement in a high number of medication metabolisms (both as a major and minor pathway). More than 100 CYP2D6 genetic variants have been identified.

CYP2C19

Discovered in the early 1980s, CYP2C19 is the second most extensively studied and well understood gene in pharmacogenomics. Over 28 genetic variants have been identified for CYP2C19, of which affects the metabolism of several classes of drugs, such as antidepressants and proton pump inhibitors.

CYP2C9

CYP2C9 constitutes the majority of the CYP2C subfamily, representing approximately 20per cent of the liver content. It is involved in the metabolism of approximately 10per cent of all drugs, which include medications with narrow therapeutic windows such as warfarin and tolbutamide. There are approximately 57 genetic variants associated with CYP2C9.

CYP3A4 and CYP3A5

The CYP3A family is the most abundantly found in the liver, with CYP3A4 accounting for 29per cent of the liver content.

These enzymes also cover between 40-50per cent of the current prescription drugs, with the CYP3A4 accounting for 40-45per cent of these medications. CYP3A5 has over 11 genetic variants identified at the time of this publication.

VKORC1

The vitamin K epoxide reductase complex subunit 1 (VKORC1) is responsible for the pharmacodynamics of warfarin. VKORC1 along with CYP2C9 are useful for identifying the risk of bleeding during warfarin administration. Warfarin works by inhibiting VKOR, which is encoded by the VKORC1 gene. Individuals with polymorphism in this have an affected response to warfarin treatment.

TPMT

Thiopurine methyltransferase (TPMT) catalyzes the S-methylation of thiopurines, thereby regulating the balance between cytotoxic thioguanine nucleotide and inactive metabolites in hematopoietic cells. TPMT is highly involved in 6-MP metabolism and TMPT activity and TPMT genotype is known to affect the risk of toxicity. Excessive levels of 6-MP can cause myelosuppression and myelotoxicity. Codeine, clopidogrel, tamoxifen, and warfarin a few examples of medications that follow the above metabolic pathways.

PREDICTIVE PRESCRIBING

Patient genotypes are usually categorized into the following predicted phenotypes:

- Extensive Metabolizer: Normal metabolic activity;
- Intermediate Metabolizer: Patients with reduced metabolic activity;
- Poor Metabolizer: Patients with little to no functional metabolic activity; and
- Ultra-Rapid Metabolizer: Patients with substantially increased metabolic activity.

The two extremes of this spectrum are the Poor Metabolizers and Ultra-Rapid Metabolizers.

Efficacy of a medication is not only based on the above metabolic statuses, but also the type of drug consumed.

Drugs can be classified into two main groups: active drugs and pro-drugs. Active drugs refer to drugs that are inactivated during metabolism, and Pro-Drugs are inactive until they are metabolized.

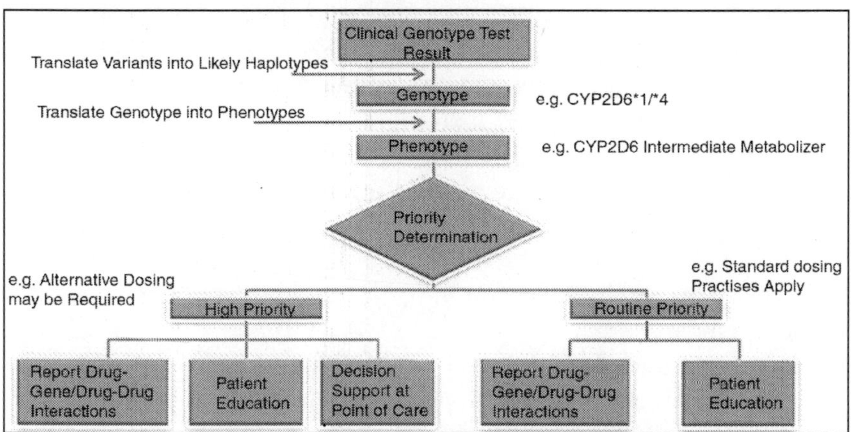

An overall process of how pharmacogenomics functions in a clinical practice. From the raw genotype results, this is then translated to the physical trait, the phenotype. Based on these observations, optimal dosing is evaluated.

For example, we have two patients who are taking codeine for pain relief. Codeine is a pro-drug, so it requires conversion from its inactive form to its active form.

The active form of codeine is morphine, which provides the therapeutic effect of pain relief. If person A receives one *1 allele each from mother and father to code for the CYP2D6 gene, then that person is considered to have an extensive metabolizer (EM) phenotype, as allele *1 is considered to have a normal-function (this would be represented as CYP2D6 *1/*1).

If person B on the other hand had received one *1 allele from the mother and a *4 allele from the father, that individual would be an Intermediate Metabolizer (IM) (the genotype would be CYP2D6 *1/*4).

Although both individuals are taking the same dose of codeine, person B could potentially lack the therapeutic benefits of codeine due to the decreased conversion rate of codeine to its active counterpart morphine.

Each phenotype is based upon the allelic variation within the individual genotype. However, several genetic events can influence a same phenotypic trait, and establishing genotype-to-phenotype relationships can thus be far from consensual with many enzymatic patterns. For instance, the influence of the CYP2D6*1/*4 allelic variant on the clinical outcome in patients treated with Tamoxifen remains debated today. In oncology, genes coding for DPD, UGT1A1, TPMT, CDA involved in the pharmacokinetics of 5-FU/capecitabine, irinotecan, 6-mercaptopurine and gemcitabine/cytarabine, respectively, have all been described as being highly polymorphic. A strong body of evidence suggests that patients affected by these genetic polymorphisms will experience severe/lethal toxicities upon drug intake, and that pre-therapeutic screening does help to reduce the risk of treatment-related toxicities through adaptive dosing strategies.

Identification of the genetic basis for polymorphic expression of a gene is done through intronic or exomic SNPs which abolishes the need for different mechanisms for explaining the variability in drug metabolism. The SNPs based variations in membrane receptors lead to multidrug resistance (MDR) and the drug–drug interactions. Even drug induced toxicity and many adverse effects can be explained by genome-wide association studies (GWAS).

APPLICATIONS

The list below provides a few more commonly known applications of pharmacogenomics:

- Improve drug safety, and reduce ADRs;
- Tailor treatments to meet patients unique genetic pre-disposition, identifying optimal dosing;
- Improve drug discovery targeted to human disease; and
- Improve proof of principle for efficacy trials.

Pharmacogenomics may be applied to several areas of medicine, including Pain Management, Cardiology, Oncology, and Psychiatry. A place may also exist in Forensic Pathology, in which pharmacogenomics can be used to determine the cause of death in drug-related deaths where no findings emerge using autopsy.

In cancer treatment, pharmacogenomics tests are used to identify which patients are most likely to respond to certain cancer drugs. In behavioural health, pharmacogenomic tests provide tools for physicians and care givers to better manage medication selection and side effect amelioration. Pharmacogenomics is also known as companion diagnostics, meaning tests being bundled with drugs. Examples include KRAS test with cetuximab and EGFR test with gefitinib. Beside efficacy, germline pharmacogenetics can help to identify patients likely to undergo severe toxicities when given cytotoxics showing impaired detoxification in relation with genetic polymorphism, such as canonical 5-FU.

In cardio vascular disorders, the main concern is response to drugs including warfarin, clopidogrel, beta blockers, and statins.

MEDICINAL CHEMISTRY

Medicinal chemistry and pharmaceutical chemistry are disciplines at the intersection of chemistry, especially synthetic organic chemistry, and pharmacology and various other biological specialties, where they are involved with design, chemical synthesis and development for market of pharmaceutical agents, or bio-active molecules (drugs).

Compounds used as medicines are most often organic compounds, which are often divided into the broad classes of small organic molecules (*e.g.*, atorvastatin, fluticasone, clopidogrel) and "biologics" (infliximab, erythropoietin, insulin glargine), the latter of which are most often medicinal preparations of proteins (natural and recombinant antibodies, hormones, etc.). Inorganic and organometallic compounds are also useful as drugs (*e.g.*, lithium and platinum-based agents such as lithium carbonate and cis-platin.

In particular, medicinal chemistry in its most common guise—focusing on small organic molecules—encompasses synthetic organic chemistry and aspects of natural products and computational chemistry in close combination with chemical biology, enzymology and structural biology, together aiming at the discovery and development of new therapeutic agents. Practically speaking, it involves chemical aspects of identification, and then systematic, thorough synthetic alteration of new chemical entities to make them suitable for therapeutic use. It includes synthetic and computational aspects of the study of existing drugs and agents in development in relation to their bioactivities (biological activities and properties), *i.e.*, understanding their structure-activity relationships (SAR). Pharmaceutical chemistry is focused on quality aspects of medicines and aims to assure fitness for purpose of medicinal products.

At the biological interface, medicinal chemistry combines to form a set of highly interdisciplinary sciences, setting its organic, physical, and computational emphases alongside biological areas such as biochemistry, molecular biology, pharmacognosy and pharmacology, toxicology and veterinary and human medicine; these, with project management, statistics, and pharmaceutical business practices, systematically oversee altering identified chemical agents such that after pharmaceutical formulation, they are safe and efficacious, and therefore suitable for use in treatment of disease.

PHARMACEUTICS

Pharmaceutics is the discipline of pharmacy that deals with the process of turning a new chemical entity (NCE) into a medication to be used safely and effectively by patients. It is also called the science of dosage form design. There are many chemicals with pharmacological properties, but need special measures to help them achieve therapeutically relevant amounts at their sites of action. Pharmaceutics helps relate the formulation of drugs to their delivery and disposition in the body. Pharmaceutics deals with the formulation of a pure drug substance into a dosage form. Branches of pharmaceutics include:

- Pharmaceutical formulation;
- Pharmaceutical manufacturing;
- Dispensing pharmacy;
- Pharmaceutical technology;
- Physical pharmacy;
- Pharmaceutical jurispundence.

Pure drug substances are usually white crystalline or amorphous powders. Historically before the advent of medicine as a science it was common for pharmacists to dispense drugs *as is*, most drugs today are administered as parts of a dosage form. The clinical performance of drugs depends on their form of presentation to the patient.

PHARMACOGNOSY

Pharmacognosy is the study of medicines derived from natural sources. The American Society of Pharmacognosy defines pharmacognosy as "the study of the physical, chemical, biochemical and biological properties of drugs, drug substances or potential drugs or drug substances of natural origin as well as the search for new drugs from natural sources." It is also defined as the study of crude drugs.

The term "pharmacognosy" was used for the first time by the Austrian physician Schmidt in 1811 and 1815 by Crr. Anotheus Seydler in a work titled *Analecta Pharmacognostica*.

Originally—during the 19th century and the beginning of the 20th century—"pharmacognosy" was used to define the branch of medicine or commodity sciences (*Warenkunde* in German) which deals with drugs in their crude, or unprepared, form. Crude drugs are the dried, unprepared material of plant, animal or mineral origin, used for medicine.

The study of these materials under the name *pharmakognosie* was first developed in German-speaking areas of Europe, while other language areas often used the older term *materia medica* taken from the works of Galen and Dioscorides. In German the term *drogenkunde* ("science of crude drugs") is also used synonymously.

As late as the beginning of the 20th century, the subject had developed mainly on the botanical side, being particularly concerned with the description and identification of drugs both in their whole state and in powder form.

Such branches of pharmacognosy are still of fundamental importance, particularly for pharmacopoeial identification and quality control purposes, but rapid development in other areas has enormously expanded the subject.

Although most pharmacognostic studies focus on plants and medicines derived from plants, other types of organisms are also regarded as pharmacognostically interesting, in particular, various types of microbes (bacteria, fungi, etc.), and, recently, various marine organisms.

In addition to the previously mentioned definition, the American Society of Pharmacognosy also defines pharmacognosy as "the study of natural product molecules (typically secondary metabolites) that are useful for their medicinal, ecological, gustatory, or other functional properties." Other definitions are more encompassing, drawing on a broad spectrum of biological subjects, including botany, ethnobotany, marine biology, microbiology, herbal medicine, chemistry, biotechnology, phytochemistry, pharmacology, pharmaceutics, clinical pharmacy and pharmacy practice.

- Medical ethnobotany: the study of the traditional use of plants for medicinal purposes;
- Ethnopharmacology: the study of the pharmacological qualities of traditional medicinal substances;
- The study of phytotherapy (the medicinal use of plant extracts); and
- Phytochemistry, the study of chemicals derived from plants (including the identification of new drug candidates derived from plant sources).
- Zoopharmacognosy, the process by which animals self-medicate, by selecting and using plants, soils, and insects to treat and prevent disease.
- Marine pharmacognosy, the study of chemicals derived from marine organisms.

At the 9th congress of Italian society of pharmacognosy it was stated that current return of phyto-therapy was clearly reflected by the increased market of such products. In 1998 the latest figures available for Europe, the total OTC market for herbal medicinal products reached a figure of $6 billion, with consumption for Germany of $2.5 billion, France $1.6 billion and Italy $600 million. In the US, where the use of herbal products has never been as prevalent as in continental Europe, the market for all herb sales reached a peak in 1998 of $700 billion. This welcomed the scientific investigation of a rigorous nature.

The plant kingdom still holds many species of plants containing substances of medicinal value which have yet to be discovered. Large numbers of plants are constantly being screened for their possible pharmacological value.

All plants produce chemical compounds as part of their normal metabolic activities. These phytochemicals are divided into (1) primary metabolites such as sugars and fats, which are found in all plants; and (2) secondary metabolites—compounds which are found in a smaller range of plants, serving a more specific function. For example, some secondary metabolites are toxins used to deter predation and others are pheromones used to attract insects for pollination. It is these secondary metabolites and pigments that can have therapeutic actions in humans and which can be refined to produce drugs—examples are inulin from the roots of dahlias, quinine from the cinchona, morphine and codeine from the poppy, and digoxin from the foxglove.

Plants synthesize a bewildering variety of phytochemicals but most are derivatives of a few biochemical motifs:

- Alkaloids are a class of chemical compounds containing a nitrogen ring. Alkaloids are produced by a large variety of organisms, including bacteria, fungi, plants, and animals, and are part of the group of natural products (also called secondary metabolites). Many alkaloids can be purified from crude extracts by acid-base extraction. Many alkaloids are toxic to other organisms. They often have pharmacological effects and are used as medications, as recreational drugs, or in entheogenic rituals. Examples are the local anesthetic and stimulant cocaine; the psychedelic psilocin; the stimulant caffeine; nicotine; the analgesic morphine; the antibacterial berberine; the anticancer compound vincristine; the antihypertension agent reserpine; the cholinomimeric galatamine; the spasmolysis agent atropine; the vasodilator vincamine; the anti-arhythmia compound quinidine; the anti-asthma therapeutic ephedrine; and the antimalarial drug quinine. Although alkaloids act on a diversity of metabolic systems in humans and other animals, they almost uniformly invoke a bitter taste.
- Polyphenols (also known as phenolics) are compounds that contain phenol rings. The anthocyanins that give grapes their purple colour, the isoflavones, the phytoestrogens from soy and the tannins that give tea its astringency are phenolics.
- Glycosides are molecules in which a sugar is bound to a non-carbohydrate moiety, usually a small organic molecule. Glycosides play numerous important roles in living organisms. Many plants store chemicals in the form of inactive glycosides. These can be activated by enzyme hydrolysis, which causes the sugar part to be broken off, making the chemical available for use. Many such plant glycosides are used as medications. In animals and humans, poisons are often bound to sugar molecules as part of their elimination from the body. An example is the cyanoglycosides in cherry pits that release toxins only when bitten by a herbivore.
- Terpenes are a large and diverse class of organic compounds, produced by a variety of plants, particularly conifers, which are often strong smelling and thus may have had a protective function. They are the major components of resin, and of turpentine produced from resin. (The name "terpene" is derived from the word "turpentine"). Terpenes are major biosynthetic building blocks within nearly every living creature. Steroids, for example, are derivatives of the triterpene

squalene. When terpenes are modified chemically, such as by oxidation or rearrangement of the carbon skeleton, the resulting compounds are generally referred to as *terpenoids*. Terpenes and terpenoids are the primary constituents of the essential oils of many types of plants and flowers. Essential oils are used widely as natural flavour additives for food, as fragrances in perfumery, and in traditional and alternative medicines such as aromatherapy. Synthetic variations and derivatives of natural terpenes and terpenoids also greatly expand the variety of aromas used in perfumery and flavours used in food additives. Vitamin A is an example of a terpene. The fragrance of rose and lavender is due to monoterpenes. The carotenoids produce the reds, yellows and oranges of pumpkin, corn and tomatoes.

A consortium of plant molecular researchers at Washington State University, the Donald Danforth Plant Science Center, the National Center for Genome Resources, and the University of Illinois at Chicago began an NIH-sponsored study of over thirty medicinal plant species late 2009. The initial work, to develop a sequence reference for the transcriptome of each, has led to the development of the Medicinal Plant Transcriptomics Database.

ISSUES IN PHYTOTHERAPY

The part of pharmacognosy focusing on use of crude extracts or semi-pure mixtures originating from nature, namely phytotherapy, is probably the best known and also the most debated area in pharmacognosy. Although phytotherapy is sometimes considered as alternative medicine, when critically conducted, it can be considered the scientific study on the effects and clinical use of herbal medicines.

Constituents and Drug Synergism

One characteristic of crude drug material is that constituents may have an opposite, moderating or enhancing effect. Hence, the final effect of any crude drug material will be a product of the interactions between the constituents and the effect of each constituent on its own. To effectively study the existence and effect of such interactions, scientific studies must examine the effect that multiple constituents, given concurrently, have on the system. Herbalists assert that as phytopharmaceuticals rely upon synergy for their activities, plants with high levels of active constituents like ginsenosides or hypericin may not correlate with the strength of the herbs. In phytopharmaceuticals or herbal medicine, the therapeutic effects of herbs cannot be determined unless its active ingredient or cofactors are identified or the herb is administered as a whole. One way to indicate strength is standardization to one or several marker compound that are believed to be mainly responsible for the biological effects. However, many herbalists believe that the active ingredient in a plant is the plant itself.

Herb and Drug Interactions

A study of herb drug interactions indicated that the vast majority of drug interactions occurred in four classes of drugs, the chief class being blood thinners, but also including protease inhibitors, cardiac glycosides and the immuno-suppressant ciclosporin.

Natural Products Chemistry

Most bioactive compounds of natural origin are secondary metabolites, *i.e.*, species-specific chemical agents that can be grouped into various categories. A typical protocol to isolate a pure chemical agent from natural origin is bioassay-guided fractionation, meaning step-by-step separation of extracted components based on differences in their physicochemical properties, and assessing the biological activity, followed by next round of separation and assaying. Typically, such work is initiated after a given crude drug formulation (typically prepared by solvent extraction of the natural material) is deemed "active" in a particular *in vitro* assay. If the end-goal of the work at hand is to identify which one(s) of the scores or hundreds of compounds are responsible for the observed *in vitro* activity, the path to that end is fairly straightforward: 1. fractionate the crude extract, *e.g.* by solvent partitioning or chromatography. 2. test the fractions thereby generated with *in vitro* assay. 3. repeat steps 1) and 2) until pure, active compounds are obtained. 4. determine structure(s) of active compound(s), typically by using spectroscopic methods. *In vitro* activity does not necessarily translate to activity in humans or other living systems.

The most common means for fractionation are solvent-solvent partitioning and chromatographic techniques such as high-performance liquid chromatography (HPLC), medium-pressure liquid chromatography, "flash" chromatography, open-column chromatography, vacuum-liquid chromatography (VLC), thin-layer chromatography (TLC), with each technique being most appropriate for a given amount of starting material. Countercurrent chromatography (CCC) is particularly well-suited for bioassay-guided fractionation because, as an all-liquid separation technique, concern about irreversible loss or denaturation of active sample components is minimized. After isolation of a pure substance, the task of elucidating its chemical structure can be addressed. For this purpose, the most powerful methodologies available are nuclear magnetic resonance spectroscopy (NMR) and mass spectrometry (MS). In the case of drug discovery efforts, structure elucidation of all components that are active *in vitro* is typically the end goal. In the case of phytotherapy research, the investigator may use *in vitro* BAGF as a tool to identify pharmacologically interesting or important components of the crude drug. The work does not stop after structural identification of *in vitro* actives, however. The task of "dissecting and reassembling" the crude drug one active component at a time, in order to achieve a mechanistic understanding of how it works in phytotherapy, is quite daunting. This is because it is simply too difficult, from cost, time, regulatory, and even scientific perspectives, to study experimental fractions of the crude drug in humans. *In vitro* assays are therefore used to identify chemical components of the crude drug that may rationally be expected to have a given pharmacological effect in humans, and to provide a rational basis for standardization of a crude drug formulation to be tested in [and sold/marketed to] humans.

Loss of Biodiversity

Farnsworth for example, has found that 25per cent of all prescriptions dispensed from community pharmacies in the United States from 1959 to 1980 contained active ingredients extracted from higher plants. In some countries in Asia and Africa 80per cent of the population relies on traditional medicine (including herbal medicine) for primary health care. Constituents of substances used by traditional healers, have rarely been incorporated into modern medicine. Quinine, physostigmine, d-tubocurarine, pilocarpine and ephedrine, have been demonstrated to have active effects Knowledge of traditional medicinal practices is disappearing, particularly in the Amazon, as native healers die out and are replaced by more modern medical practitioners. Botanists and pharmacologists are racing to learn these ancient practices, which, like the forest plants they employ, are also endangered

An explanation for some species loss is habitat lost due to invasive species introduction. Herbalist David Winston has suggested that a high proportion of nonnative species seen as invasive (kudzu, Japanese knotweed, mimosa, lonicera, St. Johnswort and purple loosestrife) may be harvested for the domestic herbal medicine market.

Species extinction is not only due to habitat loss. Overharvesting of medicinal species of plants and animals also contributes to species loss. This is particularly notable in the matter of Traditional Chinese Medicine where crude drugs of plant and animal origin are used with increasing demand. People with a stake in TCM often seek chemical and biological alternatives to endangered species because they realize that plants and animals lost from the wild are also lost to medicine forever but different cultural attitudes bedevil conservation efforts. Still conservation is not a new idea: Chinese advice against overexploitation of natural medicinal species dates from at least Mencius, a philosopher living in the 4th century BC.

Cooperation between Western conservationists and practitioners have been beset by cultural difficulties. Westerners may emphasise urgency in matters of conservation, while Chinese may wish for the products used in TCM to remain publicly available. One repeated fallacy is that rhinoceros horn is used as an aphrodisiac in TCM. It is, in fact, prescribed for fevers and convulsions by TCM practitioners. There are no peer-reviewed studies showing that this treatment is effective. In 1995 representatives of the oriental medicine communities in Asia met with conservationists at a symposium in Hong Kong, organized by TRAFFIC. The two groups established a clear willingness to cooperate through dialogue and mutual understanding. This has led to several meetings, including the 1997 First International Symposium on Endangered Species Used in Traditional East Asian Medicine where China was among 136 nations to sign a formal resolution recognising that the uncontrolled use of wild species in traditional medicine threatens their survival and the continuation of these medical practices. The resolution, drawn up by the UN Convention on International Trade in Endangered Species (CITES), aims to initiate new partnerships in conservation.

Sustainable Sources of Plant and Animal Drugs

As species face loss of habitat or overharvesting, there have been new issues to deal with in sourcing crude drugs. These include changes to the herb from farming practices, substitution of species or other plants altogether, adulteration and cross-pollination issues. For instance, ginseng which is field farmed may have significant problems with fungus, making contamination with fungicides an issue. This may be remedied with woods grown programmes, but they are insufficient to produce enough ginseng to meet demand. The wildcrafted echinacea, black cohosh and American ginseng often rely upon old growth root, often in excess of 50 years of age and it is not clear that younger stock will have the same pharmaceutical effect. Black cohosh may be adulterated with the related Chinese actea species, which is not the same. Ginseng may be replaced by ginseniodes from Jiaogulan which has been stated to have a different effect than the full panax root.

The problem may be exacerbated by the growth of pills and capsules as the preferred method of ingesting medication as they are cheaper and more available than traditional, individually tailored prescriptions of raw medicinals but the contents are harder to track. Seahorses are a case in point: Seahorses once had to be of a certain size and quality before they were accepted by practitioners and consumers. But declining availability of the preferred large, pale and smooth seahorses has been offset by the shift towards prepackaged medicines, which make it possible for TCM merchants to sell previously unused juvenile, spiny and dark-coloured animals. Today almost a third of the seahorses sold in China are prepackaged.

The farming of plant or animal species for medicinal purposes has caused difficulties. Rob Parry Jones and Amanda Vincent write:

- One solution is to farm medicinal animals and plants. Chinese officials have promoted this as a way of guaranteeing supplies as well as protecting endangered species. And there have been some successes—notably with plant species, such as American ginseng—

which is used as a general tonic and for chronic coughs. Red deer, too, have for centuries been farmed for their antlers, which are used to treat impotence and general fatigue. But growing your own is not a universal panacea. Some plants grow so slowly that cultivation in not economically viable. Animals such as musk deer may be difficult to farm, and so generate little profit. Seahorses are difficult to feed and plagued by disease in captivity. Other species cannot be cultivated at all. Even when it works, farming usually fails to match the scale of demand. Overall, cultivated TCM plants in China supply less than 20 per cent of the required 1.6 million tonnes per annum. Similarly, China's demand for animal products such as musk and pangolin scales far exceeds supply from captive-bred sources.

- Farming alone can never resolve conservation concerns, as government authorities and those who use Chinese medicine realise. For a start, consumers often prefer ingredients taken from the wild, believing them to be more potent. This is reflected in the price, with wild oriental ginseng fetching up to 32 times as much as cultivated plants. Then there are welfare concerns. Bear farming in China is particularly controversial. Around 7600 captive bears have their bile "milked" through tubes inserted into their gall bladders. World Animal Protection states that bear bile farming "causes intense, unjustified suffering to bears". Chinese officials state that 10,000 wild bears would need to be killed each year to produce as much bile, making bear farming the more desirable option. World Animal Protection, however, states that "it is commonly believed in China that the bile from a wild bear is the most potent, and so farming bears for their bile cannot replace the demand for the product extracted from wild animals".
- One alternative to farming involves replacing medical ingredients from threatened species with manufactured chemical compounds. In general, this sort of substitution is difficult to achieve because the active ingredient is often not known. In addition, most TCM users believe that TCM compounds may act synergistically so several ingredients may interact to give the required effect. Thus TCM users often prefer the wild source. Tauro ursodeoxycholic acid, the active ingredient of bear bile, can be synthesised and is used by some Western doctors to treat gallstones, but many TCM consumers reject it as being inferior to the natural substance from wild animals.

2

Thermodynamics

HEAT

FEELING AND SEEING TEMPERATURE CHANGES

Within some reasonable temperature range, we can get a rough idea how warm something is by touching it. But this can be unreliable—if you put one hand in cold water, one in hot, then plunge both of them into lukewarm water, one hand will tell you it's hot, the other will feel cold. For something too hot to touch, we can often get an impression of how hot it is by approaching and sensing the radiant heat. If the temperature increases enough, it begins to glow and we can *see* it's hot!

The problem with these subjective perceptions of heat is that they may not be the same for everybody. If our two hands can't agree on whether water is warm or cold, how likely is it that a group of people can set a uniform standard? We need to construct a device of some kind that responds to temperature in a simple, measurable way—we need a thermometer.

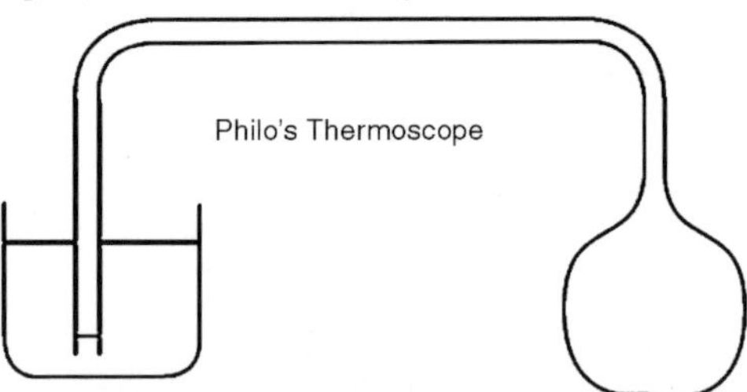

The first step on the road to a thermometer was taken by one Philo of Byzantium, an engineer, in the second century BC. He took a hollow lead sphere connected with a tight seal to one end of a pipe, the other end of the pipe being under water in another vessel.

To quote Philo: "*...if you expose the sphere to the sun, part of the air enclosed in the tube will pass out when the sphere becomes hot. This will be evident because the air will descend from the tube into the water, agitating it and producing a succession of bubbles.*

Now if the sphere is put back in the shade, that is, where the sun's rays do not reach it, the water will rise and pass through the tube ..."

"No matter how many times you repeat the operation, the same thing will happen.

In fact, if you heat the sphere with fire, or even if you pour hot water over it, the result will be the same."

Notice that Philo did what a real investigative scientist should do—he checked that the experiment was *reproducible*, and he established that the air's expansion was in response to *heat* being applied to the sphere, and was *independent of the source of the heat*.

This expansion of air on heating became widely known in classical times, and was used in various dramatic devices.For example, Hero of Alexandria describes a small temple where a fire on the altar causes the doors to open.

The altar is a large airtight box, with a pipe leading from it to another enclosed container filled with water. When the fire is set on top of the altar, the air in the box heats up and expands into a second container which is filled with water. This water is forced out through an overflow pipe into a bucket hung on a rope attached to the door hinges in such a way that as the bucket fills with water, it drops, turns the hinges, and opens the doors. The pipe into this bucket reaches almost to the bottom, so that when the altar fire goes out, the water is sucked back and the doors close again. Still, none of these ingenious devices is a *thermometer*. There was no attempt (at least none recorded) by Philo or his followers to make a *quantitative* measurement of how hot or cold the sphere was. And the "meter" in thermometer means measurement.

The First Thermometer

Galileo claimed to have invented the first thermometer. Well, actually, he called it a thermoscope, but he *did* try to measure "degrees of heat and cold" according to a colleague, and that qualifies it as a thermometer. (Technically, a *thermoscope* is a device making it possible to *see* a temperature change, a *thermometer* can *measure* the temperature change.) Galileo used an inverted narrow-necked bulb with a tubular neck, like a hen's egg with a long glass tube attached at the tip. He first heated the bulb with his hands then immediately put it into water. He recorded that the water rose in the bulb the height of "one palm". Later, either Galileo or his colleague Santorio Santorio put a paper scale next to the tube to read off changes in the water level. This definitely made it a thermometer, but who thought of it first isn't clear (they argued about it). And, in fact, this thermometer had problems.

Question: what problems? If you occasionally top up the water, why shouldn't this thermometer be good for recording daily changes in temperature?

Answer: because it's also a barometer! But—Galileo didn't know about the atmospheric pressure.

Torricelli, one of Galileo's pupils, was the first to realise, shortly after Galileo died, that the real driving force in suction was external atmospheric pressure, a satisfying mechanical explanation in contrast to the philosophical "nature abhors a vacuum". In the 1640's, Pascal pointed out that the *variability* of atmospheric pressure rendered the air thermometer untrustworthy.

Liquid-in-glass thermometers were used from the 1630's, and they were of course insensitive to barometric pressure. Meteorological records were kept from this time, but there was no real uniformity of temperature measurement until Fahrenheit, almost a hundred years later.

Newton's Anonymous Table of Temperatures

The first systematic account of a range of different temperatures, "Degrees of Heat", was written by Newton, but published anonymously, in 1701. Presumably he felt that this project lacked the timeless significance of some of his other achievements. Taking the freezing point of water as zero, Newton found the temperature of boiling water to be almost three times that of the human body, melting lead eight times as great (actually 327C, whereas 8x37=296, so this is pretty good!) but for higher temperatures, such as that of a wood fire, he underestimated considerably. He used a linseed oil liquid in glass thermometer up to the melting point of tin (232°C). Newton tried to estimate the higher temperatures indirectly. He heated up a piece of iron in a fire, then let it cool in a steady breeze. He found that, at least at the lower temperatures where he could cross check with his thermometer, the temperature dropped in a geometric progression, that is, if it took five minutes to drop from 80° above air temperature to 40° above air temperature, it took another five minutes to drop to 20° above air, another five to drop to 10° above, and so on. He then assumed this same pattern of temperature drop was true at the high temperatures beyond the reach of his thermometer, and so estimated the temperature of the fire and of iron glowing red hot. This wasn't very accurate—he (under)estimated the temperature of the fire to be about 600°C.

Fahrenheit's Excellent Thermometer

The first really good thermometer, using mercury expanding from a bulb into a capillary tube, was made by Fahrenheit in the early 1720's. He got the idea of using mercury from a colleague's comment that one should correct a *barometer* reading to allow for the variation of the density of mercury with temperature. The point that has to be borne in mind in constructing thermometers, and defining temperature scales, is that not all liquids expand at uniform rates on heating—water, for example, at first contracts on heating from its freezing point, then begins to expand at around forty degrees Fahrenheit, so a water thermometer wouldn't be very helpful on a cold day. It is also not easy to manufacture a *uniform cross section* capillary tube, but

Fahrenheit managed to do it, and demonstrated his success by showing his thermometers agreed with each other over a whole range of temperatures. Fortunately, it turns out that mercury is well behaved in that the temperature scale defined by taking its expansion to be uniform coincides very closely with the true temperature scale.

Amontons' Air Thermometer

A little earlier (1702) Amontons introduced an *air pressure thermometer*. He established that if air at atmospheric pressure (he states 30 inches of mercury) at the freezing point of water is enclosed then heated to the boiling point of water, but meanwhile kept at constant volume by increasing the pressure on it, the pressure goes up by about 10 inches of mercury. He also discovered that if he compressed the air in the first place, so that it was at a pressure of sixty inches of mercury at the temperature of melting ice, then if he raised its temperature to that of boiling water, at the same time adding mercury to the column to keep the volume of air constant, the pressure increased by 20 inches of mercury. In other words, he found that for a fixed amount of air kept in a container at constant volume, the pressure increased with temperature by about 33per cent from freezing to boiling, that percentage being *independent of the initial pressure*.

The Zeroth Law of Thermodynamics

Once the thermometer came to be widely used, more precise observations of temperature and heat flow became possible. Joseph Black, a professor at the University of Edinburgh in the 1700's, noticed that a collection of objects at different temperatures, if brought together, will all eventually reach the same temperature. As he wrote, "By the use of these instruments [thermometers] we have learned, that if we take 1000, or more, different kinds of matter, such as metals, stones, salts, woods, cork, feathers, wool, water and a variety of other fluids, although they be all at first of different heats, let them be placed together in a room without a fire, and into which the sun does not shine, the heat will be communicated from the hotter of these bodies to the colder, during some hours, perhaps, or the course of a day, at the end of which time, if we apply a thermometer to all of them in succession, it will point to precisely the same degree."

We say nowadays that bodies in "thermal contact" eventually come into "thermal equilibrium"—which means they finally attain the same temperature, after which no further heat flow takes place. This is equivalent to:

If two objects are in thermal equilibrium with a third, then they are in thermal equilibrium with each other.

The "third body" in a practical situation is just the thermometer. It's perhaps worth pointing out that this trivial sounding statement certainly wasn't obvious before the invention of the thermometer. With only the sense of touch to go on, few people would agree that a piece of wool and a bar of metal, both at 0°C, were at the same temperature.

"Flow of heat" that takes place between bodies as they move towards thermal equilibrium? For example, suppose I reproduce one of Fahrenheit's experiments, by taking 100 ccs of water at 100°F, and 100ccs at 150°F, and mix them together in an insulated jug so little heat escapes. What is the final temperature of the mix?

Of course, it's close to 125°F—not surprising, but *it does tell us something!* It tells us that the amount of heat required to raise the temperature of 100 cc of water from 100°F to 125°F is *exactly the same* as the amount needed to raise it from 125°F to 150°F.

A series of such experiments (done by Fahrenheit, Black and others) established that it *always* took the same amount of heat to raise the temperature of 1 cc of water by one degree, *independent* of the initial temperature of the water (provided it's between the freezing point and the boiling point).

This makes it possible to define a unit of heat. Perhaps unfairly to Fahrenheit, 1 calorie is the heat required to raise the temperature of 1 gram of water by 1 degree Celsius. (Celsius also lived in the early 1700's. His scale has the freezing point of water as 0°C, the boiling point as 100°C.

Fahrenheit's scale is no longer used in science, but lives on in engineering in the US, and in the British Thermal Unit, which is the heat required to raise the temperature of one pound of water by 1°F.)

Specific Heats and Calorimetry

The specific heat of a substance is the heat required in calories to raise the temperature of 1 gram by 1 degree Celsius.

As Fahrenheit continues his measurements of heat flow, it quickly became evident that for different materials, the amount of heat needed to raise the temperature of one gram by one degree could be quite different. It was natural to measure specific heats relative to that of water, the simplest and most readily available substance for calorimetric experiments. There were some surprises. For example, it had been widely thought before the measurements were made, that one cc of Mercury, being a lot heavier than one cc of water, would take more heat to raise its temperature by one degree.

This proved not to be the case—Fahrenheit himself made the measurement. In an insulating container, called a "calorimeter" he added 100ccs of water at 100°F to 100ccs of mercury at 150°F, and stirred so they quickly reached thermal equilibrium.

Question: what do you think the final temperature was?

Answer: The final temperature was, surprisingly, about 120°F. 100 cc of water evidently "contained more heat" than 100 cc of mercury, despite the large difference in weight.

The technique, called calorimetry, was widely used to find specific heats of many different substances, and at first no clear pattern emerged.

It was puzzling that the specific heat of mercury was so low compared with water. As the experiments progressed, it gradually became evident that heavier substances, paradoxically, had lower specific heats.

Meanwhile, this quantitative approach to scientific observation had spread to chemistry. Towards the end of the 1700's, Lavoisier weighed chemicals involved in reactions before and after the reaction.

This involved weighing the gases involved, so had to be carried out in closed containers, so that, for example, the weight of oxygen used and the carbon dioxide, etc., produced would accounted for in studying combustion. *The big discovery was that mass was neither created nor destroyed.*

This had not been realised before because no one had weighed the gases involved.

It made the atomic theory suddenly more plausible, with the idea that maybe chemical reactions were just rearrangements of atoms into different combinations.

Lavoisier also clarified the concept of an element, an idea that was taken up in about 1800 by John Dalton, who argues that a given compound consisted of identical molecules, made up of elementary atoms in the same proportion, such as H_2O (although that was thought initially to be HO).

This explained why, when substances reacted chemically, such as the burning of hydrogen to form water, it took exactly eight grams of oxygen for each gram of hydrogen.

(Well, you could also produce H_2O_2 under the right conditions, with exactly sixteen grams of oxygen to one of hydrogen, but the simple ratios of amounts of oxygen needed for the two reactions were simply explained by different molecular structures, and made the atomic hypothesis even more plausible.)

Much effort was expended carefully weighing the constituents in many chemical reactions, and constructing diagrams of the molecules. The important result of all this work was that it became possible to list the relative weights of the atoms involved.

For example, the data on H_2O and H_2O_2 led to the conclusion that an oxygen atom weighed sixteen times the weight of a hydrogen atom. It must be emphasized, though, that these results gave no clue as to the actual weights of atoms.

All that was known was that atoms were too small to see in the best microscopes.

Nevertheless, knowing the relative weights of some atoms in 1820 led to an important discovery.

Two professors in France, Dulong and Petit, found that for a whole series of elements *the product of atomic weight and specific heat* was the same.

Element	Specific Heat (cals/gm/ degree C)	Relative weights of the atoms	Product of relative atomic weight and specific heat
Lead	0.0293	12.95	0.3794
Tin	0.0514	7.35	0.3779
Zinc	0.0927	4.03	0.3736
Sulphur	0.1880	2.011	0.3780

The significance of this, as they pointed out, was that the "specific heat", or heat capacity, of each *atom* was the same—a piece of lead and a piece of zinc having the same number of atoms would have the same heat capacity. So heavier atoms absorbed no more heat than lighter atoms for a given rise in temperature. This partially explained why mercury had such a surprisingly low heat capacity. Of course, having no idea how big the atoms might be, they could go no further. And, indeed, many of their colleagues didn't believe in atoms anyway, so it was hard to convince them of the significance of this discovery.

Latent Heat

One of Black's experiments was to set a pan of water on a steady fire and observe the temperature as a function of time. He found it steadily increased, reflecting the supply of heat from the fire, until the water began to boil, whereupon the temperature stayed the same for a long time. The steam coming off was at the same (boiling) temperature as the water. So what was happening to the heat being supplied?

Black correctly concluded that heat needed to be supplied to change water from its liquid state to its gaseous state, that is, to steam. In fact, a lot of heat had to be supplied: 540 calories per gram, as opposed to the mere 100 calories per gram needed to bring it from the freezing temperature to boiling. He also discovered that it took 80 calories per gram to melt ice into water, with no rise in temperature. This heat is released when the water freezes back to ice, so it is somehow "hidden" in the water. He called it *latent* heat, meaning hidden heat.

THERMAL EXPANSION AND THE GAS LAW

Coefficients of Expansion

Almost all materials expand on heating—the most famous exception being water, which contracts as it is warmed from 0 degrees Celsius to 4 degrees. This is actually a good thing, because as freezing weather sets in, the coldest water, which is about to freeze, is less dense than slightly warmer water, so rises to the top of a lake and the ice begins to form there. For almost all other liquids, solidification on cooling begins at the bottom of the container. So, since water behaves in this weird way, ice skating is possible! Also, as a matter of fact, life in lakes is possible—the ice layer that forms insulates the rest of the lake water from very cold air, so fish can make it through the winter.

Linear Expansion

The coefficient of linear expansion α of a given material, for example a bar of copper, at a given temperature is defined as the fractional increase in length that takes place on heating through one degree:

Of course, α might vary with temperature (it does for water, as we just mentioned) but in fact for most materials it stays close to constant over wide temperature ranges.

For copper,

$$\alpha = 17 \times 10^{-16}.$$

Volume Expansion

For *liquids and gases*, the natural measure of expansion is the coefficient of volume expansion, β.

$$V \to V + \Delta V = (1 + \beta)V \text{ when } T \to T + 1°C$$

Of course, on heating a bar of copper, clearly the *volume* as well as the *length* increases—the bar expands by an equal fraction in all directions (this could be experimentally verified, or you could just imagine a cube of copper, in which case all directions look the same).

The volume of a cube of copper of side L is $V = L^3$. Suppose we heat it through one degree. Putting together the definitions of α, β above,

$$V \to (1 + \beta)V,\ L \to (1+\alpha)L,\ L^3 \to (1+\alpha)^3 L^3 \text{ or } V \to (1 + \alpha)^3 V.$$

So $(1 + \beta) = (1+\alpha)^3$. But remember α is very, very small—so even though $(1+\alpha)^3 = 1 + 3\alpha + 3\alpha^2 + \alpha^3$, the last two terms are *completely negligible* (check it out!) so to a fantastically good approximation:

$$\beta = 3\alpha.$$

The coefficient of volume expansion is just three times the coefficient of linear expansion.

Gas Pressure Increase with Temperature

In 1702, Amontons discovered a *linear* increase of P with T for air, and found P to increase about 33per cent from the freezing point of water to the boiling point of water. That is to say, he discovered that if a container of air were to be sealed at 0°C, at ordinary atmospheric pressure of 15 pounds per square inch, and then heated to 100°C but kept at the same volume, the air would now exert a pressure of about 20 pounds per square inch on the sides of the container. (Of course, strictly speaking, the container will also have increased in size, that would lower the effect—but it's a tiny correction, about ½per cent for copper, even less for steel and glass.) Remarkably, Amontons discovered, if the gas were initially at a pressure of *thirty* pounds per square inch at 0°C, on heating to 100°C the pressure would go to about 40 pounds per square inch—so the *percentage* increase in pressure was the same for *any* initial pressure: on heating through 100°C, the pressure would always increase by about 33per cent. Furthermore, the result turned out to be the same for different gases! Finding a Natural Temperature Scale.In class, we plotted air pressure as a function of temperature for a fixed volume of air, by making several measurements as the air was slowly heated (to give it a chance to all be at the same temperature at each stage). We found a straight line. On the graph, we extended the line backwards, to see how the pressure would presumably drop on cooling the air. We found the remarkable prediction that the pressure should drop to zero at a temperature of about –273°C. In fact, if we'd done the cooling experiment, we would have found that air doesn't actually follow the line all the way down, but condenses to a liquid at around -200°C. However, helium gas stays a gas almost to –270°C, and follows the line closely. We shall discuss the physics of gases, and the interpretation of this, much more fully in a couple of lectures. For now, the important point is that this suggests a *much more natural temperature scale* than the Celsius one: we should take –273°C as the zero of temperature. For one thing, if we do that, the pressure/temperature relationship for a gas becomes beautifully simple:

$$P \alpha T.$$

This temperature scale, in which the degrees have the same size as in Celsius, is called the Kelvin or absolute scale. Temperatures are written 300K. To get from Celsius to Kelvin, just add 273.15.

An Ideal Gas

Physicists at this point introduce the concept of an "Ideal Gas". This is like the idea of a frictionless surface: it doesn't exist in nature, but it is a very handy approximation to some real systems, and makes problems much easier to handle mathematically. The ideal gas is one for which P α T for all temperatures, so helium is close to ideal over a very wide range, and air is close to ideal at ordinary atmospheric temperatures and above.

The Gas Law

We say earlier in the course that for a gas at constant *temperature* $PV =$ constant(Boyle's Law). Now at constant *volume*,

$$P \alpha T.$$

We can put these together in one equation to find a relationship between pressure, volume and temperature:

$$PV = CT$$

where *C* is a constant. Notice, by the way, that we can immediately conclude that at fixed pressure, $V \propto T$, this is called *Charles' Law*. (*Exercise*: prove from this that the coefficient of volume expansion of a gas varies significantly with temperature.)But what is *C*? Obviously, it depends on how much gas we have—double the amount of gas, keeping the pressure and temperature the same, and the volume will be doubled, so *C* will be doubled. But notice that *C* will *not* depend on what gas we are talking about: if we have two separate one-litre containers, one filled with hydrogen, the other with oxygen, both at atmospheric pressure, and both at the same temperature, then *C* will be the same for both of them. One might conclude from this that *C* should be defined for one litre of gas at a specified temperature and pressure, such as 0°C and 1 atmosphere, and that could be a consistent scheme. It might seem more natural, though, to specify a particular *mass* of gas, since then we wouldn't have to specify a particular temperature and pressure in the definition of *C*. But that idea brings up a further problem: one gram of oxygen takes up a lot less room than one gram of hydrogen. Since we've just seen that choosing the same *volume* for the two gases gives the same constant *C* for the two gases, evidently taking the same *mass* of the two gases will give different *C*'s.

Avogadro's Hypothesis

The resolution to this difficulty is based on a remarkable discovery the chemists made two hundred years or so ago: they found that *one litre* of nitrogen could react with exactly *one litre* of oxygen to produce exactly *two liters* of NO, nitrous oxide, all volume measurements being at the same temperature and pressure. Further, one litre of oxygen combined with *two* liters of hydrogen to produce two liters of steam.

These simple ratios of interacting gases could be understood if one imagined the atoms combining to form molecules, and made the further assumption, known as Avogadro's Hypothesis (1811):

Equal volumes of gases at the same temperature and pressure contain the same number of molecules.

One could then understand the simple volume results by assuming the gases were made of diatomic molecules, H_2, N_2, O_2 and the chemical reactions were just molecular recombinations given by the equations $N_2 + O_2 = 2NO$, $2H_2 + O_2 = 2H_2O$, etc. Of course, in 1811 Avogadro didn't have the slightest idea what this number of molecules was for, say, one litre, and nobody else did either, for another fifty years. So no-one knew what an atom or molecule weighed, *but* assuming that chemical reactions were atoms combining into molecules, or rearranging from one molecular pairing or grouping to another, they could figure out the *relative* weights of atoms, such as *an oxygen atom had mass 16 times that of a hydrogen atom*—even though they had no idea how big these masses were.

This observation led to defining *the natural mass of a gas* for setting the value of the constant *C* in the gas law to be *a "mole" of gas*: hydrogen was known to be H_2 molecules, so *a mole of hydrogen was 2 grams*, oxygen was O_2, so a mole of oxygen was 32 grams, and so on. With this definition, a mole of oxygen contains the same number of molecules as a mole of hydrogen: so at the same temperature and pressure, they will occupy the same volume. At 0°C, and atmospheric pressure, the volume is 22.4 liters. So, for one mole of a gas (for example, two grams of hydrogen), we set the constant *C* equal to *R*, known as the universal gas constant, and equal to 8.3 J/(mol.K) and $PV = RT$.

For *n* moles of a gas, such as 2*n* grams of hydrogen, the law is:

$$PV = nRT$$

and this is the standard form of the Gas Law.

By the late 1700's, the experiments of Fahrenheit, Black and others had established a systematic, quantitative way of measuring temperatures, heat flows and heat capacities—but this didn't really throw any new light on just *what* was flowing. This was a time when the study of electricity was all the rage, led in America by Benjamin Franklin, who had suggested in 1747 that electricity was one (invisible) fluid (it had previously been suggested that there were two fluids, corresponding to the two kinds of electrical charging observed).

Lavoisier's Caloric Fluid Theory

Perhaps heat was another of these invisible fluids? In 1787, Lavoisier, the French founder of modern chemistry, thought so, and called it the *caloric fluid*, from the Greek word for heat. (Lavoisier was the first to attempt to list a table of *elements*, to replace the ancient elements of earth, air, water and fire. His list of thirty-three elements included hydrogen, oxygen, sulphur, charcoal, etc., but he also *included caloric*—and light.) The existence of such a fluid was really quite plausible—heat flowed from a hot body to a cold body, and the recent quantitative calorimetric experiments of Black and others seemed to establish that heat was a *conserved quantity*, as one would expect of a fluid. One could also understand some of the well-known effects of heat in terms of a fluid, and establish some of the fluid's properties. For example, since it tended to flow from hot bodies into cold bodies and spread throughout the body, presumably its particles repelled each other, just like those of the electrical fluid. However, in contrast to electricity, which had no noticeable effect on the appearance of a charged object, when heat was added to a solid things changed considerably. First the material expanded, then it changed to a liquid and finally to a gas, if sufficient heat could be delivered. Further heating expanded the gas, or increased its pressure if it was held in a fixed container. To interpret this sequence of events in terms of a caloric fluid being fed into the material, one could imagine the fluid flowing between the atoms of the solid and lessening their attraction for each other, until the solid melted into a liquid, whereupon the caloric continued to accumulate around the atoms until they were pushed apart into a gas. It was thought that in the gas each atom or molecule was surrounded by a ball of caloric, like a springy ball of wool, and these balls were packed in a container like oranges in a crate, except that the caloric balls could expand indefinitely as heat was poured in.Various other effects could be explained by the caloric theory: when a gas is suddenly compressed, it gets hotter because the same amount of caloric is now occupying a smaller volume. When two solids are rubbed together, some caloric is squeezed out at the surfaces, or perhaps tiny pieces of material are rubbed off, and lose their caloric, so heat appears. Radiant heat was presumed to be caloric particles flying through space. Recall that at that time (just before 1800) it was generally accepted that *light* was a stream of particles.

In 1769 a Lancashire wigmaker, Richard Arkwright, patented a successful cotton-spinning machine. Lancashire had been for a long time a center of the textile trade, but before Arkwright the fabrics were woven on hand looms by skilled weavers. The new machines could be operated by less skilled workers, and in fact were largely operated by children, although, in contrast to some of his competitors, Arkwright refused to employ any child younger than six. The motive power driving the machines was at first horses, but in 1771 Arkwright built a large factory containing many machines all driven by a water wheel. This was the beginning of the modern system of mass production. Prices fell, and the skilled hand weavers became impoverished. Our interest in this, however, is not the social consequences, but just the water wheel. Previously, water wheels had been used for centuries to grind flour, and for other purposes, but their efficiency had not been a major concern. In the factory, though, the more efficient the wheel, the more children could be spinning the cotton, and the bigger the profits. Twenty years earlier, John Smeaton (the first Englishman to call himself a civil engineer) had investigated different types of water wheels, and found the overshot type (in which the water pours on to the top of the wheel) to perform best.

The power output of a water wheel can be measured by using it to raise a load—in those days, it would be how many pounds could be raised through one foot per second, say (we would now just use watts, and it's amusing to note that the first unit of power, the horsepower, was proposed in 1783 by James Watt to be 33,000 foot pounds per minute). The ultimate in efficiency would be a *reversible* water wheel, which could be run backwards, to raise the water back again. This is best visualized by having a wheel with a series of buckets attached. Suppose the wheel is run for some time and its power output is used to lift a weight a given distance. Now reverse it, let the weight fall, running the wheel backwards, making sure the buckets now fill at the bottom and empty at the top. How much water is lifted back up? A truly reversible wheel would put all the water back. We know this isn't going to happen, but if the reversed wheel manages to lift half the water back, say, then it's 50per cent efficient.

In building the first factory, the water wheel was not just placed under a waterfall. The water was channeled to it for maximum efficiency. Smeaton had established that the flow of water into the buckets must be *as smooth as possible*. Turbulence was wasted effort—it didn't help the wheel go round. The water should flow onto the wheel, not fall from some height. Finally, the perfect wheel (not quite realizable in practice) would be reversible—it could be run backwards to put the water back up using the same amount of work it delivered in the first place.

Carnot's Caloric Water Wheel

Arkwright's factory was so successful that within a few years similar factories had been built wherever a water wheel could be operated economically in Northern England. The next step was to use steam power. As steam engine design improved, the English economy mushroomed far ahead of European competitors—but in contrast to the present day, these technological advances owed virtually nothing to basic science. It was all inspired tinkering.

The first attempt to analyse the steam engine in a scientific way was by a Frenchman, Sadi Carnot, in 1820—and he relied heavily an analogy with the water wheel. In the steam engine, heat is delivered to water which becomes steam and drives a piston. The piston does work, usually by turning a wheel, then waste heat is expelled. Remember that at that time heat was seen as an invisible fluid, impelled by its nature to flow from hot objects to cold objects. Carnot saw this as parallel to water which always flows from high places to low places. A water wheel placed under a waterfall will extract useful work from the falling water, work that otherwise would be wasted. Carnot concluded that the steam engine extracted work from the caloric fluid in a similar way, work which would have been lost if the heat had simply been allowed to flow from a hot object to a cold object.

By analogy with the water wheel, Carnot proved that if all friction were to be eliminated, and heat flow into and out of the steam were isothermal (this is the same as the water being fed onto the wheel at just the right height, so it doesn't fall and waste energy) then one could imagine a reversible engine. As we shall discuss in detail later, he was able to find for such an engine just how much work the engine could perform for a given heat input, and the answer was surprisingly low. Furthermore, no engine could ever be more efficient than a reversible engine, because if it were, it could be used to drive the reversible engine backwards, replacing the heat in the furnace, with energy to spare, and would be a perpetual motion machine.

Carnot's basic assumption that heat is a fluid was flawed, but his reasoning was of sufficient generality that his conclusions about efficiency were correct, and proved to be a crucial step towards understanding engines.

Count Rumford

The first real attack on the caloric theory of heat took place in a cannon factory in Bavaria, under the direction of one Count Rumford of the Holy Roman Empire. This Count was actually born Benjamin Thompson in Woburn, in the English colony of Massachusetts, in 1753, which he left in a hurry after choosing the wrong side in the Revolutionary War. He was a brilliant man, extraordinarily inventive as a scientist and engineer—but it is difficult to form a coherent picture of his character. He seemed genuinely upset by the plight of the poor in Munich and made great personal efforts for years to ensure they were properly fed and clothed. Throughout his life, he invented practical devices to make daily living better: stoves, fitted kitchens, drip coffeepots, lighting, and many more. Yet, despite this love for humanity and his clear desire to make life better for everyone, Rumford did not apparently like—or get on with—actual people. The only exceptions were those with power who might prove useful, and almost any attractive woman he met. Rumford dumped his own family unceremoniously when war broke out and he fled to England. When garrisoned on Long Island in 1782 (fighting for the British) he treated the local people horribly. He always engaged in shameless self-promotion, often with little regard for the truth. But he *did* make important contributions to many fields: food, clothing, work and education for the poor both in Bavaria and (less successfully) later in England, and all manner of engineering improvements, from the domestic devices listed above to state of the art artillery. In fact, his artillery designs were so highly regarded that by 1799 US President Adams tried to persuade him to return to America to found a Military Academy, with assurances that all was forgiven.

His father died when Benjamin was still a child, and although his mother remarried, he felt strongly that he had to take care of himself. He worked hard at school, then at age eighteen began working as a tutor for children of rich families, and after a short time became a teacher in a school in Concord, New Hampshire. At nineteen, he married a rich young widow, who decided to upgrade his appearance to fit in better with her friends. She bought him a scarlet hussar cloak, they used a two-horse chaise called a curricle, the only other curricle in the province belonging to the Royal Governor, John Wentworth. The marriage took place one day after the Governor had reviewed the troops, and the bride and groom were guests at the Governor's table. Thompson assiduously cultivated the Governor. They went together on a surveying expedition exploring the hilly country of the province. Thompson's real ambition was military, and in 1774 Governor Wentworth appointed him a major in the New Hampshire Militia. That year, the people were becoming increasingly rebellious against British rule and British taxes. Order was kept, at least in part, by the British Army. Thompson was part of a scheme to discourage desertion from that army, and when this became known to those plotting revolution, they declared him a "Rebel to the State". He moved rapidly to London, abandoning his wife and two-month-old daughter. In London, he supplied military intelligence, and was rewarded with a salaried position involving no work.

Ever the scientist (with a military bent), he spent a lot of time on gunnery experiments. He used a ballistic pendulum to find how the speed of a bullet was affected by small changes in gun design and in the gunpowder mix. He disproved the widely held view that slightly damp gunpowder was actually more effective.

He made a trip back to America in 1781. He wintered with a few hundred soldiers at Huntington, Long Island, in 1782, setting up camp in the churchyard, and forcing the local people to build fortifications for his camp using the church timbers and their rail fences. He constructed bread ovens using the tombstones. He designed a new gun carriage that could be disassembled, carried by three horses, then put together and fired in a minute and a quarter. But the war was over. He burned all the wood, rather than give it back to the people, and returned to London.

Still enthusiastic for military adventure, he decided to go to Vienna, which seemed a likely trouble spot. He first got himself promoted to full colonel, acquired the splendid uniform, and had his portrait painted by Thomas Gainsborough. When he reached Strasbourg, it happened that a military review was underway. Naturally, Thompson appeared in full regalia, impressing the reviewer, who was a nephew of the Elector of Bavaria. This landed him an important post in Munich, the capital of Bavaria. Among his other duties, he was to organize the feeding and clothing of the army. He took a practical, scientific approach. He had each garrison maintain its own vegetable garden, and gave directions on how to use them most effectively from a nutritional point of view. He ran experiments on the relative thermal conductivity of various fabrics, and found that trapped air in fabrics was the most important measure of heat insulation. He decided that uniforms should be cotton in summer, wool in winter. He invented thermal underwear.

In 1792, he became Count Rumford. It should also be mentioned that he greatly improved the city in many ways: he invented the soup kitchen for the poor, an idea which spread throughout Europe. In Switzerland, the meal tickets had Rumford's picture on them. He built workhouses, to provide work for the unemployed in making uniforms for the military. He helped design and lay out a beautiful park, where a memorial to him still stands. He also worked on many domestic improvements, such as the Rumford stove for more heat and less smoke, coffee makers, and an efficient but soft light, this last at least partly because, to quote him, "that mysterious light which comes from bodies moderately illuminated is certainly most favourable to female beauty" and Rumford was a great connoisseur of female beauty.

Rumford's Theory of Heat

The contribution to physics for which he is most remembered took place in Munich, and he stumbled into it more or less accidentally. But, as he remarks in presenting his findings to the Royal Society in 1798, "a habit of keeping the eyes open to everything that is going on in the ordinary course of the business of life has oftener led, as it were by accident, ... to sensible schemes for investigation ... than all the more intense meditations of philosophers, in the hours expressly set apart for study." What he was looking at was cannon boring, beefing up the Bavarian artillery in case of attack by the French, but what he was thinking about was whether or not Lavoisier's calorific fluid really existed. He was skeptical. Cannon were bored by turning an iron bit inside a brass cylinder, the power being supplied by horses. The friction of the iron bit on the brass generated heat. This was accounted for in the caloric theory by the pressure and movement squeezing out caloric fluid, in particular from the fragments that were sheared off. Rumford carefully collected these fragments and found them to be identical to the ordinary metal in heat capacity, etc., they didn't seem to have lost anything. Then he measured the heat production for an extended period, by having the brass cylinder immersed in water, and insulated. After extended grinding, the water (two gallons) began to boil. This was a startling event! To quote from his account:

"At 2 hours and 20 minutes it was 200°; and at 2 hours 30 minutes it Actually Boiled!

It would be difficult to describe the surprise and astonishment expressed in the countenances of the by-standers, on seeing so large a quantity of cold water heated, and actually made to boil without any fire."

Rumford goes on the analyse the whole experiment quantitatively: he gives the weight of the box, and so estimates how much heat it absorbs, as well as other parts of the apparatus which became warm, and measures the rate of cooling with the grinding stopped to estimate how much heat leaked out during the run. Taking all these factors into account, he estimated that heat production was equivalent to nine ¾ inch candles burning continuously. Long before the concept was formulated, Rumford had measures the mechanical equivalent of heat, at least approximately. In fact, many years later, Joule went over his Rumford's figures and found he was within 20per cent or so of the right answer. Rumford realised, of course, this wasn't a good way to produce heat—as he remarked, more heat could have been gained simply by burning the horses' fodder. His real interest here was in demolishing the caloric theory.

He concluded:...we must not forget to consider that most remarkable circumstance, that the source of the Heat generated by Friction, in these Experiments, appeared evidently to be *inexhaustible*. It is hardly necessary to add, that anything which any insulated body, or system of bodies, can continue to furnish without limitation, cannot possibly be a material substance: and it appears to me to be extremely difficult, if not quite impossible, to form any distinct idea of any thing, capable of being excited and communicated, in the manner the heat was excited and communicated in these Experiments, except it be Motion.

Exactly what Rumford meant by Motion has been debated, but it was some type of internal vibration of material, perhaps only distantly related to our modern, atom based, picture of heat vibrations. Still, by casting real doubt on the caloric theory, it was a step in the right direction. He had also established that if a caloric fluid really existed, it was certainly very light! He took three identical glass bottles containing equal weights of water, mercury and alcohol respectively, made them exactly equal in weight by tying small lengths of wire around the necks, then cooled them until the water froze, and weighed them again. The latent heat of freezing, and the very different heat capacities of the three fluids, should have resulted in quite different amounts of caloric fluid leaving the three bottles, yet their weights remained exactly the same, within one part in a million (the claimed accuracy of the balance).

After he returned to London in 1798, Rumford planned to repeat some of the public welfare successes in Munich. He wanted to build soup kitchens and workhouses for the poor. He also planned to found an institution which would not only facilitate the implementation of new scientific discoveries in improving living standards, but also train working class men to become mechanics. This became the Royal Institution. Unfortunately, Rumford was difficult to work with, and he did not see eye to eye with the first director, a young Cornishman called Humphry Davy. Sad to report, Rumford's idealistic notions for schooling the poor and improving living standards did not become a priority for the Institution, except for a series of lectures for the public which evolved into entertainments for the wealthy. Nevertheless, the Institution did maintain a first class laboratory in which Davy discovered new elements, including sodium and potassium, and has in fact been an excellent center of scientific research for the last two hundred years.

IDEAL GAS THERMODYNAMICS

The Kinetic Theory picture of a gas (outlined in the previous lecture) is often called the *Ideal Gas Model*. It ignores interactions between molecules, and the finite size of molecules. In fact, though, these only become important when the gas is very close to the temperature at which it become liquid, or under extremely high pressure. In this lecture, we will be analyzing the behaviour of gases in the pressure and temperature range corresponding to heat engines, and in this range the Ideal Gas Model is an excellent approximation. Essentially, our programme here is to learn how gases absorb heat and turn it into work, and *vice versa*. This heat-work interplay is called *thermodynamics*.

Julius Robert Mayer was the first to appreciate that there *is* an equivalence between heat and mechanical work. The tortuous path that led him to this conclusion is described in an earlier lecture, but once he was there, he realised that in fact the numerical equivalence—how many Joules in one calorie in present day terminology—could be figured out easily from the results of some measurements of gas specific heat by French scientists. The key was that they had measured specific heats both at constant *volume* and at constant *pressure*. Mayer realised that in the latter case, heating the gas necessarily increased its volume, and the gas therefore did work in pushing to expand its container. Having convinced himself that mechanical work and heat were equivalent, evidently the extra heat needed to raise the temperature of the gas at constant pressure was exactly the work the gas did on its container. (*Historical note*: although he did the work in 1842, he didn't publish until 1845, and at first miscalculated—but then gave a figure within 1per cent of the correct value of 4.2 joules per calorie.)

The simplest way to see what's going on is to imagine the gas in a cylinder, held in by a piston, carrying a fixed weight, able to move up and down the cylinder smoothly with negligible friction. The pressure on the gas is just the total weight pressing down divided by the area of the piston, and this total weight, of course, will not change as the piston moves slowly up or down: the gas is at *constant pressure*.

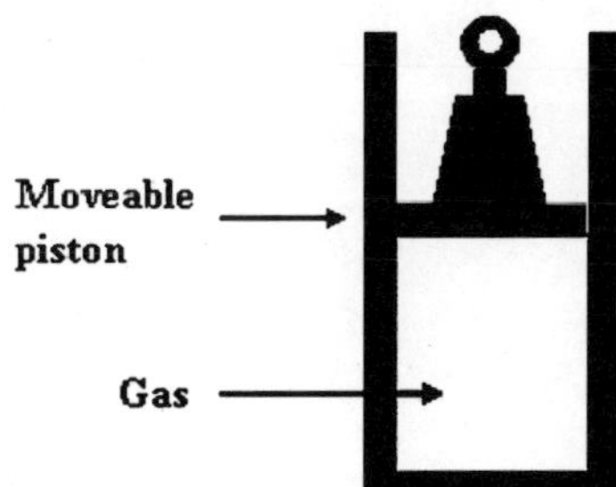

The Gas Specific Heats C_V and C_P

Consider now the two specific heats of this same sample of gas, let's say one mole:

Specific heat at constant volume, C_V (piston glued in place),

Specific heat at constant pressure, C_P (piston free to rise, no friction).

In fact, we already worked out C_V in the Kinetic Theory lecture: at temperature *T*, recall the average kinetic energy per molecule is $\frac{3}{2}kT$, so one mole of gas—Avogadro's number of molecules—will have total kinetic energy, which we'll label *internal energy*,

$$E_{\text{int}} = \frac{3}{2}kT \cdot N_A = \frac{3}{2}RT.$$

(In this simplest case, we are ignoring the possibility of the molecules having their *own* internal energy: they might be spinning or vibrating—we'll include that shortly).

That the internal energy is $\frac{3}{2}RT$ per mole immediately gives us the specific heat of a mole of gas in a fixed volume,

$$C_V = \frac{3}{2}R$$

that being the heat which must be supplied to raise the temperature by one degree.

However, if the gas, instead of being in a fixed box, is held in a cylinder at constant pressure, experiment confirms that *more* heat must be supplied to raise the gas temperature by one degree. As Mayer realised, the total heat energy that must be supplied to raise the temperature of the gas one degree *at constant pressure* is $\frac{3}{2}k$ per molecule *plus* the energy required to lift the weight. The work the gas must do to raise the weight is the force the gas exerts on the piston multiplied by the distance the piston moves. If the area of piston is A, then the gas at pressure P exerts force PA. If on heating through one degree the piston rises a distance Δh, the gas does work

$$PA.\,\Delta h = P\Delta V.$$

Now, for one mole of gas, $PV = RT$, so at constant P

$$P\Delta V = P\Delta T.$$

Therefore, the work done by the gas in raising the weight is just $R\Delta T$, the specific heat at constant pressure, the total heat energy needed to raise the temperature of one mole by one degree,

$$C_P = C_V + R.$$

In fact, this relationship is true whether or not the molecules have rotational or vibrational internal energy. (It's known as Mayer's relationship.) For example, the specific heat of oxygen at constant volume

$$C_V(O_2) = \frac{5}{2}R$$

and this is understood as a contribution of $\frac{3}{2}R$ from kinetic energy, and R from the two rotational modes of a dumbbell molecule (just why there is no contribution form rotation about the third axis can only be understood using quantum mechanics). The specific heat of oxygen at constant pressure

$$G_P(O_2) = \frac{1}{2}R.$$

It's worth having a standard symbol for the *ratio* of the specific heats:

$$\frac{C_P}{C_V} = \gamma.$$

Isotherms and Adiabats

An ideal gas in a box has three thermodynamic variables: P, V, T. But if there is a fixed mass of gas, fixing two of these variables fixes the third from $PV = nRT$ (for n moles). In a heat engine, heat can enter the gas, then leave at a different stage. The gas can expand doing work, or contract as work is done on it. To track what's going on as a gas engine transfers heat to work, say, we must follow the varying state of the gas. We do that by tracing a curve in the (P, V) plane. Supplying heat to a gas which consequently expands and does mechanical work is the key to the heat engine. But just knowing that a gas is expanding and doing work is not enough information to follow its path in the (P, V) plane. The route it follows will depend on whether or not heat is being supplied (or taken away) at the same time. There are, however, two particular ways a gas can expand reversibly—meaning that a tiny change in the external conditions would be sufficient for the gas to retrace its path in the (P, V) plane backwards. It's important to concentrate on reversible paths, because as Carnot proved and we shall discuss later, they correspond to the most efficient engines. The two sets of reversible paths are the *isotherms* and the *adiabats*.

Isothermal behaviour: The gas is kept *at constant temperature* by allowing heat flow back and forth with a very large object (a "heat reservoir") at temperature T. From $PV = nRT$, it is evident that for a fixed mass of gas, held at constant T but subject to (slowly) varying pressure, the variables P, V will trace a hyperbolic path in the (P, V) plane.

This path, $PV = nRT_1$, say is called the *isotherm* at temperature T_1. Here are two examples of isotherms:

Isotherms $PV = RT$ for One Mole at 273K, 373K

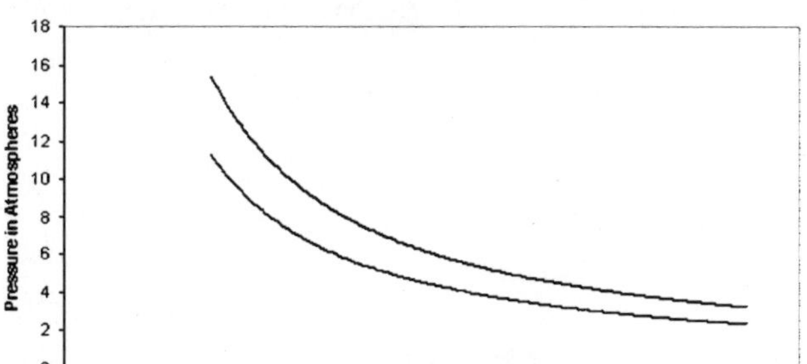

Adiabatic behaviour: "Adiabatic" means "nothing gets through", in this case *no heat gets in or out* of the gas through the walls. So all the work done in compressing the gas has to go into the internal energy E_{int}.

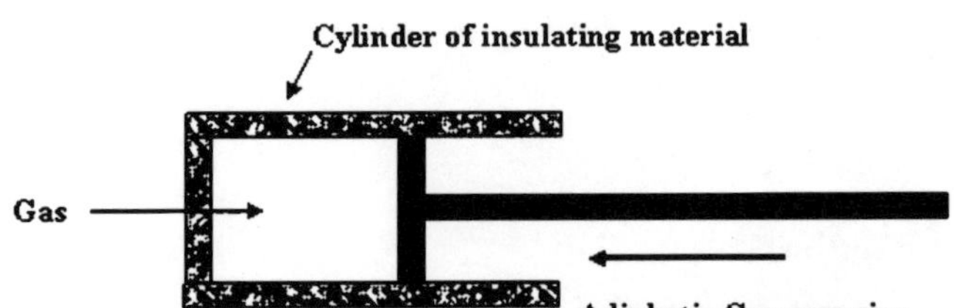

As the gas is compressed, it follows a curve in the (P, V) plane called an *adiabat*. To see how an adiabat differs from an isotherm, imagine beginning at some point on the blue 273K isotherm on the above graph, and applying pressure so the gas moves to higher pressure and lower volume. Since the gas's internal energy is increasing, but the number of molecules is staying the same, its temperature is necessarily rising, it will move towards the red curve, then above it. This means *the adiabats are always steeper than the isotherms*.

Equation for an Adiabat

What equation for an adiabat corresponds to $PV = nRT_1$ for an isotherm? On raising the gas temperature by ΔT, the change in the *internal energy*—the sum of molecular kinetic energy, rotational energy and vibrational energy (if any),

$$\Delta E_{int} = C_V \Delta T.$$

This is always true: whether or not the gas is changing volume is irrelevant, all that counts in E_{int} is the sum of the energies of the individual molecules (assuming as we do here that attractive or repulsive forces between molecules are negligible). In adiabatic compression, all the work done by the external pressure goes into this internal energy, so

$$-P\Delta V = C_V \Delta T.$$

(Compressing the gas of course gives negative ΔV, positive ΔE_{int}.)

To find the equation of an adiabat, we take the infinitesimal limit

$$-PdV = C_V dT$$

Divide the left-hand side by PV, the right-hand side by RT (since $PV = RT$, that's OK) to find

$$-\frac{R}{C_V}\frac{dV}{V} = \frac{dT}{T}.$$

Recall now that $C_P = C_V + R$,
and $C_P/C_v = \gamma$. It follows that

$$\frac{R}{C_V} = \frac{C_P - C_V}{C_V} = \gamma - 1.$$

Hence

$$-(\gamma - 1)\int \frac{dv}{v} = \int \frac{dT}{T}$$

and integrating

$$\text{In } T + (\gamma - 1)$$

$$\text{InV} = \text{const.}$$

from which the equation of an adiabat is

$$TV^{r-1} = \text{const.}$$

From $PV = RT$, the P, V equation for an adiabat can be found by multiplying the left-hand side of this equation by the constant PV/T, giving

PV^{r} = const.for an adiabat,

where $\gamma = 5/3$ for a monatomic gas, $7/5$ for a diatomic gas.

THERMODYNAMIC PROCESSES

A thermodynamic process can be defined as "an operation during which the properties of state, pressure, volume and temperature may change, with energy transfer in the form of work and/or heat flow taking place"

Whenever one or more of the properties of a system change, a change in the state of the system occurs. The path of the succession of states through which the system passes is called the thermodynamic process.

One example of a thermodynamic process is increasing the temperature of a fluid while maintaining a constant pressure. Another example is increasing the pressure of a confined gas while maintaining a constant temperature.

Second Law of Thermodynamics

One of the earliest statements of the Second Law of Thermodynamics was made by R. Clausius in 1850. He stated

"It is impossible to construct a device that operates in a cycle and produces no effect other than the removal of heat from a body at one temperature and the absorption of an equal quantity of heat by a body at a higher temperature".

The second law states that there exists a useful state variable called entropy S. The change in entropy delta S is equal to the heat transfer delta Q divided by the temperature T.

delta S = delta Q / T

For a given physical process, the combined entropy of the system and the environment remains a constant if the process can be reversed. If we denote the initial and final states of the system by "i" and "f":

Sf = Si (reversible process)

An example of a reversible process is ideally forcing a flow through a constricted pipe. Ideal means no boundary layer losses. As the flow moves through the constriction, the pressure, temperature and velocity change, but these variables return to their original values downstream of the constriction. The state of the gas returns to its original conditions and the change of entropy of the system is zero. Engineers call such a process an isentropic process. Isentropic means constant entropy.

The second law states that if the physical process is irreversible, the combined entropy of the system and the environment must increase. The final entropy must be greater than the initial entropy for an irreversible process:

$$Sf > Si \text{ (irreversible process)}$$

In a general sense, the Second Law says that the differences between systems in contact with each other tend to even out. Pressure differences, density differences, and particularly temperature differences, all tend to equalize if given the opportunity. This means that an isolated system will eventually come to have a uniform temperature. A thermodynamic engine is an engine that provides useful work from the difference in temperature of two bodies. Since any thermodynamic engine requires such a temperature difference, it follows that no useful work can be derived from an isolated system in equilibrium, there must always be energy fed from the outside. The Second Law is often invoked as the reason why perpetual motion machines cannot exist.

The Second Law can be stated in various succinct ways, including:

- It is impossible to produce work in the surroundings using a cyclic process connected to a single heat reservoir (Kelvin, 1851).
- If thermodynamic work is to be done at a finite rate, free energy must be expended.

A mathematical statement of the Second Law is: $\frac{dS}{dt} \geq 0$ on average

where

S is the entropy and

t is time.

Note that this equation does not *need* to be true, but the Second Law asserts that it is *usually* true. Entropy can decrease, but this simply tends not to happen as often. A common misconception is that the Second Law means that entropy never decreases. In fact, the Second Law asserts only a statistical tendency, hence it is only *highly unlikely* that entropy will decrease in a closed system at any given instant.

Entropy

One consequence of the second law is the development of the physical property of matter termed entropy (S). Entropy was introduced to help explain the Second Law of Thermodynamics. The change in this property is used to determine the direction in which a given process will proceed. Entropy can also be explained as a measure of the unavailability of heat to perform work in a cycle. This relates to the second law since the second law predicts that not all heat provided to a cycle can be transformed into an equal amount of work, some heat rejection must take place. The change in entropy is defined as the ratio of heat transferred during a reversible process to the absolute temperature of the system. In the early 1850s, thermodynamicist Rudolf Clausius began to put the thermodynamic concepts of energy dissipation on a mathematical footing. Clausius defined the change in entropy dS of a thermodynamic system, during a reversible process, as

$$\Delta S = dQ/T_{abs} \text{ (For a reversible process)}$$

where

S = The change in entropy of a system during some process (Btu/°R).

dQ = The amount of heat added to the system during the process (Btu).

DT_{abs} = The absolute temperature at which the heat was transferred (°R).

This expression comes from the Clausius theorem. This definition makes sense when absolute temperature has been defined. Note that the small amount d*Q* of energy transferred by heating is denoted by d*Q* rather than *dQ*, because *Q* is not a state function while the entropy is.

Clausius gave the quantity *S* the name "entropy", from the Greek word *ôñoðÞ*, "transformation". Since this definition involves only differences in entropy, the entropy itself is only defined up to an arbitrary additive constant.

When a process is irreversible, the above definition must be replaced by the statement that the entropy change is equal to the amount of energy required to return the system to its original state by a reversible transformation at a constant temperature, divided by that temperature.

Clausius' identification of *S* as a significant quantity was motivated by the study of reversible and irreversible thermodynamic transformations. A thermodynamic transformation is a change in a system's thermodynamic properties, such as temperature and volume. A transformation is reversible if it is quasistatic which means that it is infinitesimally close to thermodynamic equilibrium at all times.

Otherwise, the transformation is irreversible. To illustrate this, consider a gas enclosed in a piston chamber, whose volume may be changed by moving the piston.

If we move the piston slowly enough, the density of the gas is always homogeneous, so the transformation is reversible. If we move the piston quickly, pressure waves are created, so the gas is not in equilibrium, and the transformation is irreversible.

A heat engine is a thermodynamic system that can undergo a sequence of transformations which ultimately return it to its original state. Such a sequence is called a cyclic process, or simply a *cycle*. During some transformations, the engine may exchange energy with the environment. The net result of a cycle is

- Mechanical work done by the system (which can be positive or negative, the latter meaning that work is done *on* the engine), and
- Heat energy transferred from one part of the environment to another. By the conservation of energy, the net energy lost by the environment is equal to the work done by the engine.

If every transformation in the cycle is reversible, the cycle is reversible, and it can be run in reverse, so that the energy transfers occur in the opposite direction and the amount of work done switches sign.

Temperature

In thermodynamics, absolute temperature is *defined* in the following way. Suppose we have two heat reservoirs, which are systems sufficiently large that their temperatures do not change when energy flows into or out of them. A reversible cycle exchanges heat with the two heat reservoirs:

$$\frac{Q_1}{T_1} = \frac{Q_2}{T_2}$$

where

Q_1 is the amount of heat that the cycle absorbs from the first reservoir,

T_1 is the temperature of the first reservoir and

Q_2 is the amount of heat delivered to the second,

T_2 is the temperature of the second reservoir.

Introduce an additional heat reservoir at an arbitrary temperature T_0, as well as N cycles with the following property: the j-th such cycle operates between the T_0 reservoir and the T_j reservoir, transferring energy δQ_j to the latter. From the above definition of temperature, the energy extracted from the T_0 reservoir by the j-th cycle is

$$\delta Q_{0,j} = T_0 \frac{\delta Q_j}{T_j}$$

Now consider one cycle of the heat engine, accompanied by one cycle of each of the smaller cycles.

At the end of this process, each of the N reservoirs have zero net energy loss (since the energy extracted by the engine is replaced by the smaller cycles), and the heat engine has done an amount of work equal to the energy extracted from the T_0 reservoir,

$$W = \sum_{j=1}^{N} \delta Q_{0,j} = T_0 \sum_{j=1}^{N} \frac{\delta Qj}{T_j}$$

If this quantity is positive, this process would be a perpetual motion machine of the second kind, which is impossible. Thus,

$$\sum_{i=1}^{N} \frac{\delta Q_i}{T_i} \le 0$$

Now repeat the above argument for the reverse cycle. The result is

$$\sum_{i=1}^{N} \frac{\delta Q_i}{T_i} = 0 \text{ (reversible cycles)}$$

Now consider a reversible cycle in which the engine exchanges heats dQ_1, dQ_2,..., dQ_N with a sequence of N heat reservoirs with temperatures T_1,..., T_N. We can show that:

$$\sum_{i=1}^{N} \frac{\delta Q_i}{T_i} = 0$$

where

dQ_i is the amount of heat exchanged *from* the engine *to* the reservoir,
T_i is the temperature of each heat reservoir, and
i is an integer representing each different heat reservoir.

Since the cycle is reversible, the engine is always infinitesimally close to equilibrium, so its temperature is equal to any reservoir with which it is contact. In the limiting case of a reversible cycle consisting of a *continuous* sequence of transformations,

$$\oint \frac{\delta Q}{T} = 0 \text{ (reversible cycles)}$$

where the integral is taken over the entire cycle, and T is the temperature of the system at each point in the cycle. This is a particular case of the Clausius theorem.

State Function

We can now deduce an important fact about the entropy change during *any* thermodynamic transformation, not just a cycle. First, consider a reversible transformation that brings a system from an equilibrium state A to another equilibrium state B. If we follow this with *any* reversible transformation which returns that system to state A, our above result says that the net entropy change is zero. This implies that the entropy change in the first transformation depends *only on the initial and final states*. This allows us to define the entropy of any *equilibrium* state of a system. Choose a reference state R and call its entropy S_R. The entropy of any equilibrium state X is

$$S_X = S_R + \int_R^X \frac{\delta Q}{T}$$

Since the integral is independent of the particular transformation taken, this equation is well-defined.

Entropy Changes in Irreversible Processes

We now consider irreversible Processes. It can be shown that the entropy change during any transformation between two *equilibrium* states is

$$\Delta S \geq \int \frac{\delta Q}{T}$$

where the equality holds if the transformation is reversible.

Notice that if $dQ = 0$, then DS e≥ 0. This is the Second Law of Thermodynamics, which we have discussed earlier.

Suppose a system is thermally and mechanically isolated from the environment. For example, consider an insulating rigid box divided by a movable partition into two volumes, each filled with gas. If the pressure of one gas is higher, it will expand by moving the partition, thus performing work on the other gas. Also, if the gases are at different temperatures, heat can flow from one gas to the other provided the partition is an imperfect insulator. Our above result indicates that the entropy of the system *as a whole* will increase during these process (it could in principle remain constant, but this is unlikely.) Typically, there exists a maximum amount of entropy the system may possess under the circumstances. This entropy corresponds to a state of *stable equilibrium*, since a transformation to any other equilibrium state would cause the entropy to decrease, which is forbidden. Once the system reaches this maximum-entropy state, no part of the system can perform work on any other part. It is in this sense that entropy is a measure of the energy in a system that "cannot be used to do work".

Effect of Temperature, Volume, and Concentration on the Entropy

As discussed previously, the entropy of a substance always increases with temperature. This is due mainly to the increased number of ways that the thermal energy can be distributed amongst the allowed energy levels as the latter become accessible. The rate of increase *dS/dT* is just the ratio of the heat capacity to the temperature *C/T*. When integrated over a range of temperatures, this yields (for an ideal gas confined to a fixed volume)

$$\Delta S = C \ln\left(\frac{T_2}{T_1}\right)$$

In general, a larger volume also leads to increased entropy. For an ideal gas that expands at a constant temperature (meaning that it absorbs heat from the surroundings to compensate for the work it does during the expansion), the increase in entropy is given by

$$\Delta S = R \ln\left(\frac{V_2}{V_1}\right)$$

Because the pressure of a gas is inversely proportional to its volume, we can easily alter the above relation to express the entropy change associated with a change in the pressure of a perfect gas:

$$\Delta S = R \ln\left(\frac{P_2}{P_1}\right)$$

The pressure of a gas is directly proportional to its concentration in moles per litre, so we can re-cast this equation in terms of concentrations:

$$\Delta S = R\ln\left(\frac{C_2}{C_1}\right)$$

Although these equations strictly apply only to perfect gases and cannot be used at all for liquids and solids, it turns out that in a dilute solution, the solute can often be treated as a gas dispersed in the volume of the solution, so the last equation can actually give a fairly accurate value for the entropy of dilution of a solution.

Entropy of Mixing (Ideal Gases)

Visualize that we have a container divided into two compartments. In one compartment we have n_1 moles of an ideal gas, gas 1, at pressure, p and temperature, T. In the other compartment we have n_2 moles of another ideal gas, gas 2, at the same p and T.

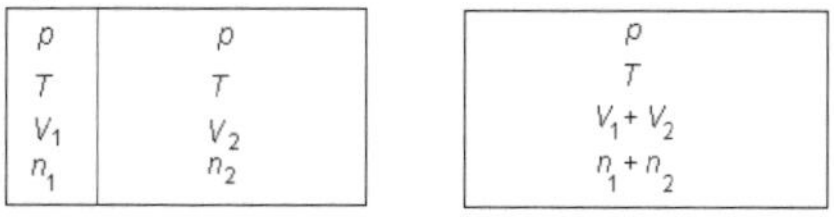

p T V_1 n_1	p T V_2 n_2	p T $V_1 + V_2$ $n_1 + n_2$

If we remove the partition the gases will begin to diffuse into each other and the system will eventually reach the state where both gases are uniformly distributed throughout the container. This is clearly an irreversibly process so that we would expect that the entropy would increase.

To calculate thc entropy change we must find a reversible path to carry out the process, even if the path is fictitious. Imagine that we can devise a process that will expand one gas reversibly and isothermally, but leave the other gas undisturbed. We know how to calculate the change in entropy for the reversible isothermal expansion of an ideal gas.

Recall that $dU = 0$ for the isothermal expansion of an ideal gas. Then,

$$dU = TdS - PdV = 0$$

So,

$$TdS = PdV$$

$$dS = \frac{P}{T}dV$$

$$= \frac{nR}{V}dV,$$

for an ideal gas. So, for gas number 1 in our fictitious isothermal expansion we have,

$$\Delta S_1 = n_1 R\ln\frac{V_1 + V_2}{V_1},$$

and for gas number 2,

$$\Delta S_2 = n_2 R \ln \frac{V_1 + V_2}{V_2},$$

The total entropy change is the sum of these two individual entropy changes,

$$\Delta S_{mix} = \Delta S_1 + \Delta S_2 = n_1 R \ln \frac{V_1 - V_2}{V_1} + n_2 R \ln \frac{V_1 + V_2}{V_2}$$

Equation 4 could be used for calculations, but it is not in the form that we will see in other contexts. To obtain the usual form factor the R out of Equation 4 and invert the argument of the logarithms,

$$\Delta S_{mix} = -R\left(n_1 \ln \frac{V_1}{V_1 + V_2} + n_2 \ln \frac{V_2}{V_1 + V_2} \right)$$

Since we are doing a calculation for ideal gases, notice that the argument of the first logarithm in Equation 5 can be written,

$$\frac{V_1}{V_1 + V_2} = \frac{\frac{n_1 RT}{p}}{\frac{n_1 RT}{p} + \frac{n_2 RT}{p}} = \frac{n_1}{n_1 + n_2} = X_1$$

where X_1 is the mole fraction of component 1. There is an equivalent expression for the argument of the second logarithm. The entropy of mixing becomes,

$$\Delta S_{mix} = -R(n_1 \ln X_1 + n_2 \ln X_2).$$

Equation 7 is also suitable for calculations, but it is not yet in the standard form. To obtain the standard form write the total number of moles $n_1 + n_2$ as n and multiply and divide equation by n. The result is

$$\Delta S_{mix} = -nR(X_1 \ln X_1 + X_2 \ln X_2).$$

Equation 8 is the same form that we will find when we derive an expression for the entropy of mixing ideal solutions and it is the same form that Shannon found for the "entropy of a message" in his famous series of papers on information theory.

If the two gases were not at the same initial pressure you would have to introduce some extra steps. Expand or compress one of the gases to bring it to the pressure of the other gas, mix the gases, and then compress or expand the mixture to bring it to the correct final volume and pressure.

If the two gases are not at the same temperature and pressure it is more complicated. You must find the final temperature using heat balance, reversibly cool and heat the two gases respectively to the same temperature, expand or contract on of the gases, mix them, and then expand or contract the mixture to the appropriate volume.

Equation 8 can easily be extended to more than two gases,

$$\Delta S_{mix} = -nR(X_1 \ln X_1 + X_2 \ln X_2 + X_3 \ln X_3 + ...)$$

Example - The Molar Entropy of Dry Air

The composition of dry air is approximately 78per cent N_2, 21per cent O_2, and 1per cent Ar by volume (which is the same as mole percent). What is the molar entropy of mixing of air?

$$\Delta S_{\text{mix,air}} = 1 \text{ mol} \times 8.314$$

$$(0.78 \ln 0.78 + 0.21 \ln 0.21 + 0.01 \ln 0.01)$$

$$= 4.7 \frac{\text{J}}{\text{K}}.$$

What Does Entropy Measure

Entropy measures disorder. If we look at the processes we have seen which have positive entropy changes we can see that in each case an increase in entropy is associated with an increase in disorder.

An isothermal expansion gives the molecules more room to move around in, the molecules are less localized.

Increasing the temperature increases the average speeds of the molecules. The molecules are said to be more disordered in "velocity space" (or momentum space).

Mixing gases (or liquids) intersperses the molecules among each other increasing the disorder.

Phase changes, such as going from a solid to a liquid or a gas, or from a liquid to a gas, increase the entropy because gases are more disordered than solids or liquids and liquids are more disordered than solids.

For example, the entropy of fusion of 1.00 mol of ice at 273.15 (heat of fusion is 6.008 kJ/mol) is

$$\Delta S_{\text{fus}} = \frac{6008\,\text{J}}{273.15\,\text{K}} = 22.0 \frac{\text{J}}{\text{K}}.$$

Vapourization of liquids has a large positive entropy of vapourization because gases are greatly disordered compared to liquids. A typical value is obtained from the vapourization of benzene at its boiling point. The heat of vapourization is 30.8 kJ at the boiling point, 353.1K. The entropy of vapourization is

$$\Delta S_{\text{vap}} = \frac{30800\,\text{J}}{353.1\,\text{K}} = 87.2 \frac{\text{J}}{\text{K}}.$$

It is interesting that the entropy of vapourization of many substances at their boiling points is close to about 86 J/K. (Water and helium are exceptions.) This phenomenon is called "Trouton's rule." It is easily understood on the basis of entropy being a measure of disorder. The vapourization process essentially "creates" a mole of disordered molecules (the gas) from a mole of highly ordered molecules (the solid or liquid). The gases are all at one atmosphere pressure because we are at their normal boiling point.

Measurement of Entropy

In real experiments, it is quite difficult to measure the entropy of a system. The techniques for doing so are based on the thermodynamic definition of the entropy, and require extremely careful calorimetry.

For simplicity, we will examine a mechanical system, whose thermodynamic state may be specified by its volume *V* and pressure *P*.

In order to measure the entropy of a specific state, we must first measure the heat capacity at constant volume and at constant pressure (denoted C_V and C_P respectively), for a successive set of states intermediate between a reference state and the desired state. The heat capacities are related to the entropy *S* and the temperature *T* by

$$C_X = T\left(\frac{\partial S}{\partial T}\right)_X$$

where the *X* subscript refers to either constant volume or constant pressure. This may be integrated numerically to obtain a change in entropy:

$$\Delta S = \int \frac{C_X}{T} dT$$

We can thus obtain the entropy of any state (P,V) with respect to a reference state (P_0,V_0). The exact formula depends on our choice of intermediate states. For example, if the reference state has the same pressure as the final state,

$$S(P,V) = S(P,V_0) + \int_{T(P,V_0)}^{T(P,V)} \frac{C_P(P,V(T,P))}{T} dT$$

In addition, if the path between the reference and final states lies across any first order phase transition, the latent heat associated with the transition must be taken into account.

The entropy of the reference state must be determined independently. Ideally, one chooses a reference state at an extremely high temperature, at which the system exists as a gas.

The entropy in such a state would be that of a classical ideal gas plus contributions from molecular rotations and vibrations, which may be determined spectroscopically.

Choosing a *low* temperature reference state is sometimes problematic since the entropy at low temperatures may behave in unexpected ways. For instance, a calculation of the entropy of ice by the latter method, assuming no entropy at zero temperature, falls short of the value obtained with a high-temperature reference state by 3.41 J/(mol·K). This is due to the "zero-point" entropy of ice mentioned earlier.

Available Useful Work

An important and revealing idealised special case is to consider applying the Second Law to the scenario of an isolated system (called the total system or universe), made up of two parts: a sub-system of interest, and the sub-system's surroundings.

These surroundings are imagined to be so large that they can be considered as an *unlimited* heat reservoir at temperature T_R and pressure P_R — so that no matter how much heat is transferred to (or from) the sub-system, the temperature of the surroundings will remain T_R; and no matter how much the volume of the sub-system expands (or contracts), the pressure of the surroundings will remain P_R.

Whatever changes dS and dS_R occur in the entropies of the sub-system and the surroundings individually, according to the Second Law the entropy S_{tot} of the isolated total system must increase:

$$dS_{\text{tot}} = dS + dS_R \geq 0$$

According to the First Law of Thermodynamics, the change dU in the internal energy of the sub-system is the sum of the heat dq added to the sub-system, *less* any work dw done *by* the sub-system, *plus* any net chemical energy entering the sub-system $\Sigma\mu_{\text{iR}} N_i$, so that:

$$dU = \delta q - \delta w + d\,(Sm_{iR}N_i)$$

where m_{iR} are the chemical potentials of chemical species in the external surroundings.

Now the heat leaving the reservoir and entering the sub-system is

$$\delta q = T_R(-dS_R) \leq T_R dS$$

where we have first used the definition of entropy in classical thermodynamics (alternatively, the definition of temperature in statistical thermodynamics); and then the Second Law inequality from above.

It therefore follows that any net work dw done by the sub-system must obey

$$\delta w \leq -dU + T_R dS + \Sigma\mu_{iR} dN_i$$

It is useful to separate the work done dw done by the subsystem into the *useful* work dw_u that can be done *by* the sub-system, over and beyond the work $P_R\, dV$ done merely by the sub-system expanding against the surrounding external pressure, giving the following relation for the useful work that can be done:

$$\delta w_u \leq -d(U - T_R S + P_R V - \Sigma\mu_{iR} N_i)$$

It is convenient to define the right-hand-side as the exact derivative of a thermodynamic potential, called the *availability* or exergy X of the subsystem,

$$\mathrm{X = U - T_R S + P_R V - \Sigma\mu_{iR} N_i}$$

The Second Law therefore implies that for any process which can be considered as divided simply into a subsystem, and an unlimited temperature and pressure reservoir with which it is in contact,

$$dX + \delta w_u \leq 0$$

i.e. the change in the subsystem's exergy plus the useful work done *by* the subsystem (or, the change in the subsystem's exergy less any work, additional to that done by the pressure reservoir, done *on* the system) must be less than or equal to zero.

Various types of thermodynamic processes are:

Cyclic Process

When a system in a given initial state goes through a number of different changes in state (going through various processes) and finally returns to its initial values, the system has undergone a cyclic process or cycle. Therefore, at the conclusion of a cycle, all the properties have the same value they had at the beginning. Steam (water) that circulates through a closed cooling loop undergoes a cycle.

Reversible Process

A reversible process for a system is defined as a process that, once having taken place, can be reversed, and in so doing leaves no change in either the system or surroundings.

In other words the system and surroundings are returned to their original condition before the process took place.

In reality, there are no truly reversible processes; however, for analysis purposes, one uses reversible to make the analysis simpler, and to determine maximum theoretical efficiencies.

Therefore, the reversible process is an appropriate starting point on which to base engineering study and calculation.

Although the reversible process can be approximated, it can never be matched by real processes. One way to make real processes approximate reversible process is to carry out the process in a series of small or infinitesimal steps.

For example, heat transfer may be considered reversible if it occurs due to a small temperature difference between the system and its surroundings. For example, transferring heat across a temperature difference of 0.00001°F "appears" to be more reversible than for transferring heat across a temperature difference of 100 °F.

Therefore, by cooling or heating the system in a number of infinitesamally small steps, we can approximate a reversible process. Although not practical for real processes, this method is beneficial for thermodynamic studies since the rate at which processes occur is not important.

Irreversible Process

An irreversible process is a process that cannot return both the system and the surroundings to their original conditions. That is, the system and the surroundings would not return to their original conditions if the process was reversed. For example, an automobile engine does not give back the fuel it took to drive up a hill as it coasts back down the hill.

There are many factors that make a process irreversible. Four of the most common causes of irreversibility are friction, unrestrained expansion of a fluid, heat transfer through a finite temperature difference, and mixing of two different substances. These factors are present in real, irreversible processes and prevent these processes from being reversible.

Adiabatic Process

An adiabatic process is one in which there is no heat transfer into or out of the system. The system can be considered to be perfectly insulated. Example:

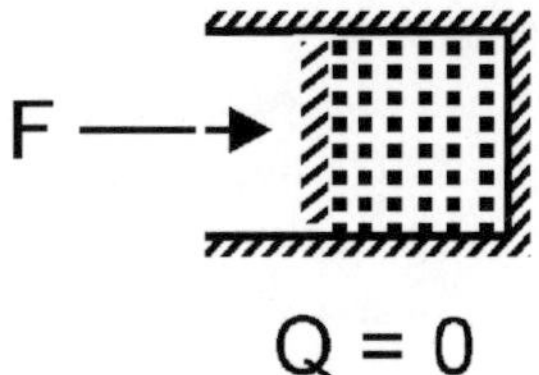

Q = 0

Fig. Compression of a Gas in an Insulated Cylinder.

In this case any change in the internal energy of the gas is due to work done on it or by it, $\Delta U = W$.

Normally if ΔU changes the temperature of a system will change. Any temperature rise or fall is due to the work done or by the gas alone and not due to heat flowing into or out of the system since $Q = 0$.

If a process is carried out fast enough the heat flow will be small and the process can be approximate as being adiabatic. This happen because heat flow is in general a slow process.

Observe that we did not say that Q is constant because it not a state variable. Q represent an energy transfer not the heat energy of the system.

In addition to the ideal gas law $PV = NkT$, the quantity PV^{γ} is constant for an ideal gas where $\gamma = c_P / c_V$, the ratio of molar specific heats. For an ideal gas the work

$$W = (P_1V_1 - P_2V_2)/(\gamma - 1)$$

Isoentropic Process

An isoentropic process is one in which the entropy of the fluid remains constant. This will be true if the process the system goes through is reversible and adiabatic. An isoentropic process can also be called a constant entropy process.

Example: A Heat Engine in which the working fluid undergoes an Adiabatic Reversible cyclic process.

T_{high}

Q_2

$\Delta S = 0$ W

Q_1

T_{low}

Any isoentropic process is also adiabatic since ΔU = ∨ dQ/T and Q = 0. However, not all adiabatic process are isoentropic. Adiabatic free expansion is not isoentropic.

For a heat engine to be reversible, not only must the change in entropy of the working fluid be zero but also the net change of the entropy of the environment (heat reservoirs) must also be zero.

Polytropic Process

When a gas undergoes a reversible process in which there is heat transfer, the process frequently takes place in such a manner that a plot of the Log P (pressure) vs. Log V (volume) is a straight line. Or stated in equation form PV^n = a constant. This type of process is called a polytropic process. An example of a polytropic process is the expansion of the combustion gasses in the cylinder of a water-cooled reciprocating engine.

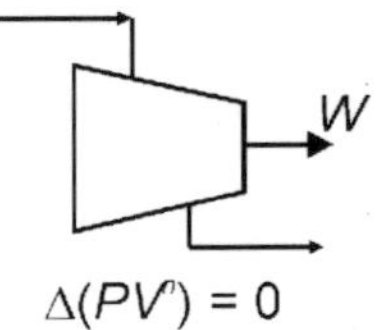

Here n can be any real number. All the process above can thought of as a special case of a polytropic process for an ideal gas.

n = 0 for Isobaric process since $PV^0 = P$ = constant.

n = 1 for Isothermal process since $PV^1 = PV = NKT$ = constant.

n = ∞ for Isovolumetric process.

n = γ for Adiabatic process.

Throttling Process

A throttling process is defined as a process in which there is no change in enthalpy from state one to state two, $h_1 = h_2$; no work is done, W = 0; and the process is adiabatic, Q = 0. To better understand the theory of the ideal throttling process let's compare what we can observe with the above theoretical assumptions. An example of a throttling process is an ideal gas flowing through a valve in midposition. From experience we can observe that:

$$P_{in} > P_{out},\ vel_{in} < vel_{out}$$

where

P = pressure

vel = velocity

These observations confirm the theory that

$$h_{in} = h_{out}$$

Remember h = u + Pv (v = specific volume), so if pressure decreases then specific volume must increase if enthalpy is to remain constant (assuming u is constant). Because mass flow is constant, the change in specific volume is observed as an increase in gas velocity, and this is verified by our observations. The theory also states W = 0. Our observations again confirm this to be true as clearly no "work" has been done by the throttling process. Finally, the theory states that an ideal throttling process is adiabatic. This cannot clearly be proven by observation since a "real" throttling process is not ideal and will have some heat transfer.

Carnot's Principle

An irreversible heat engine operating between two heat reservoirs at constant temperatures cannot have an efficiency greater than that of a reversible heat engine operating between the same two temperatures.

Another form of the Second Law of Thermodynamics or Carnot's Principle is that: It is not possible to make a heat engine whose only effect is to absorb heat from a high-temperature region and turn all that heat into work. That is, it is not possible to design a heat engine that does not exhaust heat to the environment. Or, it is not possible to design a heat engine that has an efficiency of 1.00 or 100per cent.

Carnot Cycle

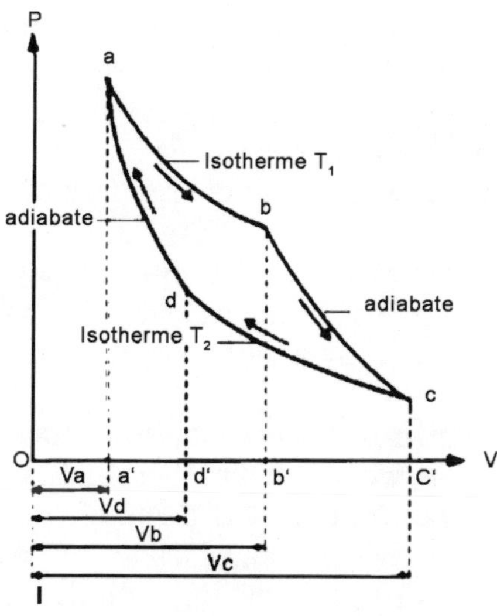

The Carnot cycle is the most efficient cycle possible. It consists of four basic reversible processes meaning that the cycle as a whole is also reversible. The four reversible processes are:

- Adiabatic compression from T_2 to T_1.
- Isothermal expansion (by placing the system in contact with a heat reservoir with temperature T_1).
- Adiabatic expansion to $T_2 < T_1$.
- Isothermal compression (by placing the system in contact with a heat reservoir with temperature T_2).

Carnot Engine

Engine using a Carnot cycle of operations. This type of engine can serve as the model for a thermic or refrigerator engine. An "animation" facilitates a better understanding of the cycle:

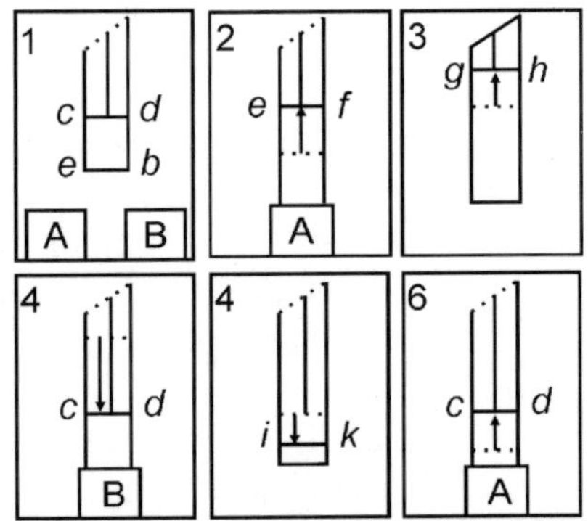

A Carnot heat engine is a hypothetical engine that operates on the reversible Carnot cycle. The basic model for this engine was developed by Nicolas Léonard Sadi Carnot in the 1824. Every thermodynamic system exists in a particular state. A thermodynamic cycle occurs when a system is taken through a series of different states, and finally returned to its initial state. In the process of going through this cycle, the system may perform work on its surroundings, thereby acting as a heat engine.

A heat engine acts by transferring energy from a warm region to a cool region of space and, in the process, converting some of that energy to mechanical work. The cycle may also be reversed. The system may be worked upon by an external force, and in the process, it can transfer thermal energy from a cooler system to a warmer one, thereby acting as a refrigerator rather than a heat engine.

In the adjacent diagram, from the original 1824 paper by Sadi Carnot entitled *On the Motive Power of Fire*, we are told to "imagine two bodies *A* and *B*, kept each at a constant temperature, that of *A* being higher than that of *B*. These two bodies, to which we can give or from which we can remove the heat without causing their temperatures to vary, exercise the functions of two unlimited reservoirs of caloric. We shall call the first the furnace and the second the refrigerator." Carnot then explains how we can obtain motive power, *i.e.* "work", by carrying a certain quantity of heat from the body A to the body B.

Carnot's Theorem

During one part of the cycle performed in an engine, some heat is absorbed from a hot reservoir. During another part, a smaller amount of heat is rejected to a cooler reservoir. The engine is therefore said to operate between these two reservoirs. It is a fact of experience that some heat is always rejected to the cooler reservoir. Because of this, the efficiency of an actual engine is never 100per cent. The processes that make up this cycle are either isothermal or adiabatic.

The Carnot Machine

We consider the standard Carnot-cycle machine, which can be thought of as having a piston moving within a cylinder, and having the following characteristics:

- A perfect seal, so that no atoms escape from the working fluid as the piston moves to expand or compress it.
- Perfect lubrication, so that there is no friction.
- An ideal-gas for the working fluid.
- Perfect thermal connection at any time either to one or to none of two reservoirs, which are at two different temperatures, with perfect thermal insulation isolating it from all other heat transfers.
- The piston moves back and forth repeatedly, in a cycle of alternating "isother-mal" and "adiabatic" expan-sions and compressions, according to the PV diagram shown:

By definition, the isothermal segments (AB and CD) occur when there is perfect thermal contact between the working fluid and one of the reservoirs, so that whatever heat is needed to maintain constant temperature will flow into or out of the working fluid, from or to the reservoir.

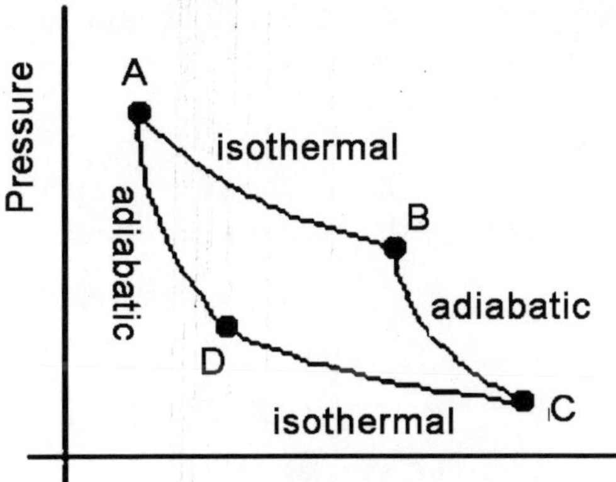

By definition, the adiabatic segments (BC and DA) occur when there is perfect thermal insulation between the working fluid and the rest of the universe, including both reservoirs, thereby preventing the flow of any heat into or out of the working fluid.

The isothermal curves (but not the adiabatic curves) are hyperbolas, according to PV = nRT. The enclosed area (and therefore the mechanical work done) will depend on the two temperatures ("height") and on the amount of heat transferred, which depends in turn on the extent of the isothermal compression or expansion ("width"), during which heat must be transferred to maintain the constant temperature.

We will denote the heat transferred to or from the high-temperature reservoir (during the transition between points A and B) as Qh.

We will denote the heat transferred to or from the low-temperature reservoir (during the transition between points C and D) as Qc.

Engine, Heat Pump or Refrigerator

If a Carnot machine cycles around the path clockwise, a high-temperature isothermal expansion from A to B, an adiabatic expansion cooling down from B to C, a low-temperature isothermal compression from C to D, and finally an adiabatic compression warming up from D to A, it functions as a heat engine, removing energy from the high-temperature reservoir as heat, transforming a portion of that energy to useful mechanical work (the enclosed area) done on the external world, and ejecting the remainder of the energy as waste heat to the low-temperature reservoir.

If a Carnot machine is driven (by an external agency, such as a motor) around the cycle counter clockwise, an adiabatic expansion cooling down from A to D, a low-temperature isothermal expansion from D to C, an adiabatic compression warming up from C to B, and finally a high temperature isothermal compression from B to A, then it functions as either a refrigerator or a heat pump, depending on whether removing heat from the low-temperature reservoir or adding heat to the high-temperature reservoir is of primary interest. The mechanical energy required to force the machine around the cycle is the work done on the machine, the area enclosed.

Efficiency

For a heat engine, the efficiency is the ratio of useful work performed to the heat energy consumed from the high-temperature reservoir:

$$Eff = \frac{W}{Q_h}$$

$$= \frac{Q_h - Q_c}{Q_h}$$

This ratio is the interesting one because you pay for the fuel to obtain Qh, in order to get the benefit of the work done, W. For a Carnot engine, this is entirely determined by the temperatures of the hot and cold reservoirs:

$$Eff = \frac{T_h - T_c}{T_h}$$

$$= 1 - \frac{T_c}{T_h}$$

This temperature dependence is a direct consequence of the second law of thermodynamics and the fact that all heat transfers occur during isothermal expansion and contraction, with no temperature difference between the heat reservoir and the working fluid, so that the entropy gained by one exactly matches the entropy lost by the other, with no net change in entropy for the system as a whole. This condition is of course an ideal one, and cannot be met in practice by any real machine. Thus, the Carnot efficiency is the best possible even theoretically; all real machines will be strictly worse than this.

For a Carnot machine functioning as a refrigerator, the "effectiveness" is the ratio of the energy removed from the low-temperature reservoir to the work required to force the machine around its cycle (the energy consumed and paid for):

$$Eff = \frac{Q_c}{W}$$

$$= \frac{Q_c}{Q_h - Q_c}$$

The effectiveness will be greater than 1 only if the absolute temperature of the cold reservoir is warmer than half that of the hot reservoir. We can see that refrigeration to extremely cold temperatures is very difficult.

For a Carnot machine functioning as a heat pump, the "effectiveness" is the ratio of the energy delivered to the high-temperature reservoir to the work required to force the machine around its cycle (the energy consumed and paid for):

$$Eff = \frac{Q_h}{W}$$

$$= \frac{Q_h}{Q_h - Q_c}$$

This effectiveness is also known as the coefficient of performance ("COP"). For heat pumps, the effectiveness is always greater than 1. Electrically powered heat pumps can make economic sense only if the effectiveness of the heat pump times the efficiency of the electrical generation and transmission process exceeds 1. Otherwise, only part of the fuel burned to produce the electricity would have to be burned to provide the heat needed. (Modern natural gas furnaces can easily transfer more than 95per cent of the combustion heat to the heated space).

As the temperature of the cold reservoir (the outside temperature) declines, the COP of the heat pump decreases towards 1. Because large electrical generators produce about one-third as much electical energy as the heat value of the fuel they consume, as soon as the COP is less than about 3, it would be cheaper to burn the original fuel directly for the heat, rather than generate electricity to operate a heat pump. This limits the geographical regions where heat pumps make economic sense.

Real Process Cycle Compared to Carnot Cycle

The most important aspect of the second law for our practical purposes is the determination of maximum possible efficiencies obtained from a power system. Actual efficiencies will always be less than this maximum. The losses (friction, for example) in the system and the fact that systems are not truly reversible preclude us from obtaining the maximum possible efficiency.

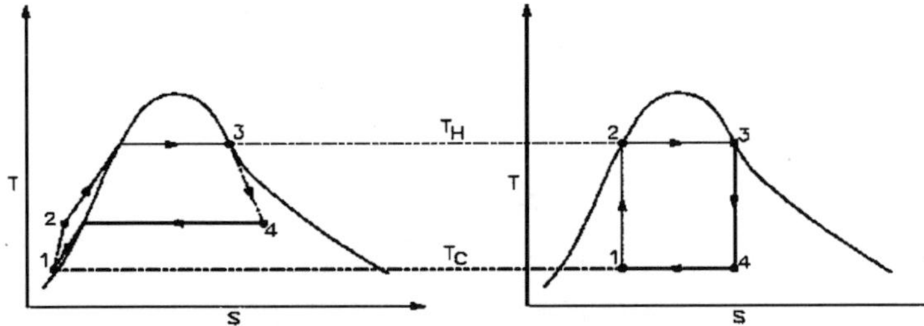

Any ideal thermodynamic process can be drawn as a path on a property diagram, such as a T-s or an h-s diagram. A real process that approximates the ideal process can also be represented on the same diagrams (usually with the use of dashed lines). In an ideal process involving either a reversible expansion or a reversible compression, the entropy will be constant. These isentropic processes will be represented by vertical lines on either T-s or h-s diagrams, since entropy is on the horizontal axis and its value does not change.

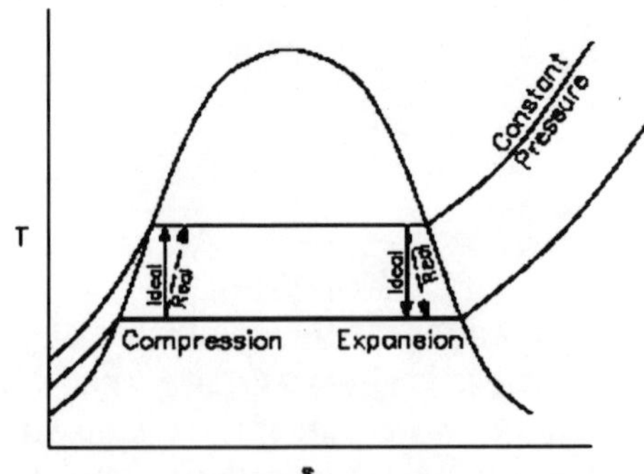

Fig. (a) Expansion and Compression Processes on T-s Diagram

A real expansion or compression process operating between the same pressures as the ideal process will look much the same, but the dashed lines representing the real process will slant slightly towards the right since the entropy will increase from the start to the end of the process. Figures shown (a and b) below shows ideal and real expansion and compression processes on T-s and h-s diagrams.

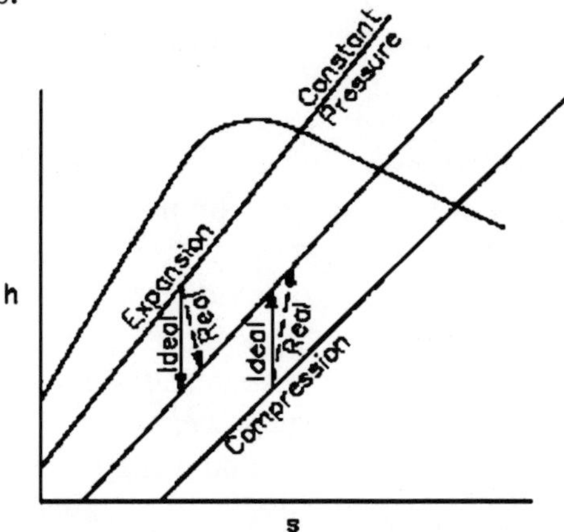

Fig. (b) Expansion and Compression Processes on h-s Diagram

Carnot cycle, opera-ting with ideal components under real world constraints, should convert almost 3/4 of the input heat into work. But, this ideal efficiency is well beyond the present capabilities of any real systems.

Early thermo-dyna-mic developments were centered around impro-ving the perfor-mance of contem-porary steam engines.

It was desirable to construct a cycle that was as close to being reversible as possible and would better lend itself to the characteristics of steam and process control than the Carnot cycle did. Towards this end, the Rankine cycle was developed.

Rankine Cycle

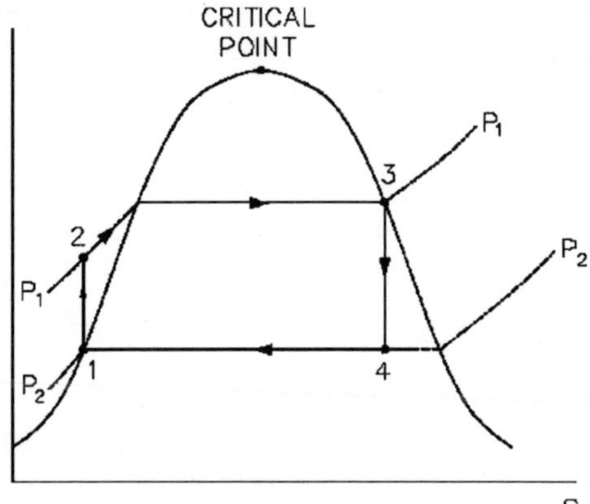

The main feature of the Rankine cycle, is that it confines the isentropic compression process to the liquid phase only. This minimizes the amount of work required to attain operating pressures and avoids the mechanical problems associated with pumping a two-phase mixture. The Rankine cycle is a thermodynamic cycle. Like other thermodynamic cycles, the maximum efficiency of the Rankine cycle is given by calculating the maximum efficiency of the Carnot cycle. It is named after William John Macquorn Rankine.

There are four processes in the Rankine cycle, each changing the state of the working fluid. These states are identified by number in the diagram above.

- *Process 1-2*: First, the working fluid is pumped (ideally isentropically) from low to high pressure by a pump. Pumping requires a power input (for example mechanical or electrical).
- *Process 2-3*: The high pressure liquid enters a boiler where it is heated at constant pressure by an external heat source to become a superheated vapour. Common heat sources for power plant systems are coal, natural gas, or nuclear power.
- *Process 3-4*: The superheated vapour expands through a turbine to generate power output. Ideally, this expansion is isentropic. This decreases the temperature and pressure of the vapour.
- *Process 4-1*: The vapour then enters a condenser where it is cooled to become a saturated liquid. This liquid then re-enters the pump and the cycle repeats.

Rankine cycles describe the operation of steam heat engines commonly found in power generation plants. In such vapour power plants, power is generated by alternately vapourizing and condensing a working fluid (in many cases water, although refrigerants such as ammonia may also be used).

The working fluid in a Rankine cycle follows a closed loop and is re-used constantly. Water vapour seen billowing from power plants is evapourating cooling water, not working fluid.

In a real Rankine cycle, the compression by the pump and the expansion in the turbine are not isentropic. In other words, these processes are non-reversible and entropy is increased during the two processes (indicated in the figure as DS). This somewhat increases the power required by the pump and decreases the power generated by the turbine.

It also makes calculations more involved and difficult. There are two main variations of the basic Rankine cycle:

Rankine Cycle with Reheat

In this variation, two turbines work in series. The first accepts vapour from the boiler at high pressure. After the vapour has passed through the first turbine, it re-enters the boiler and is reheated before passing through a second, lower pressure turbine. Among other advantages, this prevents the vapour from condensing during its expansion which can seriously damage the turbine blades.

Regenerative Rankine Cycle

The regenerative Rankine cycle is so named because after emerging from the condenser the working fluid is heated by steam tapped from the hot portion of the cycle. This increases the average temperature of heat addition which in turn increases the thermodynamic efficiency of the cycle.

Steam Cycle

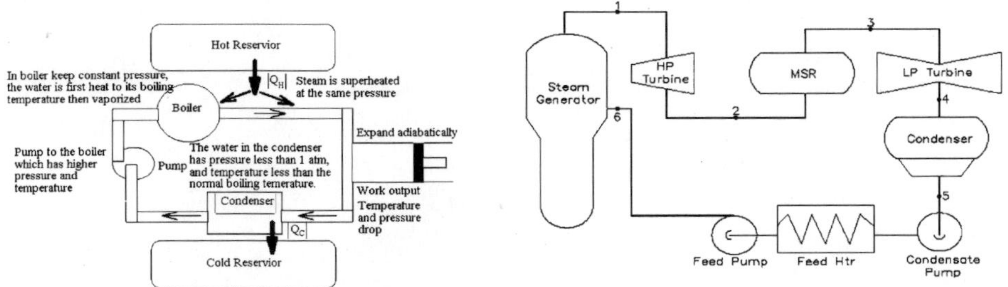

Above figure shows a simplified version of the major components of a typical steam plant cycle. This is a simplified version and does not contain the exact detail that may be found at most power plants. The following are the processes that comprise the cycle:

- 1-2: Saturated steam from the steam generator is expanded in the high pressure (HP) turbine to provide shaft work output at a constant entropy.
- 2-3: The moist steam from the exit of the HP turbine is dried and superheated in the moisture separator reheater (MSR).
- 3-4: Superheated steam from the MSR is expanded in the low pressure (LP) turbine to provide shaft work output at a constant entropy.
- 4-5: Steam exhaust from the turbine is condensed in the condenser in which heat is transferred to the cooling water under a constant vacuum condition.
- 5-6: The feedwater is compressed as a liquid by the condensate and feedwater pump and the feedwater is preheated by the feedwater heaters.
- 6-1: Heat is added to the working fluid in the steam generator under a constant pressure condition.

It must be pointed out that the cycle we have just shown is an ideal cycle and does not exactly represent the actual processes in the plant. The turbine and pumps in an ideal cycle are ideal pumps and turbines and therefore do not exhibit an increase in entropy across them. Real pumps and turbines would exhibit an entropy increase across them.

Otto Cycle

We look at the design of an Otto cycle and at how its performance can be improved by changing its volumetric compression ratio. The Otto cycle a closed cycle (where the system is a control mass), commonly used to model the cylinders of spark-ignition, internal combustion, automobile engines, *i.e.* gasoline engines.

The Otto cycle is very similar to the Diesel cycle in that both are closed cycles commonly used to model internal combustion engines. The difference between them is that the Otto cycle is a spark-ignition cycle instead of a compression-ignition cycle like the Diesel cycle. Spark-ignition cycles are designed to use fuels that require a spark to begin combustion.

Stages

Otto Cycles have four stages: expansion, cooling, compression, and combustion.

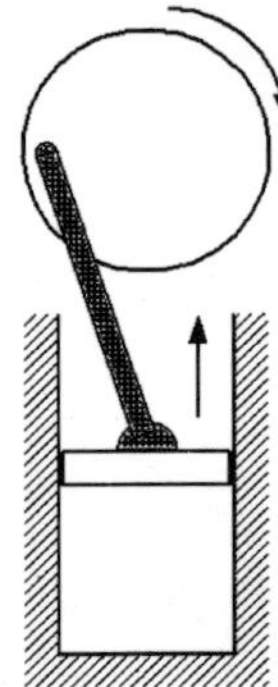

Fig. Moving up During Expansion

Expansion

In the Otto cycle, fuel is burned to heat compressed air and the hot gas expands forcing the piston to travel up in the cylinder. It is in this phase that the cycle contributes its useful work, rotating the automobile's crankshaft. We make the ideal assumption that this stage in an ideal Otto cycle is isentropic.

Piston: moving from bottom dead center to top dead center.

Cooling

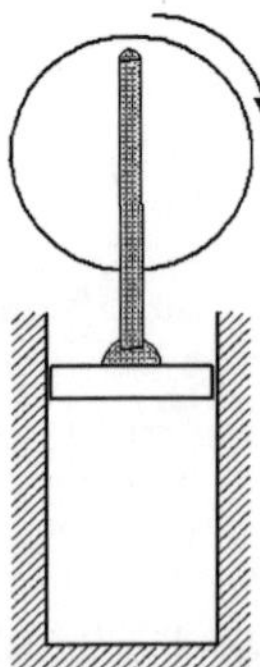

Fig. Top Dead Center During Cooling

Next, the expanded air is cooled down to ambient conditions. In an actual automobile engine, this corresponds to exhausting the air from the engine to the environment and replacing it with fresh air. Since this happens when the piston is at the top dead center position in the cycle and is not moving, we say this process is isochoric (no change in volume).

Piston: at top dead center.

Compression

In preparation for adding heat to the air, we next compress it by moving the piston down the cylinder. It is in this part of the cycle that we contribute work to the air. In the ideal Otto cycle, this compression is considered to be isentropic.

Fig. Moving Down During Compression

It is at this stage that we set the volumetric compression ratio, *r* which is the ratio of the volume of the working fluid before the compression process to its volume after. It will turn out that the efficiency of the Otto cycle (assuming that air is an ideal gas) can be described entirely in terms of this ratio.

Piston: moving from top dead center to bottom dead center.

Combustion

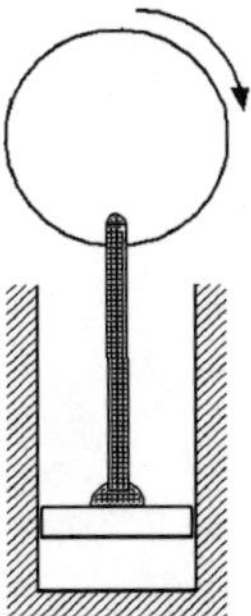

Fig. Bottom Dead Center During Combustion

Next, heat is added to the air by fuel combustion when the piston is at it bottom dead center position. Combustion is not initiated until a spark (from a spark plug, for instance) is generated in the cylinder. Because the piston is essentially immobile during this part of the cycle, we say that the heat addition is isochoric, like the cooling process.

Piston: at bottom dead center.

P-V Diagram

The P-V diagram for an Otto cycle is shown below.

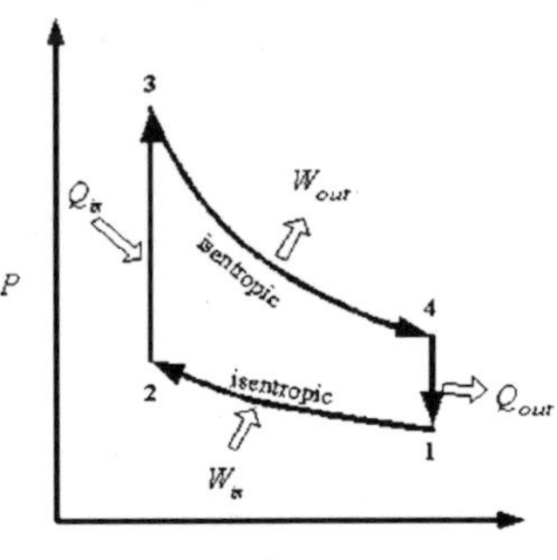

Fig. Otto Cycle P-V diagram

The Stirling Engine

In 1816, before the science of thermodynamics had been begun, a minister of the Church of Scotland named Robert Stirling designed a hot-air engine which can convert some of the heat from burning fuel into work. Advantage of this engine is low exhaust emission and high efficiencies. Disadvantage of this engine is high manufacturing costs. Idealized Stirling Engine are shown in the following, which is based on some assumptions, and they are:

- The gas is ideal,
- No leakage of gas takes place,
- No heat is lost or gained through cylinder walls,
- No heat is conducted through the regenerator,
- There is no friction.

The Stirling Cycle diagram is

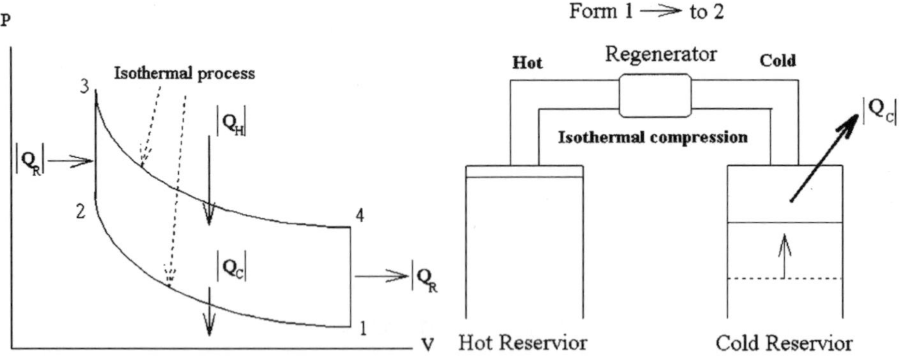

$1 2 \rightarrow$ It is an isothermal process, the piston in contact with cold reservoir is compressed isothermally, hence heat $|QC|$ has been rejected, and (isothermal compression $\rightarrow dU = 0$, W is positive and QC is negative) the heat rejected is

$$Q_C = \int_{V_1}^{V_2} PdV = nR\theta_C \ln \frac{V_2}{V_1}$$

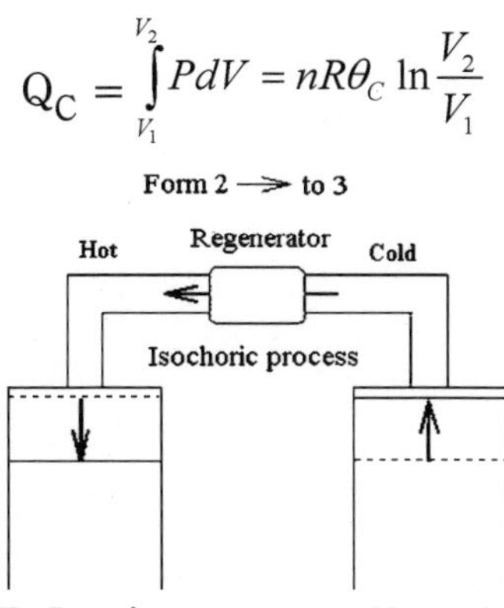

$2 \rightarrow 3$ It is an isochoric process, the left piston moves down while the right piston moves up. The volume of system is kept constant, thus no work has been done by the system, but heat QR has been input to the system by the regenerator which causes temperature to raise to θH.

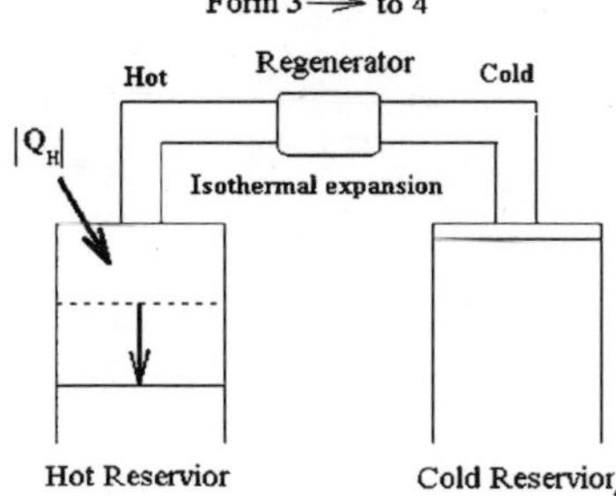

$3 \rightarrow 4$ It is an isothermal expansion process, the left piston in contact with hot reservoir expanded isothermally at temperature θH. Therefore

$$Q_H = \int_{V_3}^{V_4} PdV = nR\theta_H \ln \frac{V_4}{V_3}$$

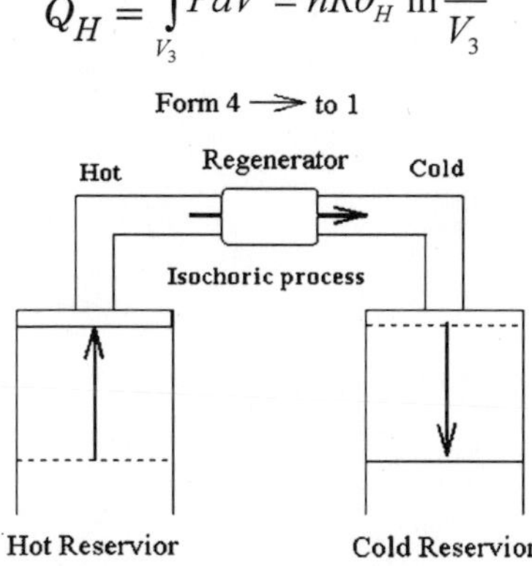

4 → 1 It is an isochoric process which is a reversed process of 2 → 3, but from θH to θC. The efficiencies of Stirling engine is

$$n = 1 - \frac{|Q_C|}{Q_H} = 1 - \frac{\theta_C}{\theta_H}$$

and work done by the system to the surroundings is $|W| = |QH| - |QC|$.

Refrigerator

Absorption some heat from cold reservoir and reject it to the hot reservoir, also a net among of work is done to the system from its surroundings. This system is called refrigerant.

The Stirling cycle is capable of being reversed, when reversed, it gives rise to one of the most useful types of refrigerator.

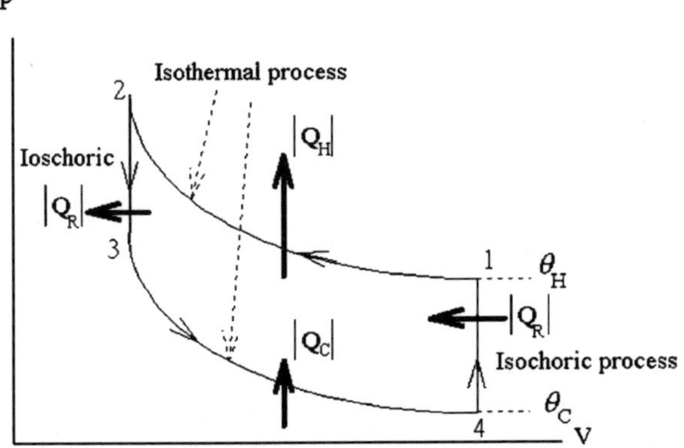

The schematic diagram for electric home refrigerators is shown below, a constant mass of refrigerant is stored in the liquid storage which have the same temperature and pressure as it in the condensor. The refrigerant go through the throttling valve, through the evapourator, into the compressor and finially back to the condensor.

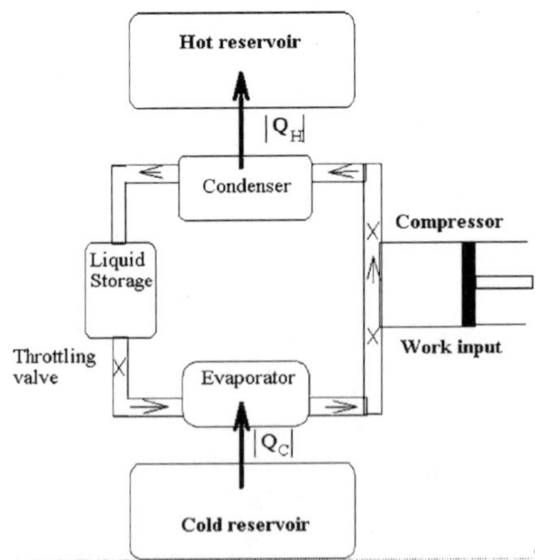

The refrigerant, while it being compressed in the condenser then stored in the liquid storage, is at a high pressure and at as low a temperature as can be obtained with air or water cooling, and it is a saturated liquid. Adiabatically undergo a throttling process, or a *Joule-Thomson* or *Joule-Kelvin expansion*, always produces cooling and partial vapourization. In the evapourator the fluid is completely vapourized, the heat to vapourize these liquid is supplied by the materials to be cooled. The vapour is then compressed adiabatically, therefore the temperature is increased. In the condenser the vapour is completely liquefied. The PV diagram of refrigerator cycle is

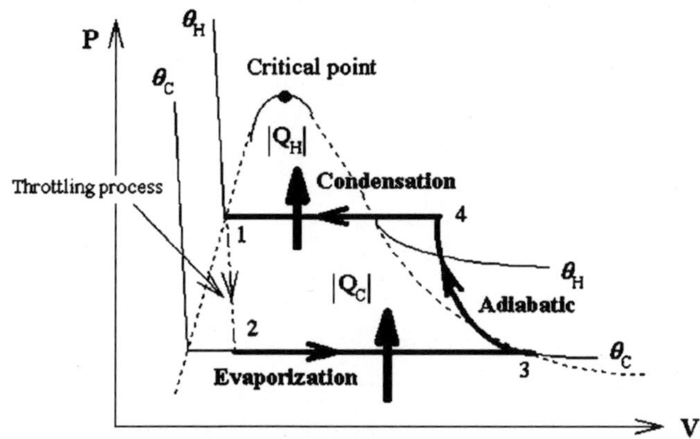

1 → 2 Throttling process involving a drop of pressure and temperature can not be represented by thermodynamic coordinates.

2 → 3 Isothermal, isobaric vapourization, and heat QC is absorbed by the refrigerant.

3 → 4 Adiabatic compression of the vapour to a temperature high than that of the condenser θH.

4 → 1 Isothermal and isobaric cooling and condensation.

Output of refrigerator: Is the heat extracted from the cold reservoir.

Input of refrigerator: Is the work done to the refrigerant by the compressor)

Coefficient of performance (or cooling energy ratio) ω

$$\omega = \frac{\text{Output}}{\text{Input}} = \frac{|Q_C|}{|W|} = \frac{|Q_C|}{|Q_H| - |Q_C|}$$

ω for commerical build refrigerator is about 2 to 7. For the case of ω = 5, that is

$$\omega = \frac{|Q_C|}{W} = 5 \Rightarrow \frac{|Q_H| - |W|}{|W|} = 5$$

which gives

$$\frac{|Q_H|}{W} = 6,$$

this means the heat liberated at the higher temperature is equal to six times the work done.

In this case, if the work is supplied by an electric motor, for every joule of electrical energy supplied, 6 J of heat will liberated, it is a very good ideal to build a heater to warm the house by refrigerating the outdoors. (In general, use resister as heater, which 1 J of electrical energy can only give 1 Joule of heat.) This heater idea is first point out by Lord Kelvin, but the first heater to heat a house is built by Haldane.

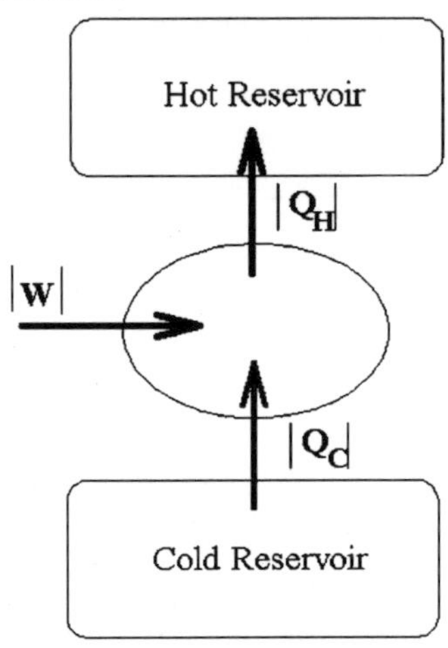

Ericsson Cycle

The Ericsson Cycle is named after inventor John Ericsson. The Ericsson cycle is very similar to what we now call the "Brayton Cycle".

The main difference is that the all Ericsson engines are externally heated and usually have a recuperator or regenerator between the compressor and the expander.

The Ericsson cycle is often compared to the Stirling Cycle because of its external combustion capabilities, use of a regenerator and the high potential efficiency.

Barber was the first to propose a similar engine in 1791 but the Barber engine lacked a regenerator/ recuperator. Ericsson invented and patented his first engine in 1833 (number 6409/1833 British).

This was 18 years before Joule and 43 years before Brayton. Brayton engines were for the most part an internal combustion version of the Ericsson Cycle which was a considerable improvement to external heating.

The "Brayton Cycle" is now known as the gas turbine cycle, which differs from the original "Brayton Cycle" in the use of a turbine compressor and expander. The gas turbine cycle is used for all modern gas turbine and turbojet engines. Ericsson eventually abandoned the open cycle in favour of the traditional closed Stirling cycle.

Causes of Inefficiency

Components

In real systems, a percentage of the overall cycle inefficiency is due to the losses by the individual components. Turbines, pumps, and compressors all behave non-ideally due to heat losses, friction and windage losses. All of these losses contribute to the non- isentropic behaviour of real equipment. These losses can be seen as an increase in the system's entropy or amount of energy that is unavailable for use by the cycle.

Cycles

In real systems, a second source of inefficiencies is from the compromises made due to cost and other factors in the design and operation of the cycle. Examples of these types of losses are: In a large power generating station the condensers are designed to subcool the liquid by 8-10°F. This subcooling allows the condensate pumps to pump the water forward without cavitation. But, each degree of subcooling is energy that must be put back by reheating the water, and this heat (energy) does no useful work and therefore increases the inefficiency of the cycle. Another example of a loss due to a system's design is heat loss to the environment, *i.e.* thin or poor insulation. Again this is energy lost to the system and therefore unavailable to do work. Friction is another real world loss, both resistance to fluid flow and mechanical friction in machines. All of these contribute to the system's inefficiency. Efficiency will be decreased by: Presence of friction, Heat losses, Cycle inefficiencies.

LAW OF THERMODYNAMICS

First, what is temperature? Let's try to clear this first. Two systems in thermal contact should exchange no heat, on average, if and only if they are at the same temperature. Let's call the two systems S1 and S2. The combined system, treating S1 and S2 together, can be S3. The important question, consideration of which will lead us to a useful quantitative definition of temperature, is "How will the energy of S3 be distributed between S1 and S2?"

With a total energy E, S has many possible internal states (microstates). The atoms of S3 can share the total energy in many ways. Let's say there are N different states.

Each state corresponds to a particular division of the total energy in the two subsystems S1 and S2. Many microstates can correspond to the same division, E1 in S1 and E2 in S2. A simple counting argument tells you that only one particular division of the energy, will occur with any significant probability. It's the one with the overwhelmingly largest number of microstates for the total system S3. That number, N(E1,E2) is just the product of the number of states allowed in each subsystem, N(E1,E2) = N1(E1)×N2(E2), and, since E1

+ E2 = E, N(E1,E2) reaches a maximum when N1 × N2 is stationary with respect to variations of E1 and E2 subject to the total energy constraint.

For convenience, physicists prefer to frame the question in terms of the logarithm of the number of microstates N, and call this the entropy, S. You can easily see from the above analysis that two systems are in equilibrium with one another when $(dS/dE)_1 = (dS/dE)_2$, *i.e.*, the rate of change of entropy, S, per unit change in energy, E, must be the same for both systems. Otherwise, energy will tend to flow from one subsystem to another as S3 bounces randomly from one microstate to another, the total energy E3 being constant, as the combined system moves towards a state of maximal total entropy. We define the temperature, T, by 1/T = dS/dE, so that the equilibrium condition becomes the very simple $T_1 = T_2$.

This statistical mechanical definition of temperature does in fact correspond to your intuitive notion of temperature for most systems. So long as dS/dE is always positive, T is always positive. For common situations, like a collection of free particles, or particles in a harmonic oscillator potential, adding energy always increases the number of available microstates, increasingly faster with increasing total energy. So temperature increases with increasing energy, from zero, asymptotically approaching positive infinity as the energy increases.

Absolute Zero

Absolute Zero is the lowest temperature theoretically possible according to kinetic theory, zero Kelvin (0 K), equivalent to –273.15°C/–459.67°F, at which molecules are in their lowest energy state.

Although the third law of thermodynamics indicates the impossibility of reaching absolute zero, in practice temperatures of less than a billionth of a degree above absolute zero have been reached. Near absolute zero, the physical properties of some materials change substantially; for example, some metals lose their electrical resistance and become superconducting. Absolute zero is the point on the thermodynamic (absolute) temperature scale where the heat energy is at a minimum, that is, no more heat can be removed from the system.

According to classical physics this temperature would correspond to zero kinetic energy of the particles of the system, in the reference frame of the system's center of mass; this, however, is now known to be false—quantum mechanics explains why the energy of a system can never drop below its zero-point energy.

By international agreement, the Celsius temperature scale starts at absolute zero with the value of exactly –273.15 °C (which approximately agrees with the original definition of the Celsius scale that was based on freezing and boiling point of water). It is approximately –459.67 °F on the Fahrenheit scale. In sciences, where SI units are in use, thermodynamic temperature is measured in kelvins where absolute zero is 0 K.

Scientists have made great advancements in achieving temperatures ever closer to absolute zero (where matter exhibits odd quantum effects). In 1994 the NIST achieved a record cold temperature of 700 nK (billionths of a kelvin). The absolute zero state was first proposed by Guillaume Amontons in 1702 who was investigating the relationship between pressure and temperature in gases. He lacked accurate and precise thermometers so his results were only semi-quantitative, but he established that the pressure of a gas increases by roughly one-third between "cold" temperatures and the boiling point of water. His work led him to speculate that a sufficient reduction in temperature would lead to the disappearance of pressure.

The problem is that all real gases liquify during the approach to absolute zero. According to kinetic theory, there should be no movement of individual molecules at absolute zero, so any material at this temperature would be solid. In a monatomic gas, most of the energy is in the form of translational motion, and the temperature can be measured in terms of the distribution of this motion, with slower speeds corresponding to lower temperatures, perhaps even down to absolute zero. But this is contrary to experimental evidence, as helium will never solidify at normal pressures, regardless of temperature. Because of quantum-mechanical effects, the speed at absolute zero is larger than zero and depends, along with the energy, on the volume within which a particle is confined.

At absolute zero, the molecules and atoms in a system are all in their ground state, the state of lowest possible energy, and a system has the least amount of kinetic energy allowed by the laws of physics. But the lowest possible zero-point energy for a confined particle in a box is not zero. Rather than being fixed and non-moving, the equation for the energy levels shows that no matter how low the temperature gets, even when the quantum number takes its minimum value of one, a particle still has some translational kinetic energy and motion. This is a reflection of Heisenberg's uncertainty principle, which states that the position and the momentum of a particle cannot both be known precisely at any given time. Similarly, using the harmonic approximation for the vibrations of a diatomic molecule, the quantum harmonic oscillator yields a positive zero-point energy even when the vibrational quantum number takes its minimum value of zero.

For polyatomic molecules, and for bodies such as crystals, whose normal mode motions can not be assigned to individual atoms or chemical bonds, the lowest-energy state is that of the system as a whole. Classically, the absolute temperature T of a system of molecules at thermodynamic equilibrium assigns an average of ½ kT to each quadratic kinetic and/or potential energy term in each mechanical degree of freedom, where k is Boltzmann's constant. But quantum mechanics shows that this is obeyed only for temperatures such that $kT > h\nu$, where h is Planck's constant and ν is a characteristic frequency. As

T decreases, the assumption that energy is continuously variable fails whenever $h\nu$ exceeds kT. For vibrational modes in crystals, this happens at room temperature, which explains the deviation of the calculated specific heats of atomic crystals from the experimental Dulong-Petit law value of 3R /mole, a fact which puzzled late 19th century physicists and physical chemists.

At 0 K, (nearly) all molecular motion ceases and $\Delta S=0$ for any adiabatic process. Pure substances can (ideally) form perfect crystals as $T \rightarrow 0$. Planck's strong form of the third law of thermodynamics states that the entropy of a perfect crystal vanishes at absolute zero. However, if the lowest energy state is degenerate (more than one microstate), this cannot be true. The original Nernst heat theorem makes the weaker and less controversial claim that the entropy change for any isothermal process approaches zero as $T \rightarrow 0$

$$\lim_{T \to 0} \Delta S = 0$$

which implies that the entropy of a perfect crystal simply approaches a constant value. The Nernst postulate identifies the isotherm T = 0 as coincident with the adiabat S = 0, although other isotherms and adiabats are distinct. As no two adiabats intersect, no other adiabat can intersect the T = 0 isotherm. Consequently no adiabatic process initiated at nonzero temperature can lead to zero temperature. An even stronger assertion is that It is impossible by any procedure to reduce the temperature of a system to zero in a finite number of operations. A perfect crystal is one in which the internal lattice structure extends uninterrupted in all directions.

The perfect order can be represented by translational symmetry along three (not usually orthogonal) axes. Every lattice element of the structure is in its proper place, whether it is a single atom or a molecular grouping. For substances which have two (or more) stable crystalline forms, such as diamond and graphite for carbon, there is a kind of "chemical degeneracy". The question remains whether both can have zero entropy at T = 0 even though each is perfectly ordered. Perfect crystals never occur in practice; imperfections, and even entire amorphous materials, simply get "frozen in" at low temperatures, so transitions to more stable states do not occur. Using the Debye model, the specific heat and entropy of a pure crystal are proportional to T^3, while the enthalpy and chemical potential are proportional to T^4. These quantities drop towards their T = 0 limiting values and approach with zero slopes. For the specific heats at least, the limiting value itself is definitely zero, as borne out by experiments to below 10K. Even the less detailed Einstein model shows this curious drop in specific heats. In fact, all specific heats vanish as absolute zero, not just those of crystals.

Likewise for the coefficient of thermal expansion. Maxwell's relations show that various other quantities also vanish. These phenomena were unanticipated. Since the relation between changes in the Gibbs free energy, the enthalpy and the entropy is

$$\Delta G = \Delta H - T\Delta S$$

it follows that as T decreases, DG and DH approach each other (so long as DS is bounded). Experimentally, it is found that most chemical reactions are exothermic and release heat in the direction they are found to be going, towards equilbirum. That is, even at room temperature T is low enough so that the fact that $(DG)_{T,P} < 0$ (usually) implies that DH < 0. (In the opposite direction, each such reaction would of course absorb heat.) More than that, the slopes of the temperature derivatives of DG and DH converge and are equal to zero at T = 0, which ensures that DG and DH are nearly the same over a considerable range of temperatures, justifying the approximate empirical Principle of Thomsen and Berthelot, which says that the equilibrium state to which a system proceeds is the one which evolves the greatest amount of heat, *i.e.*, an actual process is the most exothermic one.

As mentioned, absolute or thermodynamic temperature is conventionally measured in Kelvins (Celsius-size degrees), and increasingly rarely in the Rankine scale (Fahrenheit-size degrees). Absolute temperature is uniquely determined up to a multiplicative constant which specifies the size of the "degree", so the *ratios* of two absolute temperatures, T_2/T_1, are the same in all scales. The most transparent definition comes from the classical Maxwell-Boltzmann distribution over energies, or from the quantum analogs: Fermi-Dirac statistics (particles of half-integer spin) and Bose-Einstein statistics (particles of integer spin), all of which give the relative numbers of particles as (decreasing) exponential functions of energy over kT. On a macroscopic level, a definition can be given in terms of the efficiencies of "reversible" heat engines operating between hotter and colder thermal reservoirs.

The Third Law of Thermodynamics

A postulate related to but independent of the second law is that it is impossible to cool a body to absolute zero by any finite process. Although one can approach absolute zero as closely as one desires, one cannot actually reach this limit. The third law of thermodynamics, formulated by Walter Nernst and also known as the Nernst heat theorem, states that if one could reach absolute zero, all bodies would have the same entropy. In other words, a body at absolute zero could exist in only one possible state, which would possess a definite energy, called the zero-point energy. This state is defined as having zero entropy.

The third law of thermodynamics is usually stated as a definition:

"The entropy of a perfect crystal of an element at the absolute zero of temperature is zero".

At the absolute zero of temperature, there is zero thermal energy or heat. Since heat is a measure of average molecular motion, zero thermal energy means that the average atom does not move at all. Since no atom can have less than zero motion, the motion of every individual atom must be zero when the average molecular motion is zero. When none of the atoms which make up a perfectly ordered crystal move at all, there can be no disorder or different states possible for the crystal.

Taking the entropy of a perfect crystal of an element to be zero at the absolute zero of temperature establishes a method by which entropies of elements at any higher temperature can be determined. Since by definition dS = q_{rev}/T, the mathematical integral of dS from zero to any higher temperature T is the integral, over that temperature range, of q_{rev}/T. In other words. the difference $S - S^0$ is the integral from zero to a temperature T of (C_p/T)dT. The molar heat capacity at any temperature is a measurable quantity, and so this difference can be determined experimentally.

The third law of thermodynamics is simply the statement that S^0 is zero by definition for a pure element, and so if the heat capacity is measured under conditions of reversible heat flow, as it can be, and as a function of temperature at low temperatures, as it can be, then the entropy $S$of a pure element at any temperature T is given by:

S = the integral from zero to T of (C_p/T)dT

The values we usually write as S^0, the standard entropy of a substance, are actually the integral from zero to the standard temperature, 298.15 K, of (C_p/T)dT in order that the values of standard entropies of substances can be used with standard values for other thermodynamic functions such as enthalpy and free energy.

The value of the entropy of an element at any temperature, including 298.15 K which is the temperature of the standard entropy S^0, can be obtained from careful measurements of the heat capacity of the element from the desired temperature down to absolute zero. Experimentally, chemists have been unable to reach the absolute zero of temperature, but measurements can be and have been made down to within 0.1 K of it and the heat capacity below measurable range can be accurately estimated. The entropy of the element is obtained from integration of the heat capacity measurements. If the crystal changes form, or melts, within the temperature range desired, then the entropy of that change must also be measured and included.

The entropies of compounds can be determined from thermodynamic measurements made on the reactions which form them from the elements or dissociate them to their constituent elements once the entropies of the elements themselves are established.

The values of standard entropies of elements and compounds at 25°C given in the tables of the thermodynamic properties of pure substances are all based upon the third law of thermodynamics.

On a molar basis,

$$S = R \ln W$$

R = gas constant (units of J/mole. K)

W = the number of arrangements of the energy of atoms or molecules can take without changing the total energy in a system. This is also known as the *degeneracy*.

At absolute zero for a perfectly ordered crystalline substance, W = 1 (there is only one way to arrange the atoms in a perfect substance, hence there is only one way to distribute the energy)

This means that at T = 0, S = Rln(1) = 0.

The Third Law, then, gives us a method to find the absolute entropy for any substance: cool the substance to as close to absolute zero as possible and then measure the heat change as the substance is warmed up (remember, DS = q / T = $S_{final} - S_{initial}$, but $S_{initial}$ = 0 if we start at T = 0).

Absolute entropies for substances are tabulated at standard conditions.

The tabulated values of the absolute entropy allow us to calculate the change in entropy for chemical reactions:

$$\Delta S^o = \sum_{i=\text{products}} m_i S_i^o - \sum_{j=\text{reactants}} m_j S_j^o$$

m_i and m_j are the stoichiometric coefficients from the balanced reaction and S_i^o and S_j^o are the absolute entropies of the products and reactants.

DS° will be positive if the chemical process leads to an increase in the number of ways to disperse energy. This will happen if:

- There are more moles of products than moles of reactants (there are more ways to distribute energy because there are more particles after reaction).
- The number of moles of gaseous products is greater than the number of moles of gaseous reactants (gases can distribute energy in more ways because of the large mobility of the particles, so have a disproportionate effect on the change in entropy).
- A change in phase from *s* to *l*, *l* to *g*, or *s* to *g*.

Absolute entropies

Energy values, as you know, are all relative, and must be defined on a scale that is completely arbitrary; there is no such thing as the absolute energy of a substance, so we can arbitrarily define the enthalpy or internal energy of an element in its most stable form at 298K and 1 atm pressure as zero.

The same is not true of the entropy; since entropy is a measure of the "dilution" of thermal energy, it follows that the less thermal energy available to spread through a system (that is, the lower the temperature), the smaller will be its entropy. In other words, as the absolute temperature of a substance approaches zero, so does its entropy.

This principle is the basis of the Third law of thermodynamics, which states that the entropy of a perfectly-ordered solid at 0° K is zero.

The absolute entropy of a substance at any temperature above 0°K must be determined by calculating the increments of heat q required to bring the substance from 0°K to the temperature of interest, and then summing the ratios q / T. Two kinds of experimental measurements are needed:

1. The enthalpies associated with any phase changes the substance may undergo within the temperature range of interest. Melting of a solid and vapourization of a liquid correspond to sizeable increases in the number of microstates available to accept thermal energy, so as these processes occur, energy will flow into a system, filling these new microstates to the extent required to maintain a constant temperature (the freezing or boiling point); these inflows of thermal energy correspond to the heats of fusion and vapourization. The entropy increase associated with melting, for example, is just $\Delta H_{fusion} / T_m$.
2. The heat capacity C of a phase expresses the quantity of heat required to change the temperature by a small amount ΔT, or more precisely, by an infinitessimal amount dT. Thus the entropy increase brought about by warming a substance over a range of temperatures that does not encompass a phase transition is given by the sum of the quantities C dT/T for each increment of temperature dT. This is of course just the integral.

$$S_{0^0 \to T^0} = \int_{0^0}^{T^0} \frac{C}{T} dT$$

Because the heat capacity is itself slightly temperature dependent, the most precise determinations of absolute entropies require that the functional dependence of C on T be used in the above integral in place of a constant C. For rough determinations, one can simply plot the enthalpy increment C DT as a function of temperature and measure the area under the curve.

It is possible, though exceedingly difficult, to calculate the entropy of any system under any conditions of interest from the equation

$$S = R \ln W$$

It is also possible, using more advanced theoretical thermodynamics, to determine S experimentally by measuring heat capacities and enthalpies of phase transitions. Values of S determined experimentally, often referred to as "absolute" entropies, have been tabulated for many materials at many temperatures, and a few examples are given in table. We treat these values as observations and attempt to understand these in the context of equation.

There are several interesting generalities observed in table. First, in comparing the entropy of the gaseous form of a substance to either its liquid or solid form at the same temperature, we find that the gas always has substantially greater entropy. This is easy to understand from equation: the molecules in the gas phase occupy a very much larger volume. There are very many more possible locations for each gas molecule and thus very many more arrangements of the molecules in the gas. It is intuitively clear that W should be larger for a gas, and therefore the entropy of a gas is greater than that of the corresponding liquid or solid.

Table. Absolute Entropies of Specific Substances.

	T (°C)	S (J/mol°C)
$H_2O(g)$	25	188.8
$H_2O(l)$	25	69.9
$H_2O(l)$	0	63.3
$H_2O(s)$	0	41.3
$NH_3(g)$	25	192.4
$HN_3(l)$	25	140.6
$HN_3(g)$	25	239.0
$O_2(g)$	25	205.1
$O_2(g)$	50	207.4
$O_2(g)$	100	211.7
$CO(g)$	25	197.7
$CO(g)$	50	200.0
$CO_2(g)$	24	213.7
$CO_2(g)$	50	216.9
$Br_2(l)$	25	152.2
$Br_2(g)$	25	245.5
$I_2(s)$	25	116.1
$I_2(g)$	25	260.7
$CaF_2(s)$	25	68.9
$CaCl_2(s)$	25	104.6
$CaBr_2(s)$	25	130
$C_8H_{18}(s)$	25	361.1

Second, we observe that the entropy of a liquid is always greater than that of the corresponding solid. This is understandable from our kinetic molecular view of liquids and solids. Although the molecules in the liquid occupy a comparable volume to that of the molecules in the solid, each molecule in the liquid is free to move throughout this entire volume. The molecules in the solid are relatively fixed in location. Therefore, the number of arrangements of molecules in the liquid is significantly greater than that in the solid, so the liquid has greater entropy by equation 1.

Third, the entropy of a substance increases with increasing temperature. The temperature is, of course, a measure of the average kinetic energy of the molecules. In a solid or liquid, then, increasing the temperature increases the total kinetic energy available to the molecules.

The greater the energy, the more ways there are to distribute this energy amongst the molecules. Although we have previously only referred to the range of positions for a molecule as affecting W, the range of energies available for each molecule similarly affects W. As a result, as we increase the total energy of a substance, we increase W and thus the entropy.

Fourth, the entropy of a substance whose molecules contain many atoms is greater than that of a substance composed of smaller molecules. The more atoms there are in a molecule, the more ways there are to arrange those atoms. With greater internal flexibility, W is larger when there are more atoms, so the entropy is greater.

Fifth, the entropy of a substance with a high molecular weight is greater than that of substance with a low molecular weight.

This result is a harder to understand, as it arises from the distribution of the momentum of the molecules rather than the positions and energies of the molecules. It is intuitively clear that the number of arrangements of the molecules is not affected by the mass of the molecules.

However, even at the same temperature, the range of momentum available for a heavier molecule is greater than for a lighter one. To see why, recall that the momentum of a molecule is $p=mv$ and the kinetic energy is $KE = mv^2/2 = p^2/2m$. Therefore, the maximum momentum available at a fixed total kinetic energy KE is:

$$p = \sqrt{2KE}$$

Since this is larger for larger mass molecules, the range of momentum is greater for heavier particles, thus increasing W and the entropy.

Helmholtz Free Energy

In thermodynamics, the Helmholtz free energy is a thermodynamic potential which measures the "useful" work obtainable from constant temperature, constant volume thermodynamic systems.

For a simple system, with a fixed number of particles, the negative of the difference in the Helmholtz energy is equal to the maximum amount of work extractable from a thermodynamic process in which temperature is held constant.

The Helmholtz free energy was developed by Hermann von Helmholtz and is denoted by the letter A or the letter F. The Helmholtz free energy as goes by the name Helmholtz energy or Helmholtz function among others.

The Helmholtz energy is defined as:

$$A = U - TS$$

where

- A is the Helmholtz energy (SI: joules, CGS: ergs),
- U is the internal energy of the system (SI: joules, CGS: ergs),
- T is the absolute temperature (kelvins),
- S is the entropy (SI: joules per kelvin, CGS: ergs per kelvin).

In earlier times the theory of heat, *i.e.* that heat is a form of energy having relation to vibratory motion, was beginning to supplant both the caloric theory, *i.e.* that heat is a fluid, and the four element theory in which heat was the lightest of the four elements. Many textbooks and teaching articles during these centuries presented these theories side by side.

Similarly, during these years, heat was beginning to be distinguished into different classification categorize, such as "free heat", "combined heat", "radiant heat", specific heat, heat capacity, "absolute heat", "latent caloric", "free" or "perceptible" caloric, among others. In 1780, for example, Laplace and Lavoisier stated: "In general, one can change the first hypothesis into the second by changing the words 'free heat, combined heat, and heat released' into 'vis viva, loss of vis viva, and increase of vis viva.'"

In this manner, the total mass of caloric in a body, called *absolute heat*, was regarded as a mixture of two components; the free or perceptible caloric could affect a thermometer while the other component, the latent caloric, could not. The use of the words "latent heat" implied a similarity to latent heat in the more usual sense; it was regarded as chemically bound to the molecules of the body.

In the adiabatic compression of a gas, the absolute heat remained constant by the observed rise of temperature indicated that some latent caloric had become "free" or perceptible.During the early 19th century, the concept of perceptible or free caloric began to be referred to as "free heat" or heat set free. In 1824, for example, the French physicist Sadi Carnot, in his famous "Reflections on the Motive Power of Fire", speaks of quantities of heat 'absorbed or set free' in different transformations.

In 1882, the German physicist and physiologist Hermann von Helmholtz coined the phrase 'free energy' for the expression $E - TS$, in which the change in F (or G) determines the amount of energy 'free' for work under the given conditions. In modern use, we attach the term "free" to Gibbs free energy, *i.e.* for systems at constant pressure and temperature, or to Helmholtz free energy, *i.e.* for systems at constant volume and temperature, to mean 'available in the form of useful work.

With reference to the Gibbs free energy, we add the qualification that it is the energy free for non-volume work. To note, some books do not include the attachment "free", referring to G as simply Gibbs energy. This is the influence of a 1988 IUPAC meeting designed to unified terminologies between the USA, Europe, and other countries, in which descriptive 'free' was supposedly banished. This ruling, however, is still far from accepted and the majority of published articles and books still use the descriptive 'free' for both historical, informative, and for clarification reasons.

The Helmholtz free energy is defined by

$$A = U - TS(1)$$

where E is the energy, T is the temperature, and S is the entropy. When a system changes its thermodynamic state, the change in Helmholtz free energy is therefore given by

$$dA = dU - TdS - SdT(2)$$

If T and V are constant, the (2) reduces to

$$dA = dU - TdS$$

But the combined law of thermodynamics states that

$$dU - TdS + PdV \leq 0$$

and, since we have stipulated dV = 0, this becomes

$$dU - TdS \leq 0$$

Therefore

$$dA \leq 0$$

The Helmholtz free energy is intimately related to the equilibrium constant at constant volume A_V

$$A = -Kt \ln A_V$$

where k is Boltzmann's constant.

A system with fixed external parameters in thermal contact with a heat reservoir at equilibrium has a minimum Helmholtz free energy, commonly denoted A_0

Gibbs Free Energy

Useful energy, or energy available to do work, is of central interest because there is never a shortage of useful work to be done, and usually an insufficiency of useful energy to do it. Chemical reactions can be made to do work, or to serve as pathways for the conversion of heat into work. Energy which is, or which can be, available to do useful work is called Gibbs free energy or more often simply free energy. Free energy is called Gibbs free energy and given the symbol G in honour of Josiah Willard Gibbs, a professor of chemistry at Harvard University who almost singlehandedly developed both the concept and the quantitative equations which describe it.

Free energy is a state function because it is formally defined only in terms of state functions, the state functions enthalpy and entropy, and the state variable temperature. The definition of free energy is:

$$G = H - TS$$

where (in SI units)

- G is the Gibbs energy (joules)
- H is the enthalpy (joules)
- T is the temperature (kelvins)
- S is the entropy (joules per kelvin)

A change in free energy dG would then be given by:

$$dG = dH - d(TS)$$

Since temperature is a state variable and entropy is a state function they are separable, and so:

$$dG = dH - TdS - SdT$$

However, at constant temperature the change in temperature dT is zero, so the term SdT is zero also. For any constant-temperature (isothermal) change, then $dG = dH - TdS$. Rearrangement of this equation gives, for larger changes, the Gibbs-Helmholtz equation:

$$DH = DG + TDS$$

Total energy available as heat = DG + energy not available for doing work

It therefore follows that DG must be the energy which is available for doing work. This free or available energy which can do useful work is then a most useful thing to know or to have.

The conventions of heat flow q are also those of enthalpy change. When DH is negative, heat is evolved (or given off) in the exothermic process or reaction, while when DH is positive, heat is absorbed in the endothermic process or reaction from the surroundings. Free energy change also follows the same conventions.

When DG is negative, energy is evolved (given up) in the process or reaction and the change can do useful work on something else. This is a spontaneous process, and is sometimes called an exergonic (energy-giving) process.

When DG is positive, energy is absorbed in the process or reaction and useful work must be done on the materials so that the reaction will occur. This is a nonspontaneous process, and is sometimes called an endergonic (energy-requiring) process.

Derivation

Let S_{tot} be the total entropy of an isolated system, that is, a system which cannot exchange heat or mass with its surroundings. By the second law of thermodynamics:

$$S\Delta S_{tot} \geq 0$$

and if $\Delta S_{tot} = 0$ then the process is reversible.

The heat transfer Q vanishes for an adiabatic system. Any adiabatic process is reversible and isentropic.

$$\left(\frac{\Delta q}{T} = \Delta S = 0\right)$$

Now consider diabatic systems, having internal entropy S_{int}. Such a system is thermally connected to its surroundings, which have entropy S_{ext}.

The entropy form of the second law does not apply directly to the diabatic system, it only applies to the closed system formed by both the system and its surroundings. Therefore a process is possible if

$$\Delta S_{int} + \Delta S_{ext} \geq 0 .$$

We will try to express the left side of this equation entirely in terms of state functions. DS_{ext} is defined as:

$$DS_{ext} = -\frac{\Delta q}{T}$$

Temperature T is the same for two systems in thermal equilibrium. (By the zeroeth law of thermodynamics, if a system is in thermal equilibrium with a second and a third system, the latter two are in equilibrium as well.) Also, Dq_{rev} is heat transferred *to* the system, so -Dq_{rev} is heat transferred to the surroundings, and DQ/T is entropy gained by the surroundings. We now have:

$$\Delta S_{int} - \frac{\Delta q}{T} \geq 0$$

Multiply both sides by T:

$$T\Delta S_{int} - \Delta q \geq 0$$

DQ is heat transferred *to* the system; if the process is now assumed to be isobaric, then Dq_p = DH:

$$T\Delta S_{int} - \Delta H \geq 0$$

DH is the enthalpy change of reaction (for a chemical reaction at constant pressure and temperature). Then

$$\Delta H - T\Delta S_{int} \geq 0$$

for a possible process. Let the change DG in Gibbs energy be defined as

$$\Delta G = \Delta H - T\Delta S_{int} \,(1)$$

Notice that it is not defined in terms of any external state functions, such as DS_{ext} or DS_{tot}. Then the second law becomes:

DG < 0 favoured reaction

DG = 0 reversible reaction

DG > 0 disfavoured reaction

Also, the sign of Delta G tells us about the spontaneity of the reaction.

DG < 0 Spontaneous

DG = 0 Equilibrium

DG > 0 Nonspontaneous

Gibbs energy G itself is defined as

$$G = H - T\,S_{\text{int}} \quad (2)$$

but notice that to obtain equation (2) from equation (1) we must assume that T is constant.

Thus, Gibbs energy is most useful for thermochemical processes at constant temperature and pressure: both isothermal and isobaric. Such processes don't move on a P-T diagram, such as phase change of a pure substance, which takes place at the saturation pressure and temperature. However, chemical reactions do undergo changes in chemical potential, which is a state function.

Thus, thermodynamic processes are not confined to the two dimensional P-V diagram. There is a third dimension for n, the quantity of gas. Naturally for the study of explosive chemicals, the processes are not necessarily isothermal and isobaric. For these studies, Helmholtz free energy is used.

Use of Gibbs Free Energy: Phase Transitions

We are interested in the cases where two phases of the same substance can coexist. An example is ice in water at 0°C: if no heat is exchanged with the surroundings, the mixture will persist indefinitely.

In practical cases we are interested in charting the behaviour of the substance as a function of external temperature and pressure. For most choices, only one phase will persist at equilibrium - water, or ice, or vapour, for example. But for certain choices, two or even three phases may coexist. The phase diagram for water is shown below.

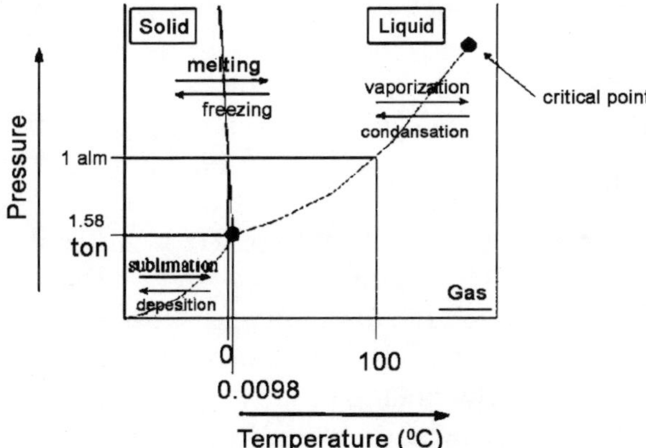

It differs from a generic substance in the backward slope of the ice-water coexistence line: putting ice under pressure may cause it to melt, whereas most liquids close to their freezing point will freeze under pressure.

What determines the lines of phase coexistence?

Consider a system of two phases, 1 (say gas) and 2 (say liquid) at a fixed pressure and temperature.

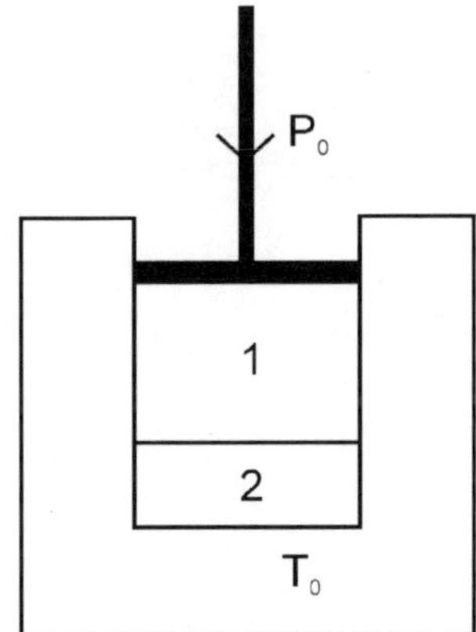

From the fact that the system will minimize its Gibbs free energy, we can derive the following condition for phase coexistence: The Gibbs free energy per unit mass in each phase is the same.

At temperatures and pressures not on the coexistence line the Gibbs free energy of one phase will be lower than the other, and only the phase with the lower energy will be present at equilibrium.

Suppose we know the location of one point on a coexistence line (for instance the melting point at atmospheric pressure). Can we discover other points - for instance, the melting point at a higher or lower pressure? The answer is yes, for very small changes: in fact we can discover the slope of the line:

$$\frac{dP}{dT} = \frac{L}{T\Delta V}$$

where L is the latent heat of the transition for some quantity of the substance, and DV is the volume change of the same quantity as it undergoes the transition. This is called the Clausius-Clapeyron equation.

We can use this equation to estimate the boiling point of water at the top of Mount Everest, where the pressure is only about a third of that at sea-level, to be 82°C.

(Input data: pressure at the top of Everest is 0.36 atmospheres, the density of water vapour at 100°C is 0.598 kg/m^3 and the latent heat is 2.257 × 103 J/g.)

Of course this estimate requires assuming that the phase coexistence line has negligible curvature over a fairly large range, so it is no surprise that the result is only approximate. By looking at the phase diagram above you should be able to say if the true temperature is higher or lower.

Heat Capacity

The heat capacity of a substance is a measure of how well the substance stores heat. Whenever we supply heat to a material, it will necessarily cause an increase in the material's temperature. The heat capacity is defined as the amount of heat required per unit increase in temperature, so that

Heat added = Heat capacity × (Change in temperature)

Thus, materials with large heat capacities, like water, hold heat well - their temperature won't rise much for a given amount of heat - whereas materials with small heat capacities, like copper, don't hold heat well - their temperature will rise significantly when heat is added.

Heat capacity (usually denoted by a capital C, often with subscripts) is a measurable physical quantity that characterizes the ability of a body to store heat as it changes in temperature. It is defined as the rate of change of temperature as heat is added to a body at the given conditions and state of the body (foremost its temperature).

In the International System of Units, heat capacity is expressed in units of joules per kelvin. It is termed an "extensive quantity" because it is sensitive to the size of the object (for example, a bathtub of water has a greater heat capacity than a cup of water). Dividing heat capacity by the body's mass yields a specific heat capacity (also called more properly "mass-specific heat capacity" or more loosely "specific heat"), which is an "intensive quantity," meaning it is no longer dependent on amount of material, and is now more dependent on the type of material, as well as the physical conditions of heating.

Heat capacity is mathematically defined as the ratio of a small amount of heat dQ added to the body, to the corresponding small increase in its temperature dT:

$$C = \left(\frac{\delta Q}{dT}\right)_{cond.} = T\left(\frac{dS}{dT}\right)_{cond.}$$

For thermodynamic systems with more than one physical dimension, the above definition does not give a single, unique quantity unless a particular infinitesimal path through the system's phase space has been defined (this means that one needs to know at all times where all parts of the system are, how much mass they have, and how fast they are moving). This information is used to account for different ways that heat can be stored as kinetic energy (energy of motion) and potential energy (energy stored in force fields), as an object expands or contracts.

For all real systems, the path though these changes must be explicitly defined, since the value of heat capacity depends on which path from one temperature to another, is chosen. Of particular usefulness in this context are the values of heat capacity for constant volume, CV, and constant pressure, CP. These will be defined below.

Heat Capacity of Fluids

The state of a simple fluids with fixed mass is described by two thermodynamic parameters such as temperature T and pressure P. Therefore as mentioned above, one may distinguish between heat capacity at constant volume, C_V, and heat capacity at constant pressure, C_P:

$$C_V = \left(\frac{\delta Q}{dT}\right)_V = T\left(\frac{\partial S}{\partial T}\right)_V$$

$$C_P = \left(\frac{\delta Q}{dT}\right)_P = T\left(\frac{\partial S}{\partial T}\right)_P$$

where dQ is the infinitesimal amount of heat added, and dT is the subsequent rise in temperature.

The increment of internal energy is the heat added and the work added:

$$dU = T\,dS - P\,dV$$

So the heat capacity at constant volume is

$$C_V = \left(\frac{\partial U}{\partial T}\right)_V$$

The enthalpy is defined by H = U + PV. The increment of enthalpy is

$$dH = dU + (PdV + VdP)$$

which at dP=0, reduces to:

$$dH = T\,dS + V\,dP$$

So the heat capacity at constant pressure is

$$C_P = \left(\frac{\partial H}{\partial T}\right)_P$$

Note that this last "definition" is a bit circular, since the concept of "enthalpy" itself was invented to be a measure of heat absorbed or produced at constant pressures (the conditions in which chemists usually work). As such, enthalpy merely accounts for the extra heat which is produced or absorbed by pressure-volume work at constant pressure.

Thus, it is not surprising that constant-pressure heat capacities may be defined in terms of enthalpy, since "enthalpy" was defined in the first place to make this so.

Specific Heat Capacity

The specific heat capacity of a material is

$$c = \frac{\partial C}{\partial m}$$

which in the absence of phase transitions is equivalent to

$$c = c_m = \frac{C}{m} = \frac{C}{\rho V}$$

- C is the heat capacity of a body made of the material in question ($J \cdot K^{-1}$)
- m is the mass of the body (kg).

- V is the volume of the body (m^3)
- $\delta = mV^{-1}$ is the density of the material ($kg \cdot m^{-3}$)

For gases, and also for other materials under high pressures, there is need to distinguish between different boundary conditions for the processes under consideration (since values differ significantly between different conditions). Typical processes for which a heat capacity may be defined include isobaric (constant pressure, dP = 0) and isochoric (constant volume, dV = 0) processes, and one conventionally writes for gases:

$$c_P = \left(\frac{\partial C}{\partial m}\right)_P$$

$$c_V = \left(\frac{\partial C}{\partial m}\right)_V$$

Units shown are SI units but, of course, any consistent set of units may be used.

A related parameter to c is CV–1, the volumetric heat capacity, (J·m–3·K–1 in SI units). In engineering practice, cV for solids or liquids often signifies a volumetric heat capacity, rather than a constant-volume one. In such cases, the mass-specific heat capacity (specific heat) is often explicitly written with the subscript m, as cm. Of course, from the above relationships, for solids one writes:

$$c_m = \frac{C}{m} = \frac{c_V}{\rho}$$

Dimensionless Heat Capacity

The dimensionless heat capacity of a material is

$$C^* = \frac{C}{nR} = \frac{C}{Nk}$$

where

- C is the heat capacity of a body made of the material in question ($J \cdot K^{-1}$)
- n is the amount of matter in the body (mol)
- R is the gas constant ($J \cdot K^{-1} \cdot mol^{-1}$)
- nR=Nk is the amount of matter in the body ($J \cdot K^{-1}$)
- N is the number of molecules in the body. (dimensionless)
- k is Boltzmann's constant ($J \cdot K^{-1} \cdot molecule^{-1}$)

Gas Phase

According to the equipartition theorem from classical statistical mechanics, for a system made up of independent and quadratic degrees of freedom, any input of energy into a closed system composed of N molecules is evenly divided among the degrees of freedom available to each molecule. It can be shown that, in the classical limit of statistical mechanics, for each independent and quadratic degree of freedom, that

$$E_i = \frac{k_B T}{2}$$

where

E_i is the mean energy (measured in joules) associated with degree of freedom i.

T is the temperature (measured in Kelvin)

k_B is Boltzmann's constant, (1.380 6505(24) × 10^{-23} J K^{-1})

In the case of a monatomic gas such as helium under constant volume, if it assumed that no electronic or nuclear quantum excitations occur, each atom in the gas has only 3 degrees of freedom, all of a translational type. No energy dependence is associated with the degrees of freedom which define the position of the atoms. While, in fact, the degrees of freedom corresponding to the momenta of the atoms are quadratic, and thus contribute to the heat capacity. There are N atoms, each of which has 3 components of momentum, which leads to 3N total degrees of freedom. This gives:

$$C_V = \left(\frac{\partial U}{\partial T}\right)_V = \frac{3}{2} N k_B = \frac{3}{2} n R$$

$$C_{V}, m = \frac{C_V}{n} = \frac{3}{2} R = 1.5R$$

where

C_V is the heat capacity at constant volume of the gas

$C_{V,m}$ is the molar heat capacity at constant volume of the gas

N is the total number of atoms present in the container

n is the number of moles of atoms present in the container (n is the ratio of N and Avogadro's number)

R is the ideal gas constant, (8.314570[70] J $K^{-1}mol^{-1}$). R is equal to the product of Boltzmann's constant k_B and Avogadro's number

In the somewhat more complex case of an ideal gas of diatomic molecules, the presence of internal degrees of freedom are apparent. In addition to the three translational degrees of freedom, there are rotational and vibrational degrees of freedom. In general, the number of degrees of freedom, f, in a molecule with n_a atoms is $3n_a$:

$$f = 3n_a$$

Mathematically, there are a total of three rotational degrees of freedom, one corresponding to rotation about each of the axes of three dimensional space. However, in practice we shall only consider the existence of two degrees of rotational freedom for linear molecules. This approximation is valid because the moment of inertia about the internuclear axis is vanishingly small with respect other moments of inertia in the molecule (this is due to the extremely small radii of the atomic nuclei, compared to the distance between them in a molecule). Quantum mechanically, it can be shown that the interval between successive rotational energy eigenstates is inversely proportional to the moment of inertia about that axis. Because the moment of inertia about the internuclear axis is vanishingly small relative to the other two rotational axes, the energy spacing can be considered so high that no excitations of the rotational state can possibly occur unless the temperature is extremely high. We can easily calculate the expected number of vibrational degrees of freedom (or vibrational modes). There are three degrees of translational freedom, and two degrees of rotational freedom, therefore

$$f_{\text{vib}} = f - f_{\text{trans}} - f_{\text{rot}} = 6 - 3 - 2 = 1$$

Each rotational and translational degree of freedom will contribute R/2 in the total molar heat capacity of the gas. Each vibrational mode will contribute R to the total molar heat capacity, however. This is because for each vibrational mode, there is a potential and kinetic energy component. Both the potential and kinetic components will contribute R/2 to the total molar heat capacity of the gas. Therefore, we expect that a diatomic molecule would have a molar constant-volume heat capacity of

$$C_{\text{V,m}} = \frac{3R}{2} + R + R = \frac{7R}{2} = 3.5R$$

where the terms originate from the translational, rotational, and vibrational degrees of freedom, respectively. However, as the atoms composing the molecules become heavier, the heat capacities move closer to their expected values. One of the reasons for this phenomenon is the quantization of vibrational, and to a lesser extent, rotational states. In fact, if it is assumed that the molecules remain in their lowest energy vibrational state because the inter-level energy spacings are large, the predicted molar constant volume heat capacity for a diatomic molecule becomes

$$C_{\text{V,m}} = \frac{3R}{2} + R = \frac{5R}{2} = 2.5R$$

which is a fairly close approximation of the heat capacities of the lighter molecules in the above table.

If the quantum harmonic oscillator approximation is made, it turns out that the quantum vibrational energy level spacings are actually inversely proportional to the square root of the reduced mass of the atoms composing the diatomic molecule.

Therefore, in the case of the heavier diatomic molecules, the quantum vibrational energy level spacings become finer, which allows more excitations into higher vibrational levels at a fixed temperature.

Solid Phase

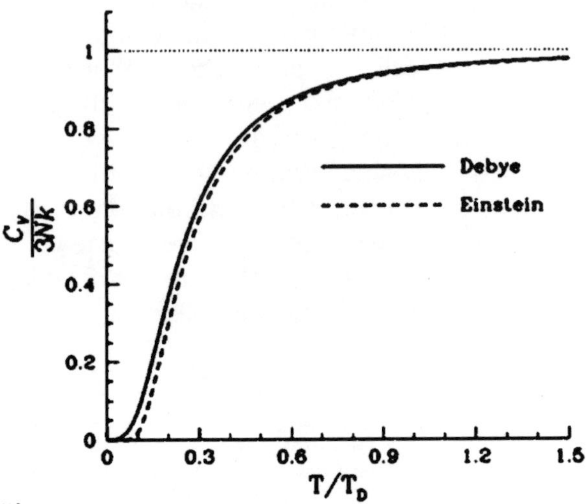

The dimensionless heat capacity divided by three, as a function of temperature as predicted by the Debye model and by Einstein's earlier model. The horizontal axis is the temperature divided by the Debye temperature. Note that, as expected, the dimensionless heat capacity is zero at absolute zero, and rises to a value of three as the temperature becomes much larger than the Debye temperature. The red line corresponds to the classical limit of the Dulong-Petit law

For matter in a crystalline solid phase, the Dulong-Petit law, which was discovered empirically, states that the dimensionless specific heat capacity assumes the value 3. Indeed, for solid metallic chemical elements at room temperature, heat capacities range from about 2.8 to 3.4 (beryllium being a notable exception at 2.0).

The theoretical maximum heat capacity for larger and larger multi-atomic gases at higher temperatures, also approaches the Dulong-Petit limit of 3R, so long as this is calculated per mole of atoms, not molecules. The reason is that gases with very large molecules, in theory have almost the same high-temperature heat capacity as solids, lacking only the (small) heat capacity contibution that comes from potential energy that cannot be stored between separate molecules in a gas.

The Dulong-Petit "limit" results from the equipartition theorem, and as such is only valid in the classical limit of a microstate continuum, which is a high temperature limit. For light and non-metallic elements, as well as most of the common molecular solids based on carbon compounds at standard ambiant temperature, quantum effects may also play an important role, as they do in multi-atomic gases. These effects usually combine to give heat capacities lower than 3 R per mole of atoms in the solid, although heat capacities calculated per mole of molecules in molecular solids may be more than 3 R. For example, the heat capacity of water ice at the melting point is about 4.6 R per mole of molecules, but only 1.5 R per mole of atoms. The lower number results from the "freezing out" of possible vibration modes for light atoms at suitably low temperatures, just as in many gases. These effects are seen in solids more often than liquids: for example the heat capacity of liquid water is again close to the theoretical 3 R/mole of atoms of the Dulong-Petit theoretical maximum.

Heat Capacity at Absolute Zero

From the definition of entropy

$$TdS = \delta Q$$

we can calculate the absolute entropy by integrating from zero temperature to the final temperature T_f

$$S(T_f) = \int_{T=0}^{T_f} \frac{\delta Q}{T} = \int_0^{T_f} \frac{\delta Q}{dT}\frac{\delta T}{T} = \int_0^{T_f} C(T)\frac{dT}{T}$$

The heat capacity must be zero at zero temperature in order for the above integral not to yield an infinite absolute entropy, thus violating the third law of thermodynamics. One of the strengths of the Debye model is that (unlike the preceding Einstein model) it predicts an approach of heat capacity towards zero as zero temperature is approached, and also predicts the proper mathematical form of this approach.

Standard States

Changes in energy content of a system are most easily compared if everyone agrees on a set of reference conditions.

There are several conventions, but the commonly used set refers changes in chemical systems to defined standard states. The primary reference is to the standard states of the elements.

The Standard State and the Zero Reference Energy Level

Elements in their standard states are considered to have chemical potentials and enthalpies of 0, or

$$\mu^o{}_{\text{element}} = 0$$

The standard state of an element is its natural state at 1 atms pressure, 25°C.

By defining the free energy of the elements in this way, we can regard any compound as having a chemical potential (partial free enrgy), or an enthalpy of formation, composed of the sum of all changes in chemical potential (or of enthalpy) for the reactions leading to its formation, by any convenient path. Since free energy and enthalpy are variables of state, the value is a unique function of the state, so this approach can be used to define the the relative energy content of any chemical system by reference to the work needed to get there starting from the elements.

Standard states of Solutes and Gases, and Free Energy Changes of Reaction

In order to compare free energies for chemical processes, it is convenient to normalize free energy changes so as to eliminate differences in reaction volume. This is achieved by using DG°, the molar free energy change, and a standard state for reactants in solution. Under normal temperature and pressure (NTP) of 25°C and1 atms pressure:

- Solutes are in their standard states when they have an activity of 1 M.
- Gases are in their standard states when they are at a pressure of 1 atms.

Standard State of the Solvent

Treatment of the solvent represents a tricky issue. By convention, the solvent is assumed to have a standard state of 1 M (the units being necessary to avoid dimensions in logaritmic terms), which does not change under the conditions of biochemical reaction (solutes at dilute solution). In the case of aqueous solutions, this may seem odd, because the activity of liquid water is 55.35 M (at NTP). This convention is adopted because the interactions with the solvent are subsumed under the standard chemical potentials of the solutes (which are referred to the standard state of a 1 M solution), and under the activity coefficients relating activities to concentrations. For reactions, the interactions are subsumed under DG°, since this is derived by summation of values for μ^o. The convention allows one to ignore interactions between solute and solvent; this is usually appropriate since they are not significantly affected by changes in the solvent. In effect, for biochemical reactions in which water is a substrate or product (mainly hydrolysis and lyase reactions), water is omitted from the thermodynamic equation. Thus for ATP hydrolysis:

$$ATP + H_2O \Leftrightarrow ADP + Pi$$

$$\Delta G' = \Delta G^{0'} + RT \ln \frac{(ADP).(Pi)}{(ATP)}$$

THE THERMODYNAMICS OF FLUIDS

GRAPHICAL METHODS

Although geometrical representations of propositions in the thermodynamics of fluids are in general use, and have done good service in disseminating clear notions in this science, yet they have by no means received the extension in respect to variety and generality of which they are capable. So far as regards a general graphical method, which can exhibit at once all the thermodynamic properties of a fluid concerned in reversible processes, and serve like for the demonstration of general theorems and the numerical solution of particular problems, it is the general if not the universal practice to use diagrams in which the rectilinear co-ordinates represent volume and pressure. The object of this article is to call attention to certain diagrams of different construction, which afford graphical methods coextensive in their applications with that in ordinary use, and preferable to it in many cases in respect of distinctness or of convenience.

Quantities and Relations

We have to consider the following quantities:

v, the volume,
p, the pressure,
t, the (absolute) temperature, of a given body in any state,
å, the energy,
ç, the entropy,
W, the work done, by the body in passing from one state and
H, the heat received, to another.

These are subject to the relations expressed by the following differential equations:—

$$dW = \alpha p dv,$$

$$d\text{å} = \hat{A} dH - dW,$$

$$\text{dh} = \frac{dH^{*}}{t}$$

Where á and Â are constants depending upon the units by which v, p, W and H are measured. We may suppose our units so chosen that á = 1 and Â = 1, and write our equations in the simpler form,

$$d\text{å} = dH - dW,$$

$$dW = p dv,$$

$$dH = t d\text{ç}.$$

Eliminating dW and dH, we have

$$d\text{å} = t d\text{ç} - p dv.$$

The quantities v, p, t, å, and ç are determined when the state of the body is given, and it may be permitted to call them *functions of the state of the body*. The state of a body, in the sense in which the term is used in the thermodynamics of fluids, is capable of two independent variations, so that between the five quantities v, p, t, å, and ç there exist relations expressible by three finite equations, different in general for different substances, but always such as to be in harmony with the differential equation. This equation evidently signifies that if å be expressed as function of v and ç, the partial differential co-efficients of this function taken with respect to v and to ç will be equal to - p and to t respectively.

On the other hand W and H are not functions of the state of the body (or functions of any of the quantities v, p, t, å, and ç), but are determined by the whole series of states through which the body is supposed to pass.

Fundamental Idea and General Properties

Now if we associate a particular point in a plane with every separate state, of which the body is capable, in any continuous manner, so that states differing infinitely little are associated with points which are infinitely near to each other, the points associated with states of equal volume will form lines, which may be called *lines of equal volume*, the different lines being distinguished by the numerical value of the volume (as lines of volume 10, 20, 30, etc.). In the same way we may conceive of *lines of equal pressure, of equal temperature, of equal energy, and of equal entropy*. These lines we may also call *isometric, isopiestic, isothermal, isodynamic, isentropic*, and if necessary use these words as substantives.

Suppose the body to change its state, the points associated with the states through which the body passes will form a line, which we may call the path of the body. The conception of a path must include the idea of direction, to express the order in which the body passes through the series of states. With every such change of state there is connected in general a certain amount of work done, W, and of heat received, H, which we may call the *work* and the *heat* of the *path*. The value of these quantities may be calculated from equations,

$$dW = pdv,$$

$$dH = td\text{ç},$$

$$i.e., W = + \int pdv,$$

$$H = + \int td\eta$$

The integration being carried on from the beginning to the end of the path. If the direction of the path is reversed, W and H change their signs, remaining the same in absolute value.

If the changes of state of the body form a cycle, *i.e.*, if the final state is the same as the initial, the path becomes a *circuit*, and the work done and heat received are equal, as may be seen from equation, which when integrated for this case becomes $0 = H - W$.

The circuit will enclose a certain area, which we may consider as positive or negative according to the direction of the circuit which circumscribes it. The direction in which areas must be circumscribed in order that their value may be positive, is of course arbitrary. In other words, if x and y are the rectangular co-ordinates, we may define an area either as $+\int ydx$, or as $+\int xdy$.

If an area be divided into any number of parts, the work done in the circuit bounding the whole area is equal to the sum of the work done in all the circuits bounding the partial areas. This is evident from the consideration, that the work done in each of the lines which separate the partial areas appears twice and with contrary signs in the sum of the work done in the circuits bounding the partial areas. Also the heat received in the circuit bounding the whole area is equal to the sum of the heat received in all the circuits bounding the partial areas.

If all the dimensions of a circuit are infinitely small, the ratio of the included area to the work or heat of the circuit is independent of the shape of the circuit and the direction in which it is described, and varies only with its position in the diagram.

That this ratio is independent of the direction in which the circuit is described, is evident from the consideration that a reversal of this direction simply changes the sign of both terms of the ratio. To prove that the ratio is independent of the shape of the circuit, let us suppose the area ABCDE divided up by an infinite number of isometrics $v_1 v_1$, $v_2 v_2$, etc., with equal differences of volume dv, and an infinite number of isopiestics $p_1 p_1$, $p_2 p_2$, etc., with equal differences of pressure dp. Now from the principle of continuity, as the whole figure is infinitely small, the ratio of the area of one of the small quadrilaterals into which the figure is divided to the work done in passing around it is approximately the same for all the different quadrilaterals.

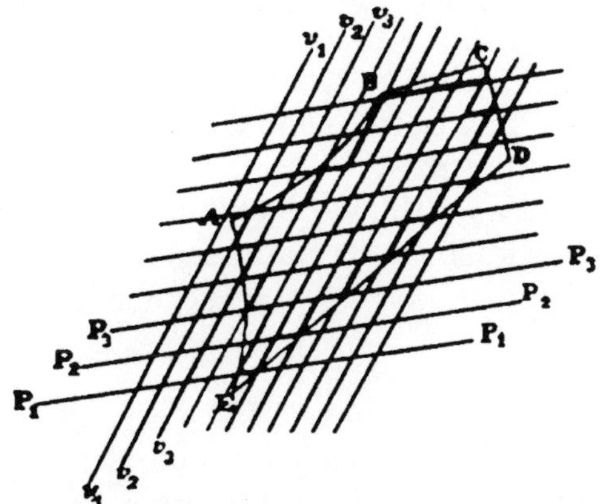

Therefore the area of the figure composed of all the complete quadrilaterals which fall within the given circuit has to the work done in circumscribing this figure the same ratio, which we will call ã. But the area of this figure is approximately the same as that of the given circuit, and the work done in describing this figure is approximately the same as that done in describing the given circuit. Therefore the area of the given circuit has to the work done or heat received in that circuit this ratio ã, which is independent of the shape of the circuit.

Now if we imagine the systems of equidifferent isometrics and isopiestics, which have just been spoken of, extended over the whole diagram, the work done in circumscribing one of the small quadrilaterals, so that the increase of pressure directly precedes the increase of volume, will have in every part of the diagram a constant value, viz, the product of the differences of volume and pressure ($dv \times dp$), as may easily be proved by applying equation successively to its four sides. But the area of one of these quadrilaterals, which we could consider as constant within the limits of the infinitely small circuit, may vary for different parts of the diagram, and will indicate proportionally the value of ã, which is equal to the area divided by $dv \times dp$.

In like manner, if we imagine systems of isentropics and isothermals drawn throughout the diagram for equal differences *d*ç and *dt*, the heat received in passing around one of the small quadrilaterals, so that the increase of *t* shall directly precede that of ç, will be the constant product *d*ç × *dt*, as may be proved by equation, and the value of ã, which is equal to the area divided by the heat, will be indicated proportionally by the areas.

This quantity ã, which is the ratio of the area of an infinitely small circuit to the work done or heat received in that circuit, and which we may call the scale on which work and heat are represented by areas, or more briefly, the *scale of work and heat*, may have a constant value throughout the diagram or it may have a varying value.

The diagram in ordinary use affords an example of the first case, as the area of a circuit is everywhere proportional to the work or heat. There are other diagrams which have the same property, and we may call all such *diagrams of constant scale*.

In any case we may consider the scale of work and heat as known for every point of the diagram so far as we are able to draw the isometrics and isopiestics or the isentropics and isothermals.

If we write ä*W* and ä*H* for the work and heat of an infinitesimal circuit, and ä*A* for the area included, the relations of these quantities are thus expressed:

$$\delta W = \delta H = \frac{1}{\gamma}\delta A .$$

We may find the value of *W* and *H* for a circuit of finite dimensions by supposing the included area *A* divided into areas ä*A* infinitely small in all directions, for which therefore the above equation will hold, and taking the sum of the values of ä*H* or ä*W* for the various areas ä*A*. Writing W^c and H^c for the work and heat of the circuit *C*, and Ó for a summation or integration performed within the limits of this circuit, we have

$$W^c = H^c = \sum c \frac{1}{\gamma}\delta A$$

We have thus an expression for the value of the work and heat of a circuit involving an integration extending over an area instead of one extending over a line, as in equations.

Similar expressions may be found for the work and the heat of a path which is not a circuit. For this case may be reduced to the preceding by the consideration that $W = 0$ for a path on an isometric or on the line of no pressure, and $H = 0$ for a path on an isentropic or on the line of absolute cold. Hence the work of any path S is equal to that of the circuit formed of S, the isometric of the final state, the line of no pressure and the isometric of the initial state, which circuit may be represented by the notation $[S, v'' \cdot p^0, v']$. And the heat of the same path is the same as that of the circuit $[S, ç'', t^0, ç']$. Therefore using W^s and H^s to denote the work and heat of any path S, we have

$$W^s = \sum^{\left[S,V'',p^0,v'\right]} \frac{1}{\gamma}\delta A \,,$$

$$H^s = \sum^{\left[s,n'',t^0,n'\right]} \frac{1}{\gamma}\delta A$$

Where as before the limits of the integration are denoted by the expression occupying the place of an index to the sign Ó. These equations evidently include equation as a particular case.

It is easy to form a material conception of these relations. If we imagine, for example, mass inherent in the plane of the diagram with a varying (superficial) density represented by

$$\frac{1}{\gamma}$$

, then

$$\sum \frac{1}{\gamma}\delta A$$

Will evidently denote the mass of the part of the plane included within the limits of integration, this mass being taken positively or negatively according to the direction of the circuit. Thus far we have made no supposition in regard to the nature of the law, by which we associate the points of a plane with the states of the body, except a certain condition of continuity.

Whatever law we may adopt, we obtain a method of representation of the thermodynamic properties of the body, in which the relations existing between the functions of the state of the body are indicated by a net-work of lines, while the work done and the heat received by the body when it changes its state are represented by integrals extending over the elements of a line, and also by an integral extending over the elements of certain areas in the diagram, or, if we choose to introduce such a consideration, by the mass belonging to these areas.

The different diagrams which we obtain by different laws of association are all such as may be obtained from one another by a process of *deformation*, and this consideration is sufficient to demonstrate their properties from the well-known properties of the diagram in which the volume and pressure are represented by rectangular coordinates.

For the relations indicated by the net-work of isometrics, isopiestics etc are evidently not altered by deformation of the surface upon which they are drawn, and if we conceive of mass as belonging to the surface, the mass included within given lines will also not be affected by the process of deformation. If, then, the surface upon which the ordinary diagram is drawn has the uniform superficial density 1, so that the work and heat of a circuit, which are represented in this diagram by the included area, shall also be represented by the mass included, this latter relation will hold for any diagram formed from this by deformation of the surface on which it is drawn.

The choice of the method of representation is of course to be determined by considerations of simplicity and convenience, especially in regard to the drawing of the lines of equal volume, pressure, temperature, energy and entropy, and the estimation of work and heat. There is an obvious advantage in the use of diagrams of constant scale, in which the work and heat are represented simply by areas.

Such diagrams may of course be produced by an infinity of different methods, as there is no limit to the ways of deforming a plane figure without altering the magnitude of its elements. Among these methods, two are especially important,—the ordinary method in which the volume and pressure are represented by rectilinear co-ordinates, and that in which the entropy and temperature are so represented. A diagram formed by the former method may be called, for the sake of distinction, a *volume-pressure* diagram,—one formed by the latter, an *entropytemperature* diagram. That the latter as well as the former satisfies the condition that ã = 1 throughout the whole diagram.

The Entropy-temperature

As the general equations are not altered by interchanging v, —p and — W with ç, t and H respectively, it is evident that, so far as these equations are concerned, there is nothing to choose between a volume-pressure and an entropy-temperature diagram. In the former, the work is represented by an area bounded by the path which represents the change of state of the body, two ordinates and the axis of abscissas. The same is true of the heat received in the latter diagram.

Again, in the former diagram, the heat received is represented by an area bounded by the path and certain lines, the character of which depends upon the nature of the body under consideration. Except in the case of an ideal body, the properties of which are determined by assumption, these lines are more or less unknown in a part of their course, and in any case the area will generally extend to an infinite distance. Very much the same inconveniences attach themselves to the areas representing work in the entropy temperature diagram.

There is, however, a consideration of a general character, which shows an important advantage on the side of the entropy-temperature diagram. In thermodynamic problems, heat received at one temperature is by no means the equivalent of the same amount of heat received at another temperature. For example, a supply of a million calories at 150^c is a very different thing from a supply of a million calories at 50^c. But no such distinction exists in regard to work. This is a result of the general law, that heat can only pass from a hotter to a colder body, while work can be transferred by mechanical means from one fluid to any other, whatever may be the pressures.

Hence, in thermodynamic problems, it is generally necessary to distinguish between the quantities of heat received or given out by the body at different temperatures, while as far as work is concerned, it is generally sufficient to ascertain the total amount performed. If, then, several heat-areas and one work-area enter into the problem, it is evidently more important that the former should be simple in form, than that the latter should be so. Moreover, in the very common case of a circuit, the work-area is bounded entirely by the path, and the form of the isometrics and the line of no pressure are of no especial consequence.

It is worthy of notice that the simplest form of a perfect thermodynamic engine, so often described in treatises on thermodynamics, is represented in the entropy-temperature diagram by a figure of extreme simplicity, viz: a rectangle of which the sides are parallel to the co-ordinate axes.

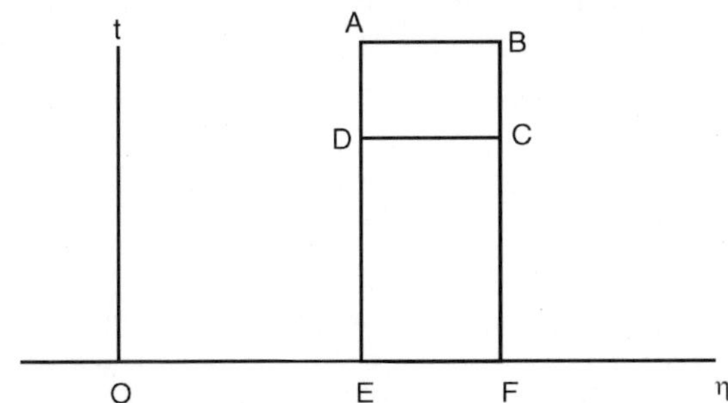

Thus, the circuit ABCD may represent the series of states through which the fluid is made to pass in such an engine, the included area representing the work done, while the area ABFE represents the heat received from the heater at the highest temperature AE, and the area CDEF represents the heat transmitted to the cooler at the lowest temperature DE.

There is another form of the perfect thermodynamic engine, viz: one with a perfect regenerator as defined by Rankine, the representation of which becomes peculiarly simple in the entropy-temperature diagram. The circuit consists of two equal straight lines AB and CD parallel to the axis of abscissas, and two precisely similar curves of any form BC and AD.

The included area ABCD represents the work done, and the areas ABba and CDdc represent respectively the heat received from the heater and that transmitted to the cooler. The heat imparted by the fluid to the regenerator in passing from B to C, and afterwards restored to the fluid in its passage from D to A, is represented by the areas BCcb and DAad.

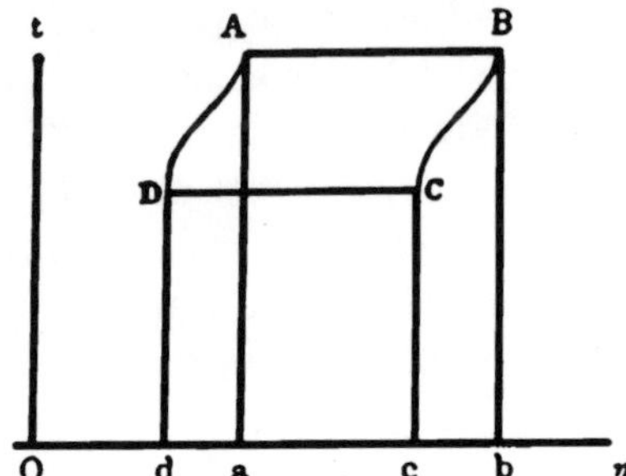

Fig. It is often a matter of the first importance in the study of any thermodynamic engine, to compare it with a perfect engine. Such a comparison will obviously be much facilitated by the use of a method in which the perfect engine is represented by such simple forms.

The method in which the co-ordinates represent volume and pressure has a certain advantage in the simple and elementary character of the notions upon which it is based, and its analogy with Watt's indicator has doubtless contributed to render it popular. On the other hand, a method involving the notion of *entropy*, the very existence of which depends upon the second law of thermodynamics, will doubtless seem to many far-fetched, and may repel beginners as obscure and difficult of comprehension.

This inconvenience is perhaps more than counterbalanced by the advantages of a method which makes the second law of thermodynamics so prominent, and gives it so clear and elementary an expression. The fact, that the different states of a fluid can be represented by the positions of a point in a plane, so that the ordinates shall represent the temperatures, and the heat received or given out by the fluid shall be represented by the area bounded by the line representing the states through which the body passes, the ordinates drawn through the extreme points of this line, and the axis of abscissas,—this fact, clumsy as its expression in words may be, is one which presents a clear image to the eye, and which the mind can readily grasp and retain.

If, then, it is more important for purposes of instruction and the like to familiarize the learner with the second law, than to defer its statement as long as possible, the use of the entropy-temperature diagram may serve a useful purpose in the popularizing of this science.

The foregoing considerations are in the main of a general character, and independent of the nature of the substance to which the graphical method is applied. On this, however, depend the forms of the isometrics, isopiestics and isodynamics in the entropy-temperature diagram, and of the isentropics, isothermals and isodynamics in the volume-pressure diagram. As the convenience of a method depends largely upon the ease with which these lines can be drawn, and upon the peculiarities of the fluid which has its properties represented in the diagram, it is desirable to compare the methods under consideration in some of their most important applications. We will commence with the case of a perfect gas.

Case of a Perfect Gas

A perfect or ideal gas may be defined as such a gas, that for any constant quantity of it the product of the volume and the pressure varies as the temperature, and the energy varies as the temperature, *i.e.*,

$$pv = at,$$

$$å = ct.$$

The significance of the constant a is sufficiently indicated by equation. The significance of c may be rendered more evident by differentiating equation and comparing the result

$$då = cdt$$

With the general equations and, *viz*:

$$då = dH - dW, dW = pdv.$$

If

$$dv = 0, dW = 0, \text{ and } dH = cdt, \text{ i.e.}$$

$$\left(\frac{dH}{dt}\right)_v = c,$$

i.e., c is the quantity of heat necessary to raise the temperature of the body one degree under the condition of constant volume. It will be observed, that when different quantities of the same gas are considered, a and c both vary as the quantity, and $c \div a$ is constant; also, that the value of $c \div a$ for different gases varies as their specific heat determined for equal volumes and for constant volume.

Any other equations which subsist between v, p, t, å and ç may be derived from the three independent equations (A), (B) and (D). If we eliminate å from (B) and (D), we have

$$ç = a \log v + c \log t + c \log c.$$

Eliminating v from equation, we have

$$ç = (a + c) \log t - a \log p + c \log c + a \log a.$$

Eliminating t, we have

$$\eta = (\alpha + c)\log v + c \log p + c \log \frac{c}{a}.$$

If v is constant, equation becomes

$$ç = c \log t + \text{Const.},$$

i.e., the isometrics in the entropy-temperature diagram are logarithmic curves identical with one another in form,—a change in the value of v having only the effect of moving the curve parallel to the axis of ç. If p is constant, equation (F) becomes

$$ç = (a + c) \log t + \text{Const.},$$

So that the isopiestics in this diagram have similar properties. This identity in form diminishes greatly the labour of drawing any considerable number of these curves. For if a card or thin board be cut in the form of one of them, it may be used as a pattern or ruler to draw all of the same system.

The isodynamics are straight in this diagram (eq B).

To find the form of the isothermals and isentropics in the volume pressure diagram, we may make t and ç constant in equations (A) and (G) respectively, which will then reduce to the well-known equations of these curves:—

$$pv = \text{Const.},$$

$$\text{and } p^{c}v^{a+c} = \text{Const.}$$

The equation of the isodynamics is of course the same as that of the isothermals. None of these systems of lines have that property of identity of form, which makes the systems of isometrics and isopiestics so easy to draw in the entropy-temperature diagram.

Case of Condensable Vapours

The case of bodies which pass from the liquid to the gaseous condition is next to be considered. It is usual to assume of such a body, that when sufficiently superheated it approaches the condition of a perfect gas.

If, then, in the entropy-temperature diagram of such a body we draw systems of isometrics, isopiestics and isodynamics, as if for a perfect gas, for proper values of the constants a and c, these will be asymptotes to the true isometrics, etc., of the vapour, and in many cases will not vary from them greatly in the part of the diagram which represents vapour unmixed with liquid, except in the vicinity of the line of saturation. In the volume-pressure diagram of the same body, the isothermals, isentropics and isodynamics, drawn for a perfect gas for the same values of a and c, will have the same relations to the true isothermals, etc.

In that part of any diagram which represents a mixture of vapour and liquid, the isopiestics and isothermals will be identical, as the pressure is determined by the temperature alone. In both the diagrams which we are now comparing, they will be straight and parallel to the axis of abscissas.

The form of the isometrics and isodynamics in the entropy-temperature diagram, or that of the isentropics and isodynamics in the volume-pressure diagram, will depend upon the nature of the fluid, and probably cannot be expressed by any simple equations. The following property, however, renders it easy to construct equidifferent systems of these lines, viz: any such system will divide any isothermal (isopiestic) into equal segments.

It remains to consider that part of the diagram which represents the body when entirely in the condition of liquid.

The fundamental characteristic of this condition of matter is that the volume is very nearly constant, so that variations of volume are generally entirely inappreciable when represented graphically on the same scale on which the volume of the body in the state of vapour is represented, and both the variations of volume and the connected variations of the connected quantities may be, and generally are, neglected by the side of the variations of the same quantities which occur when the body passes to the state of vapour.

Let us make, then, the usual assumption that v is constant, and see how the general equations,are thereby affected.

We have first,

$$dv = 0,$$

Then

$$dW = 0,$$

and

$$d\text{å} = td\text{ç}.$$

If we add

$$dH = td\text{ç},$$

These four equations will evidently be equivalent to the three independent equations, combined with the assumption which we have just made. For a liquid, then, å, instead of being a function of two quantities v and ç, is a function of ç alone,—t is also a function of ç alone, being equal to the differential co-efficient of the function å; that is, the value of one of the three quantities t, å and ç, is sufficient to determine the other two.

The value of v, moreover, is fixed without reference to the values of t, å and ç (so long as these do not pass the limits of values possible for liquidity); while p does not enter into the equations, *i.e.*, p may have any value (within certain limits) without affecting the values of t, å, ç or v.

If the body change its state, continuing always liquid, the value of W for such a change is 0, and that of H is determined by the values of any one of the three quantities t, å and ç.

It is, therefore, the relations between t, å, ç and H, for which a graphical expression is to be sought; a method, therefore, in which the co-ordinates of the diagram are made equal to the volume and pressure, is totally inapplicable to this particular case; v and p are indeed the only two of the five functions of the state of the body, v, p, t, å, and ç, which have no relations either to each other, or to the other three, or to the quantities W and H, to be expressed. The values of v and p do not really determine the state of an incompressible fluid,—

the values of *t*, å, and ç are still left undetermined, so that through every point in the volume-pressure diagram which represents the liquid there must pass (in general) an infinite number of isothermals, isodynamics and isentropics. The character of this part of the diagram is as follows:—the states of liquidity are represented by the points of a line parallel to the axis of pressures, and the isothermals, isodynamics and isentropics, which cross the field of partial vapourization and meet this line, turn upward and follow its course.

The line of liquidity is a curve AB determined by the relation between *t* and ç. This curve is also an isometric. Every point of it has a definite volume, temperature, entropy and energy. The latter is indicated by the isodynamics $_1E_1$, E_2E_2, etc., which cross the region of partial vapourization and terminate in the line of liquidity. (They do not in this diagram turn and follow the line.)

If the body pass from one state to another, remaining liquid, as from M to N in the figure, the heat received is represented as usual by the area MNnm That the work done is nothing, is indicated by the fact that the line AB is an isometric. Only the isopiestics in this diagram are superposed in the line of fluidity, turning downward where they meet this line and following its course, so that for any point in this line the pressure is undetermined. This is, however, no inconvenience in the diagram, as it simply expresses the fact of the case, that when all the quantities *v*, *t*, å, and ç are fixed, the pressure is still undetermined.

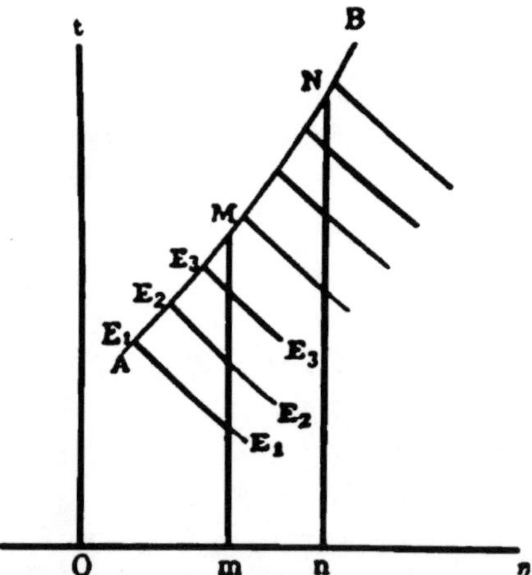

Fig. Diagram in which the Isometrics, Isopiestics, Isothermals, Isodynamics and Isentropics of a Perfect Gas are all Straight Lines

There are many cases in which it is of more importance that it should be easy to draw the lines of equal volume, pressure, temperature, energy and entropy, than that work and heat should be represented in the simplest manner. In such cases it may be expedient to give up the condition that the scale (ã) of work and heat shall be constant, when by that means it is possible to gain greater simplicity in the form of the lines just mentioned.

In the case of a perfect gas, the three relations between the quantities v, p, t, å, and ç are given, equations. These equations may be easily transformed into the three

$$\text{Log}\, p + \log v - \log t = \log a,$$

$$\text{Log å} - \log t = \log c,$$

$$\text{ç} - c \log \text{å} - a \log v = 0;$$

so that the three relations between the quantities log v, log p, log t, log å and ç are expressed by linear equations, and it will be possible to make the five systems of lines all rectilinear in the same diagram, the distances of the isometrics being proportional to the differences of the logarithms of the volumes, the distances of the isopiestics being proportional to the differences of the logarithms of the pressures, and so with the isothermals and the isodynamics,—the distances of the isentropics, however, being proportional to the differences of entropy simply.

The scale of work and heat in such a diagram will vary inversely as the temperature. For if we imagine systems of isentropics and isothermals drawn throughout the diagram for equal small differences of entropy and temperature, the isentropics will be equidistant, but the distances of the isothermals will vary inversely as the temperature, and the small quadrilaterals into which the diagram is divided will vary in the same ratio: ã $\geq 1 \div$ t.

So far, however, the form of the diagram has not been completely defined. This may be done in various ways: *e.g.*, if x and y be the rectangular co-ordinates, we may make

$$x = \log v,$$

$$y = \log p;$$

or

$$x = \text{ç}, y = \log t;$$

or

$$x = \log v, y = \text{ç}; \text{ etc.}$$

Or we may set the condition that the logarithms of volume, of pressure and of temperature, shall be represented in the diagram on the same scale. (The logarithms of energy are necessarily represented on the same scale as those of temperature). This will require that the isometrics, isopiestics and isothermals cut one another at angles of 60°.

The general character of all these diagrams, which may be derived from one another by projection by parallel lines, may be illustrated by the case in which $x = \log v$, and $y = \log p$.

Through any point A of such a diagram let there be drawn the isometric vv', the isopiestic pp', the isothermal tt', and the isentropic çç'. The lines pp' and vv' are of course parallel to the axes.

$$\tan tAp = \left(\frac{dy}{dx}\right)_t = \left(\frac{d\log p}{d\log v}\right)_t = -1$$

The Volume-entropy Diagram

The method of representation, in which the co-ordinates of the point in the diagram are made equal to the volume and entropy of the body, presents certain characteristics which entitle it to a somewhat detailed consideration, and for some purposes give it substantial advantages over any other method. We might anticipate some of these advantages from the simple and symmetrical form of the general equations of thermodynamics, when volume and entropy are chosen as independent variables, viz:—

$$p = -\frac{d\in}{dv}, t = \frac{d\in}{d\eta}$$

$$dW = pdv,$$

$$dH = tdn.$$

Eliminating p and t we have also

$$dW = -\frac{d\in}{dv}dv, dH = \frac{d\in}{d\eta}d\eta,$$

The geometrical relations corresponding to these equations are in the volume-entropy diagram extremely simple. To fix our ideas, let the axes of volume and entropy be horizontal and vertical respectively, volume increasing towards the right and entropy upward. Then the pressure taken negatively will equal the ratio of the difference of energy to the difference of volume of two adjacent points in the same horizontal line, and the temperature will equal the ratio of the difference of energy to the difference of entropy of two adjacent points in the same vertical line.

Or, if a series of isodynamics be drawn for equal infinitesimal differences of energy, any series of horizontal lines will be divided into segments inversely proportional to the pressure, and any series of vertical lines into segments inversely proportional to the temperature.

We see by equations and, that for a motion parallel to the axis of volume, the heat received is 0, and the work done is equal to the decrease of the energy, while for a motion parallel to the axis of entropy, the work done is 0, and the heat received is equal to the increase of the energy. These two propositions are true either for elementary paths or for those of finite length. In general, the work for any element of a path is equal to the product of the pressure in that part of the diagram into the horizontal projection of the element of the path, and the heat received is equal to the product of the temperature into the vertical projection of the element of the path.

If we wish to estimate the value of the integrals + ∫*pdv* and + ∫*tdç*, which represent the work and heat of any path, by means of measurements upon the diagram, or if we wish to appreciate readily by the eye the approximate value of these expressions, or if we merely wish to illustrate their meaning by means of the diagram; for any of these purposes the diagram which we are now considering will have the advantage that it represents the differentials *dv* and *dç* more simply and clearly than any other.

But we may also estimate the work and heat of any path by means of an integration extending over the elements of an area, viz: by the formula,

$$W^c = H^c = \sum{}^c \frac{1}{\gamma}\delta A$$

$$W^s = \sum{}^{\left[s,v'',p^0,v'\right]} \frac{1}{\gamma}\delta A$$

$$H^s = \sum{}^{\left[s,n'',t^0,n'\right]} \frac{1}{\gamma}\delta A$$

In regard to the limits of integration in these formula, we see that for the work of any path which is not a circuit, the bounding line is composed of the path, the line of no pressure and two vertical lines, and for the heat of the path, the bounding line is composed of the path, the line of absolute cold and two horizontal lines.

As the sign of *ã*, as well as that of *äA*, will be indeterminate until we decide in which direction an area must be circumscribed in order to be considered positive, we will call an area positive which is circumscribed in the direction in which the hands of a watch move. This choice, with the positions of the axes of volume and entropy which we have supposed, will make the value of *ã* in most cases positive

The value of *ã*, in a diagram drawn according to this method, will depend upon the properties of the body for which the diagram is drawn. In this respect, this method differs from all the others which have been discussed in detail in this article. It is easy to find an expression for *ã* depending simply upon the variations of the energy, by comparing the area and the work or heat of an infinitely small circuit in the form of a rectangle having its sides parallel to the two axes.

Let $N_1 N_2 N_3 N_4$ be such a circuit, and let it be described in the order of the numerals, so that the area is positive. Also let $å_1$, $å_2$, $å_3$, $å_4$ represent the energy at the four corners. The work done in the four sides in order commencing at N_1, will be $å_1 - å_2$, 0, $å_3 - å_4$, 0. The total work, therefore, for the rectangular circuit is

$$å_1 - å_2 + å_3 - å_4.$$

Now as the rectangle is infinitely small, if we call its sides *dv* and *dç*, the above expression will be equivalent to

$$-\frac{d^2 \in}{dvd\eta}dvd\eta$$

Dividing by the area *dv dç*, and writing *ãv,ç* for the scale of work and heat in a diagram of this kind, we have

$$\frac{1}{\gamma_{v,\eta}} = -\frac{d^2 \in}{dvd\eta} = \frac{dp}{d\eta} = -\frac{dt}{dv}$$

The two last expressions for the value of 1 ÷ *ãv,ç* indicate that the value of *ãv,ç* in different parts of the diagram will be indicated proportionally by the segments into which vertical lines are divided by a system of equidifferent isopiestics, and also by the segments into which horizontal lines are divided by a system of equidifferent isothermals.

As, in almost all cases, the pressure of a body is increased when it receives heat without change of volume, $\frac{dp}{d\eta}$ is in general positive, and the same will be true of *ãv,ç* under the assumptions which we have made in regard to the directions of the axes and the definition of a positive area.

In the estimation of work and heat it may often be of use to consider the deformation necessary to reduce the diagram to one of constant scale for work and heat. Now if the diagram be so deformed that each point remains in the same vertical line, but moves in this line so that all isopiestics become straight and horizontal lines at distances proportional to their differences of pressure, it will evidently become a volume-pressure diagram. Again, if the diagram be so deformed that each point remains in the same horizontal line, but moves in it so that isothermals become straight and vertical lines at distances proportional to their differences of temperature, it will become an entropy-temperature diagram. These considerations will enable us to compute numerically the work or heat of any path which is given in a volume-entropy diagram, when the pressure and temperature are known for all points of the path, in a manner analogous to that explained.

The ratio of any element of area in the volume-pressure or the entropy-temperature diagram, or in any other in which the scale of work and heat is unity, to the corresponding element in the volume entropy diagram is represented by $\frac{1}{\gamma_{v,n}}$ or $-\frac{d^2 \in}{dvd\eta}$ The cases in which this ratio is 0, or changes its sign, demand especial attention, as in such cases the diagrams of constant scale fail to give a satisfactory representation of the properties of the body, while no difficulty or inconvenience arises in the use of the volume-entropy diagram.

As, $-\frac{d^2 \in}{dv d\eta} = \frac{dp}{d\eta}$ value is evidently zero in that part of the diagram which represents the body when in part solid, in part liquid, and in part vapour. The properties of such a mixture are very simply and clearly exhibited in the volume-entropy diagram.

Let the temperature and the pressure of the mixture, which are independent of the proportions of vapour, solid and liquid, be denoted by *t'* and *p'*. Also let V, L and S be points of the diagram which indicate the volume and entropy of the body in three perfectly defined states, viz: that of a vapour of temperature *t2* and pressure *p2,* that of a liquid of the same temperature and pressure, and that of a solid of the same temperature and pressure. And let v_v, ς_v, v_L, ς_L, v_s, ς_s denote the volume and entropy of these states. The position of the point which represents the body, when part is vapour, part liquid, and part solid, these parts being as $\grave{\imath}$, v, and $1 - \grave{\imath} - v$, is determined by the equations

$$v = \grave{\imath}\ _v + v v_L + (1 - \grave{\imath} - v) v_s,$$

$$\varsigma = \grave{\imath}\, \varsigma_v + v \varsigma_L + (1 - \grave{\imath} - v) \varsigma_s,$$

Where v and ς are the volume and entropy of the mixture. The truth of the first equation is evident. The second may be written

$$\varsigma - \varsigma_s = \grave{\imath}\,(\varsigma_v - \varsigma_s) + v(\varsigma_L - \varsigma_s),$$

Or multiplying by *t2,*

$$t'(\varsigma - \varsigma s) = \grave{\imath}\, t'(\varsigma_v - \varsigma_s) + v t'(\varsigma_L - \varsigma_s).$$

The first member of this equation denotes the heat necessary to bring the body from the state S to the state of the mixture in question under the constant temperature *t',* while the terms of the second member denote separately the heat necessary to vapourize the part $\grave{\imath}$, and to liquefy the part v of the body.

The values of v and ς are such as would give the centre of gravity of masses $\grave{\imath}$, v and $1 - \grave{\imath} - v$ placed at the points V, L and S. Hence the part of the diagram which represents a mixture of vapour, liquid and solid, is the triangle VLS. The pressure and temperature are constant for this triangle, *i.e.*, an isopiestic and also an isothermal here expand to cover a space. The isodynamics are straight and equidistant for equal differences of energy. For $\frac{d \in}{dv} = -p'$ and $\frac{d \in}{d\eta} = t'$, both of which are constant throughout the triangle.

This case can be but very imperfectly represented in the volume pressure, or in the entropy-temperature diagram. For all points in the same vertical line in the triangle VLS will, in the volume-pressure diagram, be represented by a single point, as having the same volume and pressure.

And all the points in the same horizontal line will be represented in the entropy-temperature diagram by a single point, as having the same entropy and temperature. In either diagram, the whole triangle reduces to a straight line. It must reduce to a line in any diagram whatever of constant scale, as its area must become 0 in such a diagram.

This must be regarded as a defect in these diagrams, as essentially different states are represented by the same point. In consequence, any circuit within the triangle VLS will be represented in any diagram of constant scale by two paths of opposite directions superposed, the appearance being as if a body should change its state and then return to its original state by inverse processes, so as to repass through the same series of states. It is true that the circuit in question is like this combination of processes in one important particular, viz: that $W = H = 0$, *i.e.*, there is no transformation of heat into work. But this very fact, that a circuit without transformation of heat into work is possible, is worthy of distinct representation.

A body may have such properties that in one part of the volume entropy diagram $\frac{1}{\gamma_{v,\eta}}$ *i.e.*, $\frac{dp}{d\eta}$ is positive and in another negative. These parts of the diagram may be separated by a line, in which $\frac{dp}{d\eta} = 0$, or by one in which $\frac{dp}{d\eta}$ changes abruptly from a positive to a negative value. (In part, also, they may be separated by an area in which $\frac{dp}{d\eta} = 0$.) In the representation of such cases in any diagram of constant scale, we meet with a difficulty of the following nature.

Let suppose that on the right of the line LL in a volume entropy diagram, $\frac{dp}{d\eta}$ is positivc, and on the left negative. Then, if we draw any circuit ABCD on the right side of LL, the direction being that of the hands of a watch, the work and heat of the circuit will be positive. But if we draw any circuit EFGH in the same direction on the other side of the line LL, the work and heat will be negative. For

$$W = H = \sum \frac{1}{\gamma_{v,\eta}} \delta A = \sum \frac{dp}{d\eta} \delta A$$

And the direction of the circuits makes the areas positive in both cases. Now if we should change this diagram into any diagram of constant scale, the areas of the circuits, as representing proportionally the work done in each case, must necessarily have opposite signs, ie., the direction of the circuits must be opposite. We will suppose that the work done is positive in the diagram of constant scale, when the direction of the circuit is that of the hands of a watch. Then, in that diagram, the circuit ABCD would have that direction and the circuit EFGH the contrary direction.

Now if we imagine an indefinite number of circuits on each side of LL in the volume-entropy diagram, it will be evident that to transform such a diagram into one of constant scale, so as to change the direction of all the circuits on one side of LL, and of none on the other the diagram must be *folded over* along that line; so that the points on one side of LL in a diagram of constant scale do not represent any states of the body, while on the other side of this line, each point, for a certain distance at least, represents two different states of the body, which in the volume-entropy diagram are represented by points on opposite sides of the line LL.

We have thus in a part of the field two diagrams superposed, which must be carefully distinguished. If this be done, as by the help of different colours, or of continuous and dotted lines, or otherwise, and it is remembered that there is no continuity between these superposed diagrams, except along the bounding line LL, all the general theorems which have been developed in this article can be readily applied to the diagram. But to the eye or to the imagination, the figure will necessarily be much more confusing than a volume-entropy diagram.

If

$$\frac{dp}{d\eta} = 0$$

for the line LL, there will be another inconvenience in the use of any diagram of constant scale, viz: in the vicinity of the line LL,

$\frac{dp}{d\eta}$, *i.e.*, $1 \div \tilde{a}_{v}$, ç will have a very small value, so that areas will be very greatly reduced in the diagram of constant scale, as compared with the corresponding areas in the volume-entropy diagram. Therefore, in the former diagram, either the isometrics, or the isentropics, or both, will be crowded together in the vicinity of the line LL, so that this part of the diagram will be necessarily indistinct.

It may occur, however, in the volume-entropy diagram, that the same point must represent two different states of the body. This occurs in the case of liquids which can be vapourized. Let MM be the line representing the states of the liquid bordering upon vapourization. This line will be near to the axis of entropy, and nearly parallel to it. If the body is in a state represented by a point of the line MM, and is compressed without addition or subtraction of heat, it will remain of course liquid. Hence, the points of the space immediately on the left of MM represent simple liquid.

On the other hand, the body being in the original state, if its volume should be increased without addition or subtraction of heat, and if the conditions necessary for vapourization are present (conditions relative to the body enclosing the liquid in question, etc.), the liquid will become partially vapourized, but if these conditions are not present it will continue liquid.

Hence, every point on the right of MM and sufficiently near to it represents two different states of the body in one of which it is partially vapourized, and in the other it is entirely liquid. If we take the points as representing the mixture of vapour and liquid, they form one diagram, and if we take them as representing simple liquid, they form a totally different diagram superposed on the first. There is evidently no continuity between these diagrams except at the line MM; we may regard them as upon separate sheets united only along MM. For the body cannot pass from the state of partial vapourization to the state of liquid except at this line.

The reverse process is indeed possible; the body can pass from the state of superheated liquid to that of partial vapourization, if the conditions of vapourization alluded to above are supplied, or if the increase of volume is carried beyond a certain limit, but not by gradual changes or reversible processes.

After such a change, the point representing the state of the body will be found in a different position from that which it occupied before, but the change of state cannot be properly represented by any path, as during the change the body does not satisfy that condition of uniform temperature and pressure which has been assumed throughout this article, and which is necessary for the graphical methods under discussion.

Of the two superposed diagrams, that which represents simple liquid is a continuation of the diagram on the left of MM. The isopiestics, isothermals and isodynamics pass from one to the other without abrupt change of direction or curvature. But that which represents a mixture of vapour and liquid will be different in its character, and its isopiestics and isothermals will make angles in general with the corresponding lines in the diagram of simple liquid. The isodynamics of the diagram of the mixture, and those of the diagram of simple liquid, will differ in general in curvature at the line MM, but not in direction, $\frac{d\in}{dv}=-p$ for and $\frac{d\in}{d\eta}=t$.

The case is essentially the same with some substances, as water, for example, about the line which separates the simple liquid from a mixture of liquid and solid.

In these cases the inconvenience of having one diagram superposed upon another cannot be obviated by any change of the principle on which the diagram is based. For no distortion can bring the three sheets, which are united along the line MM (one on the left and two on the right), into a single plane surface without superposition. Such cases, therefore, are radically distinguished from those in which the superposition is caused by an unsuitable method of representation.

To find the character of a volume-entropy diagram of a perfect gas, we may make å constant in equation (D), which will give for the equation of an isodynamic and isothermal

$$\varsigma = a \log v + \text{Const.},$$

And we may make p constant in equation (G), which will give for the equation of an isopiestic

$$\varsigma = (a + c) \log v + \text{Const.}$$

It will be observed that all the isodynamics and isothermals can be drawn by a single pattern and so also with the isopiestics.

The case will be nearly the same with vapours in a part of the diagram. In that part of the diagram which represents a mixture of liquid and vapour, the isothermals, which of course are identical with the isopiestics, are straight lines. For when a body is vapourized under constant pressure and temperature, the quantities of heat received are proportional to the increments of volume; therefore, the increments of entropy are proportional to the increments of volume.

As $\dfrac{d\epsilon}{dv} = -p$ and $\dfrac{d\epsilon}{d\eta} = t$, any isothermal is cut at the same angle by all the isodynamics, and is divided into equal segments by equidifferent isodynamics. The latter property is useful in drawing systems of equidifferent isodynamics.

The Isometric, Isopiestic, Isothermal and Isentropic

The arrangement of the isometric, the isopiestic, the isothermal and the isentropic drawn through any same point, in respect to the order in which they succeed one another around that point, and in respect to the sides of these lines towards which the volume, pressure, temperature and entropy increase, is not altered by any deformation of the surface on which the diagram is drawn, and is therefore independent of the method by which the diagram is formed. This arrangement is determined by certain of the most characteristic thermodynamic properties of the body in the state in question, and serves in turn to indicate these properties. It is determined, namely, by the value of $\left(\dfrac{dp}{d\eta}\right)_v$ as positive, negative, or zero, *i.e.*, by the effect of heat as increasing or diminishing the pressure when the volume is maintained constant, and by the nature of the internal thermodynamic equilibrium of the body as stable or neutral,—an unstable equilibrium, except as a matter of speculation, is of course out of the question.

Let us first examine the case in which $\left(\dfrac{dp}{d\eta}\right)_v$ is positive and the equilibrium is stable. As $\left(\dfrac{dp}{d\eta}\right)_v$ does not vanish at the point in question, there is a definite isopiestic passing through that point, on one side of which the pressures are greater, and on the other less, than on the line itself. As $\left(\frac{dt}{dv}\right)_\eta = -\left(\frac{dp}{d\eta}\right)_v = -$, the case is the same with the isothermal. It will be convenient to distinguish the sides of the isometric, isopiestic, etc., on which the volume, pressure, etc., increase, as the *positive* sides of these lines.

The condition of stability requires that, when the pressure is constant, the temperature shall increase with the heat received,—therefore with the entropy.

His may be written $[dt{:}d\varsigma]_p > 0$. It also requires that, when there is no transmission of heat, the pressure should increase as the volume diminishes, *i.e.*, that $[dp{:}dv] < 0$. Through the point in question, A, let there be drawn the isometric *vv'* and the isentropic *çç'*, and let the positive sides of these lines be indicated as in the figure. The conditions $\left(\frac{dp}{d\eta}\right)_v > 0$ and $[dp{:}\ dv]_\varsigma < 0$ require that the pressure at v and at *ç* shall be greater than at A, and hence, that the isopiestic shall fall as pp2 in the figure, and have its positive side turned as indicated.

Again, the conditions $\left(\frac{dt}{dv}\right)_\eta < 0$ and $[dt{:}\ d\varsigma]_p > 0$ require that the temperature at *ç* and at p shall be greater than at A, and hence, that the isothermal shall fall as tt2 and have its positive side turned as indicated. As it is not necessary that $\left(\frac{dt}{d\eta}\right)_p > 0$,, the lines pp2 and tt2 may be tangent to one another at A, provided that they cross one another, so as to have the same order about the point A as is represented in the figure; *i.e.*, they may have a contact of the second (or any even) order. But the condition that $\left(\frac{dp}{d\eta}\right)_v > 0$, and hence $\left(\frac{dt}{dv}\right)_\eta < 0$, does not allow pp2 to be tangent to vv2, nor tt2 to *çç2*.

If $\left(\frac{dp}{d\eta}\right)_v$ be still positive, but the equilibrium be neutral, it will be possible for the body to change its state without change either of temperature or of pressure; *i.e.*, the isothermal and isopiestic will be identical. The lines will fall, except that the isothermal and isopiestic will be superposed.

In like manner, if $\left(\frac{dp}{d\eta}\right)_v < 0$, it may be proved that the lines will fall for stable equilibrium, and in the same way for neutral equilibrium, except that pp2 and tt2 will be superposed.

The case that $\left(\frac{dp}{d\eta}\right)_v = 0$ includes a considerable number of conceivable cases, which would require to be distinguished. It will be sufficient to mention those most likely to occur.

In a field of stable equilibrium it may occur that $\left(\frac{dp}{d\eta}\right)_v = 0$ along a line, on one side of which $\left(\frac{dp}{d\eta}\right)_v > 0$, and on the other side $\left(\frac{dp}{d\eta}\right)_v < 0$. At any point in such a line the isopiestics will be tangent to the isometrics and the isothermals to the isentropics. In a field of neutral equilibrium representing a mixture of two different states of the substance, where the isothermals and isopiestics are identical, a line may occur which has the threefold character of an isometric, an isothermal and an isopiestic. For such a line $\left(\frac{dp}{d\eta}\right)_v = 0$. If $\left(\frac{dp}{d\eta}\right)_v$ has opposite signs on opposite sides of this line, it, will be an isothermal of maximum or minimum temperature.

The case in which the body is partly solid, partly liquid and partly vapours has already been sufficiently discussed.

The arrangement of the isometric, isopiestic, etc., will indicate directly the sign of any differential co-efficient of the form $\left(\frac{du}{dw}\right)_z$, where u, w and z may be any of the quantities $v, p, t,$ ç (and å, if the isodynamic be added in the figure). The value of such a differential co-efficient will be indicated, when the rates of increase of v, p, etc., are indicated, as by isometrics, etc., drawn both for the values of v, etc., at the point A, and for values differing from these by a small quantity. For example, the value of $\left(\frac{dp}{dv}\right)_\eta$ will be indicated by the ratio of the segments intercepted upon an isentropic by a pair of isometrics and a pair of isopiestics, of which the differences of volume and pressure have the same numerical value. The case in which W or H appears in the numerator or denominator instead of a function of the state of the body, can be reduced to the preceding by the substitution of pdv for dW, or that of *tdç* for dH.

In the foregoing discussion, the equations which express the fundamental principles of thermodynamics in an analytical form have been assumed, and the aim has only been to show how the same relations may be expressed geometrically.

It would, however, be easy, starting from the first and second laws of thermodynamics as usually enunciated, to arrive at the same results without the aid of analytical formula,—to arrive, for example, at the conception of energy, of entropy, of absolute temperature, in the construction of the diagram without the analytical definitions of these quantities, and to obtain the various properties of the diagram without the analytical expression of the thermodynamic properties which they involve. Such a course would have been better fitted to show the independence and sufficiency of a graphical method, but perhaps less suitable for an examination of the comparative advantages or disadvantages of different graphical methods.

The possibility of treating the thermodynamics of fluids by such graphical methods as have been described evidently arises from the fact that the state of the body considered, like the position of a point in a plane, is capable of two and only two independent variations. It is, perhaps, worthy of notice, that when the diagram is only used to demonstrate or illustrate general theorems, it is not necessary, although it may be convenient, to assume any particular method of forming the diagram; it is enough to suppose the different states of the body to be represented continuously by points upon a sheet.

3

Enzymes Kinetics

DESCRIPTION

The use of enzymes in the diagnosis of disease is one of the important benefits derived from the intensive research in biochemistry since the 1940's. Enzymes have provided the basis for the field of clinical chemistry. It is, however, only within the recent past few decades that interest in diagnostic enzymology has multiplied. Many methods currently on record in the literature are not in wide use, and there are still large areas of medical research in which the diagnostic potential of enzyme reactions has not been explored at all.

This section has been prepared by Worthington Biochemical Corporation as a practical introduction to enzymology. Because of its close involvement over the years in the theoretical as well as the practical aspects of enzymology, Worthington's knowledge covers a broad spectrum of the subject. Enzymes are very large, complex protein molecules consisting of intertwined chains of amino acids. They are formed within the cells of all living creatures, including humans, animals, plants, fungi, bacteria, and microscopic single cell organisms. Although enzymes are found in all living cells, they are inanimate chemical compounds that are highly biodegradable, posing no threat to the environment. They are catalysts for chemical reactions, at work in nature, in our bodies, and in industry.

Enzymes control many vital functions - such as the metabolic processes which convert nutrients into energy - and they are highly efficient at increasing the reaction rate of biochemical processes. Each enzyme has a highly specific target, breaking down or synthesizing certain compounds, and operating under specific temperature, pH and pressure.

Because there are so many different enzymes, they are categorized according to the compounds they interact with to produce a reaction. Commonly used enzymes include lipases which split fats into glycerol and fatty acids; amylases which break starch down to produce simple sugars; proteases which break down proteins; and cellulases which break down cellulose. Enzymes can be manufactured for commercial purposes by superheating a fermentation broth under aseptic conditions to form a completely sterile nutrient medium. The nutrient is then converted into a desired enzyme by using a carefully selected microorganism - such as Dyadic's C1 - in the presence of oxygen. The use of the broth, microorganism, nutrients and operating conditions determine the type and yield of each enzyme. Once fermentation is completed, various centrifugal, filtration, and precipitation processes separate the enzyme from the fermentation broth.

Utilizing its proprietary technology, Dyadic has manufactured and sold enzymes for the textiles, animal feed, starch, pulp and paper and food industries, since 1994. Dyadic's global market reach and manufacturing capabilities, paired with its large scale 150,000 litre fermenters in the USA and Europe, enable it to market and sell over 50 products to customers in more than 35 countries.

Having dedicated and knowledgeable sales personnel located in North and South America, Europe, and Asia allows Dyadic to provide its customers with excellent service and support. Through the placement of inventory in strategically located high volume ports, Dyadic is able to provide the customer with superior delivery service. Dyadic continues to evolve its ability to serve various markets through innovation and listening to customer needs.

By continuing to leverage its evolving biotechnology infrastructure, Dyadic is expanding its product offerings within the $1.8 billion enzyme market. Dyadic's integrated C1 technology platform enables the company to continue discovering and developing innovative enzyme products, thereby providing customers with value-added solutions for their pressing business needs.

CELLS FUNCTION OF ENZYMES

Life is a dynamic process that involves constant changes in chemical composition. These changes are regulated by catalytic reactions, which are regulated by enzymes. At one time, the cell was actually concieved of as a sac of enzymes. It was believed that if we knew all of the reactions and their rates of action, we could define the cell, and indeed, life itself. Few biologists continue to think of this as a simple task, but we know that life as we know it could not exist without the function of enzymes. Ideally, we would examine enzymes within an intact cell, but this is difficult to control. Consequently, enzymes are studied in vitro after extraction from cells. In this exercise, we will extract the enzyme tyrosinase and study its kinetic parametres. It is only one of thousands of enzymes working in concert within cells, but it is one but which readily demonstrates the main features of enzyme kinetics.

Since all enzymes are proteins, and proteins are differentially soluble in salt solutions, enzyme extraction procedures often begin with salt (typically, ammonium sulfate) precipitation. On the simplest level, proteins can be divided into albumins and globulins on the basis of their solubility in dilute salts. Albumins are considered to be soluble while globulins are insoluble. Solubility is relative, however, and as the salt concentration is increased, most proteins will precipitate.

Thus, if we homogenize a tissue in a solution that retains the enzyme in its soluble state, the enzyme can be subsequently separated from all insoluble proteins by centrifugation or filtration. The enzyme will be impure, since it will be in solution with many other proteins. If aliquots of a concentrated ammonium sulfate solution are then added serially, individual proteins will begin to precipitate according to their solubility. By careful manipulation of the salt concentrations, we can produce fractions which contain purer solutions of enzymes, or at least are enriched for a given enzyme. Fortunately, absolute purity of an enzyme extract is seldom required, but when it is, the fractions must be subjected to further procedures designed for purification (such as electrophoresis and/or column chromatography).

In order to determine the effectiveness of the purification, each step in the extraction procedure must be monitored for enzyme activity. That monitoring can be accomplished in many ways, but usually involves a measurement of the decrease in substrate, or the increase in product specific to the enzyme. One of the important concepts of metabolism is that enzymes from differing sources may have the same function (*i.e.* the same substrate and product), but possess significantly different Km values. Since biological function is as dependent on the rate of a reaction as it is on the direction of a reaction, it becomes necessary to measure the Km value for any enzyme under study.

Enzymes act as catalysts because of their three dimensional protein structure. This structure is controlled by many factors, but is particularly sensitive to changes in pH, salts and temperature. Small changes in the temperature of a reaction can significantly alter the reaction rate, and extremely high temperatures can irreversibly alter both the three dimensional structure of the enzyme and its activity. It may even render the enzyme non-functional; that is, to denature the enzyme. Salts can also cause denaturation, but the effects of ammonium sulfate are usually reversible. Heavy metal salts, by contrast, usually irreversibly alter the structure of the protein, and thus their routine use as fixatives in histological work.

ACTIVE SITES

An enzyme works by binding to a given substrate in such a geometrical fashion that the substrate is able to undergo its inherent reaction at a more rapid rate. This type of reaction is commonly referred to as the lock and key mode for enzyme action. It implies that there is a particular part of the enzyme structure, the active site, which specifically binds sterically to a substrate. The enzyme does not actually react with the substrate but merely brings the substrate into the proper alignment or configuration for it to react spontaneously or in conjunction with another substance. Since a reaction proceeds normally by a random kinetic action of molecules bumping into each other, any time molecules are aligned, they will react faster. Thus, for any given enzyme there will be a best fit configuration to the protein in order to align the substrate and to facilitate the reaction. When the enzyme is in its ideal configuration, the reaction will proceed at its maximum rate, and the overall rate of activity will be dependent upon substrate concentration.

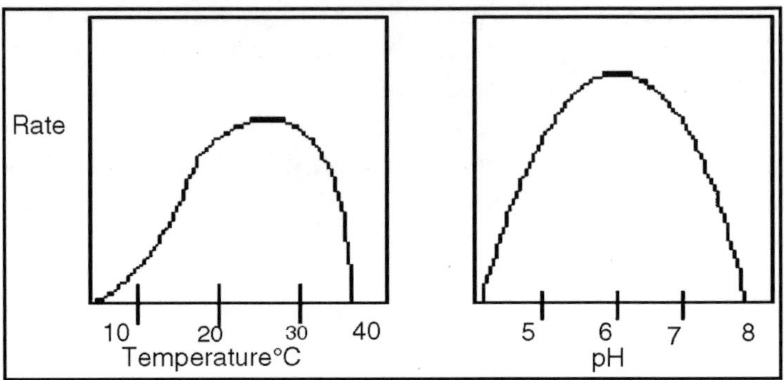

Fig. Hypothetical Effect of Temperature and pH.

Maximum reaction rate assumes that an optimal pH, salt environment and temperature have been established. Figure demonstrates some typical effects of temperature and pH on the rate of an enzyme catalysed reaction. Maximum rate further assumes the presence of any co-enzymes and/or cofactors that the enzyme requires. Co-enzymes are organic molecules which must bind to the protein portion of the enzyme in order to form the correct configuration for a reaction. Cofactors are inorganic molecules which do the same.

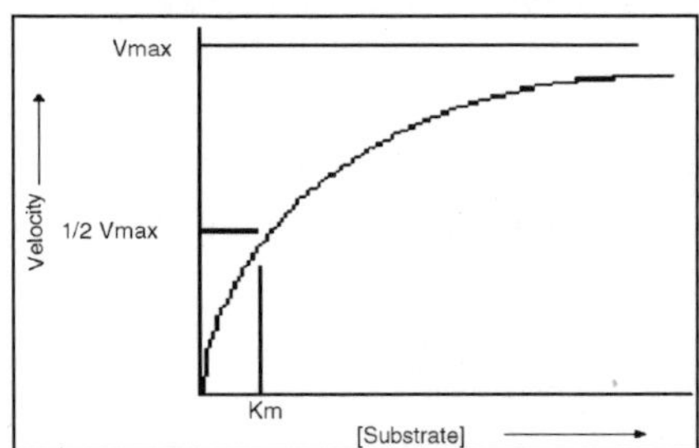

Fig. Michaells-Menten Plot of Enzyme Activity.

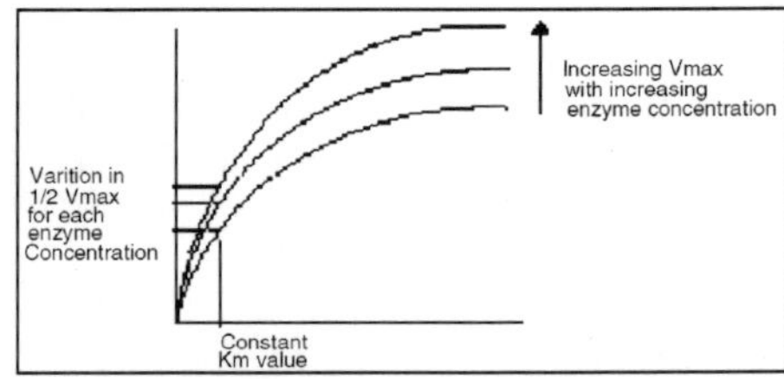

Fig. Effect of Increasing Enzyme Concentration.

Now, if we measure the concentration of an enzyme via its rate of activity (*i.e.* the velocity of the catalysed reaction), we must control the reaction for the effects of temperature, pH, salt concentration, co-enzymes, cofactors, and substrate concentration. Each of these parametres affects the rate of an enzyme reaction. Thus, each must be carefully controlled if we attempt to study the affects of changes in the enzyme itself. For example, alterations in the rate of a reaction are directly dependent upon the concentration of functional enzyme molecules only when the enzyme is the limiting factor in the reaction. There must be sufficient substrate to saturate all enzyme molecules in order for this criterion to be met. If the substrate concentration is lowered to the point where it becomes rate limiting, it is impossible to accurately measure the enzyme concentration, because there will be two variables at work.

The relationship between substrate concentration and enzyme concentration was mathematically established by pioneering work of two biochemists, L. Michaelis and M.L. Menten in 1913. In recognition of their work, the plots of enzyme activity vs. substrate concentration are known as Michaelis-Menten plots. These are relatively simple plots in which the substrate concentration is on the x-axis, and the velocity of reaction is on the y-axis. The plot demonstrates that as the substrate increases, the velocity increases hyperbolically, and approaches a maximum rate known as V_{max}. This is dependent upon saturation of the enzyme. At V_{max}, all enzyme molecules are complexed with substrate, and thus any additional substrate added to the reaction has no effect on the rate of reaction.

However, this situation becomes more complex: as you change the enzyme concentration, V_{max} will also change. Thus, V_{max} is not a constant value, but is constant only for a given enzyme concentration. Consequently, the value of V_{max} can not be used directly to infer enzyme concentration. It is dependent upon at least two variables, enzyme concentration and substrate concentration (assuming temperature, pH and cofactors have all been controlled). What Michaelis and Menten discovered was a simple means of solving the equations for two variables. If multiple plots of enzyme activity vs. substrate concentration are made with increasing enzyme concentration, the value of V_{max} continues to increase, but the substrate concentration which corresponds to 1/2 V_{max} remains constant. This concentration is the Michaelis Constant for an enzyme. As mentioned, it is designated as Km and is operationally the concentration of substrate which will give exactly 1/2 V_{max} when reacted with an enzyme with maximum pH, temperature and cofactors.

According to the Michaelis-Menten equation:

$$V = \frac{V_{max}(S)}{Km + (S)}$$

This equation is derived from the formula for a hyperbola (c=xy) where

$$Km = (S)(V_{max} / v-1)$$

When $v = V_{max} / 2$, $Km = (S)(V_{max}/(V_{max}/ 2)-1) = (S)$ confirming that the units of this constant are those of concentration.

A Michaelis-Menten plot thus can give us an easy way to measure the rate constant for a given enzyme. An immediate difficulty is apparent, however, when Michaelis-Menten plots are used. V_{max} is an asymptote. Its value can only be certain if the reaction is run at an infinite concentration of substrate. Obviously, this is an impossible prospect in lab. In 1934, two individuals,

Lineweaver and Burke made a simple mathematical alteration in the process by plotting a double inverse of substrate concentration and reaction rate (velocity).

The Lineweaver/Burke equation is:

$$\frac{1}{V} = \frac{Km + (S)}{V_{max}(S)}$$

This equation fits the general form of a straight line, y=mx+b, where m is the slope of the line and b is the intercept. Thus, the Lineweaver/Burke Plot for an enzyme is more useful than Michaelis-Menten, since as velocity reaches infinity, $1/V_{max}$ approaches 0. Moreover, since the plot results in a straight line, the slope is equal to Km/V_{max}, the y intercept equals $1/V_{max}$ (1/S=0). Projection of the line back through the x axis yields the value –1/Km (when 1/V=0). These values can easily be determined by using a linear regression plot and calculating the corresponding values for x=0 and y=0. The inverse of the intercept values will then yield V_{max} and Km.

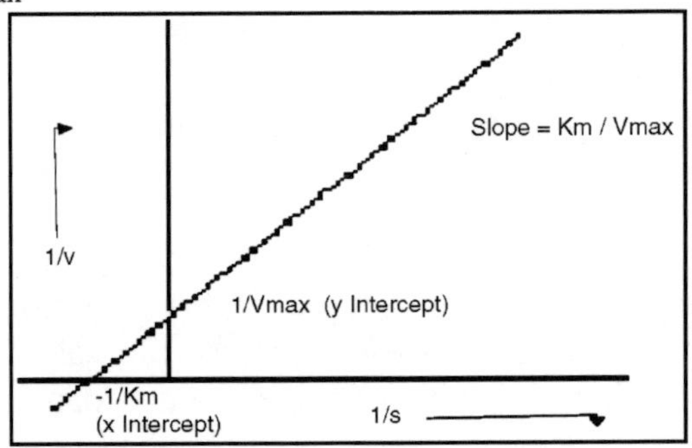

Fig. Lineweaver-Burke plot of Enzyme Activity.

Remember that the point of all of these calculations is to determine the true activity and thus the concentration of the enzyme. If the reaction conditions are adjusted so that the substrate concentration is at Km, then alterations in the rate of reaction are linear and due to alterations in enzyme concentration. Kinetic analysis is the only means of accurately determining the concentration of active enzyme.

SPECIFIC ACTIVITY

This brings us to a definition for enzyme activity. specific activity is defined in terms of enzyme units per mg enzyme protein. An enzyme unit is the amount of substrate converted to product per unit time under specific reaction conditions for pH and temperature. As generally accepted, an enzyme unit is defined as that which catalyses the transformation of 1 micromole of substrate per minute at 30° C and optimal chemical environment (pH and Substrate concentration). Specific Activity relates the enzyme units to the amount of protein in the sample. While it is relatively easy to measure the protein content of a cell fraction, there may be a variable relationship between the protein content and a specific enzyme function. Remember that the initial extraction of an enzyme is accomplished by differential salt precipitation. Many proteins will precipitate together due to their solubility, but have no other common characteristics. To determine both protein content and enzyme activity requires two different procedures. We can measure the amount of protein, or we can kinetically measure the enzyme activity. Combining the two will give us the specific activity.

ENZYME INHIBITION

Finally, before studying a specific enzyme, let's examine the problem of enzyme inhibition. Remember that enzymes function by sterically binding to a substrate. If a molecule interferes with that binding, it will hinder or inhibit the activity of the enzyme. If the inhibitor molecule binds to the same active site as the substrate, then the reaction is known as competitive inhibition because the two molecules, substrate and inhibitor, compete for the same reaction site on the enzyme molecule. With this type of inhibition, V_{max} will not change because V_{max} is a function of all enzyme molecules uniting with substrate (thus having no effective competition). Km, on the other hand, will alter with changes in the concentration of a competitive inhibitor, because it requires larger concentrations of substrate to overcome the direct competition of the inhibitor for the active site.

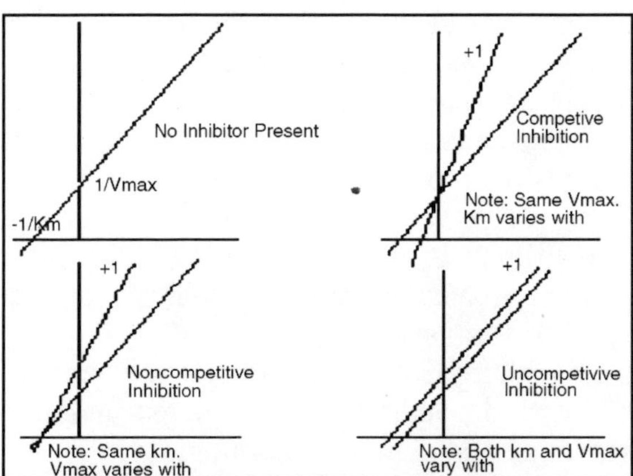

Fig. Inhibitor Effects on L-B plots.

If, however, the inhibitor binds to a site on the enzyme other than the active site, then the inhibition is known as allosteric, or non-competitive inhibition. In this instance, the substrate and inhibitor bind to different parts of the enzyme molecule and thus are not in competition. An allosteric inhibitor alters the structure of the enzyme or physically blocks access to the active site. With non-competitive inhibition, V_{max} will change because, in effect, enzyme is being removed from the reaction. Its kinetic effects are equivalent to lowering the enzyme concentration. Km will not change, however, since this value is constant regardless of the effective enzyme concentration. Finally, there is a third class of inhibitor which can best be defined by its effect on V_{max} and Km. Known as uncompetitive, it alters both of these values. It has effects on both the active site and allosteric sites. The graphic representation of the three types of enzyme inhibition are show in Figure.

TYROSINASE

This exercise involves the isolation (extraction) of the enzyme tyrosinase from potatoes and subsequent measurement of its activity. Tyrosinase is the common name for an enzyme that is formally termed Monophenol Monooxygenase and is listed as Enzyme #1.14.18.1 in the standard Enzyme Nomenclature. 1 It is also known as phenolase, monophenol oxidase and as cresolase. It is, functionally, an oxygen oxidoreductase enzyme.

This nomenclature points out another difficulty of working with enzymes. Their names are derived from the known activities. Enzymes isolated from different sources and measured for their catalytic activity with varying substrates can turn out to be the same protein. Thus, the enzyme tyrosinase, discovered in animal systems, was named for its action on the amino acid tyrosine, and specifically for its ability to form dopaquinone, an intermediate metabolite in the production of melanin.

The same enzyme isolated from plant materials had been examined for its ability to oxidize phenolic residues, and thus the names phenolase, monophenol oxidase and cresolase. Since it has been extensively studied in melanin production, we will continue to use the common name of tyrosinase.

The enzyme tyrosinase is fairly ubiquitous; that is, it is found in nearly all cells. In research, it has been purified from the fungus N. crassa 2 by freezing kilogram quantities of the fungal mycelia in liquid nitrogen, homogenizing the frozen tissue with a French Press, precipitating the proteins in ammonium sulfate, and purifying the enzyme chromato-graphically on Sephadex and Celite columns. A fairly complex undertaking.

Tyrosinase has been extracted from hamster melanomas by modifications of this technique and with the addition of acetone extractions as well as DEAE-cellulose chromatography and alumina treatments.

3 Tyrosinase has also been separated from many plant tissues utilizing a far simpler technique based principally on ammonium sulfate precipitation of proteins.

The catalytic action of this enzyme is the conversion of tyrosine + O_2 to yield dihydroxyphenylalanine (DOPA), which is then converted to dopaquinone + H_2O. Dopaquinone in turn can be readily converted to dopachrome, an orange to red pigment (found in human red hair), which can then be converted to the black/brown melanin pigments (found in virtually all human pigments).

$$\text{Tyrosine} + 1/2\ O_2 \rightarrow \text{DOPA}$$

$$2DOPA + O_2 \rightarrow 2Dopaquinone + 2H_2O$$

$$Dopaquinone \rightarrow Leukodopachrome$$

$$Leukodopachrome + Dopaquinone \rightarrow Dopachrome + DOPA$$

The enzyme catalyses the first two of these reactions, namely the conversion of tyrosine and the conversion of DOPA. The formation of dopachrome from dopaquinone is spontaneous.

We can now monitor the activity of the enzyme by analyzing the disappearance of tyrosine and/or DOPA as substrates, the appearance of leukodopachrome or dopachrome as products, or by monitoring the use of oxygen. Physiologists and chemists have long preferred the manometric determination of gaseous oxygen exchange, but far simpler is the determination of dopachrome, a natural pigment with an absorbance maximum at 475 nm. This absorbance allows us to use standard spectrophotometric analysis by analyzing the formation rate of dopachrome from the substrate DOPA. The summary reaction for tyrosinase activity, as used in this exercise is,

$$DOPA + 1/2\ O_2 \rightarrow Dopachrome$$

ENZYMES AND LIFE PROCESSES

The living cell is the site of tremendous biochemical activity called metabolism. This is the process of chemical and physical change which goes on continually in the living organism. Build-up of new tissue, replacement of old tissue, conversion of food to energy, disposal of waste materials, reproduction - all the activities that we characterize as "life."

This building up and tearing down takes place in the face of an apparent paradox. The greatest majority of these biochemical reactions do not take place spontaneously. The phenomenon of catalysis makes possible biochemical reactions necessary for all life processes. Catalysis is defined as the acceleration of a chemical reaction by some substance which itself undergoes no permanent chemical change.

The catalysts of biochemical reactions are enzymes and are responsible for bringing about almost all of the chemical reactions in living organisms. Without enzymes, these reactions take place at a rate far too slow for the pace of metabolism.

The oxidation of a fatty acid to carbon dioxide and water is not a gentle process in a test tube - extremes of pH, high temperatures and corrosive chemicals are required. Yet in the body, such a reaction takes place smoothly and rapidly within a narrow range of pH and temperature.

In the laboratory, the average protein must be boiled for about 24 hours in a 20per cent HCl solution to achieve a complete breakdown. In the body, the breakdown takes place in four hours or less under conditions of mild physiological temperature and pH.

It is through attempts at understanding more about enzyme catalysts - what they are, what they do, and how they do it - that many advances in medicine and the life sciences have been brought about.

EARLY ENZYME DISCOVERIES

The existence of enzymes has been known for well over a century. Some of the earliest studies were performed in 1835 by the Swedish chemist Jon Jakob Berzelius who termed their chemical action catalytic. It was not until 1926, however, that the first enzyme was obtained in pure form, a feat accomplished by James B. Sumner of Cornell University. Sumner was able to isolate and crystallize the enzyme urease from the jack bean. His work was to earn him the 1947 Nobel Prize. John H. Northrop and Wendell M. Stanley of the Rockefeller Institute for Medical Research shared the 1947 Nobel Prize with Sumner. They discovered a complex procedure for isolating pepsin. This precipitation technique devised by Northrop and Stanley has been used to crystallize several enzymes.

CHEMICAL NATURE OF ENZYMES

All known enzymes are proteins. They are high molecular weight compounds made up principally of chains of amino acids linked together by peptide bonds.

Peptide Bond

$R-CH(NH_2)-CO-NH-CH(COOH)-R'$

where:

$R'-CH(NH_2)-COOH$

and

$R-CH(NH_2)-COOH$

Represent two typical amino acids

Fig. Typical Protein Structure -two Amino Acids Joined by a Peptide Bond.

Enzymes can be denatured and precipitated with salts, solvents and other reagents. They have molecular weights ranging from 10,000 to 2,000,000.

Many enzymes require the presence of other compounds - cofactors - before their catalytic activity can be exerted. This entire active complex is referred to as the holoenzyme; *i.e.*, apoenzyme (protein portion) plus the cofactor (coenzyme, prosthetic group or metal-ion-activator) is called the holoenzyme.

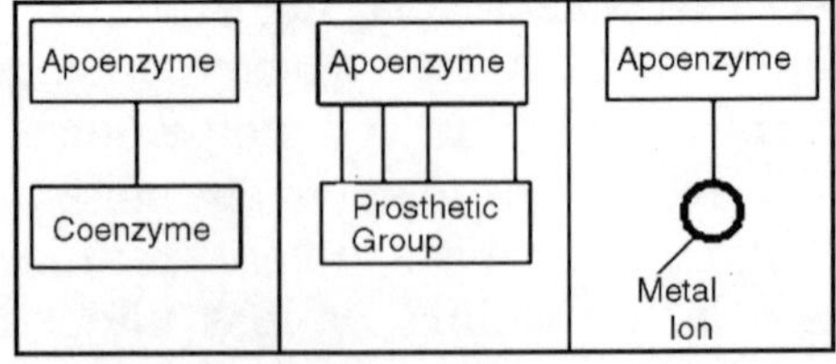

Fig. Holoenzymes - Apoenzymes Plus Various Types of Cofactors.

Apoenzyme + Cofactor = Holoenzyme

According to Holum, the cofactor may be:

- A coenzyme - a non-protein organic substance which is dialyzable, thermostable and loosely attached to the protein part.
- A prosthetic group - an organic substance which is dialyzable and thermostable which is firmly attached to the protein or apoenzyme portion.
- A metal-ion-activator - these include K^{+}, Fe^{++}, Fe^{+++}, Cu^{++}, Co^{++}, Zn^{++}, Mn^{++}, Mg^{++}, Ca^{++}, and Mo^{+++}.

SPECIFICITY OF ENZYMES

One of the properties of enzymes that makes them so important as diagnostic and research tools is the specificity they exhibit relative to the reactions they catalyse. A few enzymes exhibit absolute specificity; that is, they will catalyse only one particular reaction. Other enzymes will be specific for a particular type of chemical bond or functional group. In general, there are four distinct types of specificity:

- *Absolute specificity*: The enzyme will catalyse only one reaction.
- *Group specificity*: The enzyme will act only on molecules that have specific functional groups, such as amino, phosphate and methyl groups.
- *Linkage specificity*: The enzyme will act on a particular type of chemical bond regardless of the rest of the molecular structure.
- *Stereochemical specificity*: The enzyme will act on a particular steric or optical isomer.

Though enzymes exhibit great degrees of specificity, cofactors may serve many apoenzymes. For example, nicotinamide adenine dinucleotide (NAD) is a coenzyme for a great number of dehydrogenase reactions in which it acts as a hydrogen acceptor. Among them are the alcohol dehydrogenase, malate dehydrogenase and lactate dehydrogenase reactions.

NAMING AND CLASSIFICATION

Except for some of the originally studied enzymes such as pepsin, rennin, and trypsin, most enzyme names end in "ase". The International Union of Biochemistry (I.U.B.) initiated standards of enzyme nomenclature which recommend that enzyme names indicate both the substrate acted upon and the type of reaction catalysed.

Under this system, the enzyme uricase is called urate: O_2 oxidoreductase, while the enzyme glutamic oxaloacetic transaminase (GOT) is called L-aspartate: 2-oxoglutarate aminotransferase. Enzymes can be classified by the kind of chemical reaction catalysed:

- Addition or removal of water
  - Hydrolases these include esterases, carbo-hydrases, nucleases, deaminases, amidases, and proteases

  - Hydrases such as fumarase, enolase, aconitase andcarbonic anhydrase
- Transfer of electrons
  - Oxidases
  - Dehydrogenases
- Transfer of a radical
  - *Transglycosidases*: Of monosaccharides
  - *Transphosphorylases and phosphomutases*: of a phosphate group
  - *Transaminases*: of amino group
  - *Transmethylases*: of a methyl group
  - *Transacetylases*: of an acetyl group
- Splitting or forming a C-C bond
  - Desmolases
- Changing geometry or structure of a molecule
  - Isomerases
- Joining two molecules through hydrolysis of pyrophosphate bond in ATP or other tri-phosphate
  - Ligases

BASIC ENZYME REACTIONS

Enzymes are catalysts and increase the speed of a chemical reaction without themselves undergoing any permanent chemical change. They are neither used up in the reaction nor do they appear as reaction products. The basic enzymatic reaction can be represented as follows,

$$S + E \rightarrow P + E$$

where E represents the enzyme catalyzing the reaction, S the substrate, the substance being changed, and P the product of the reaction.

ENZYME KINETICS: ENERGY LEVELS

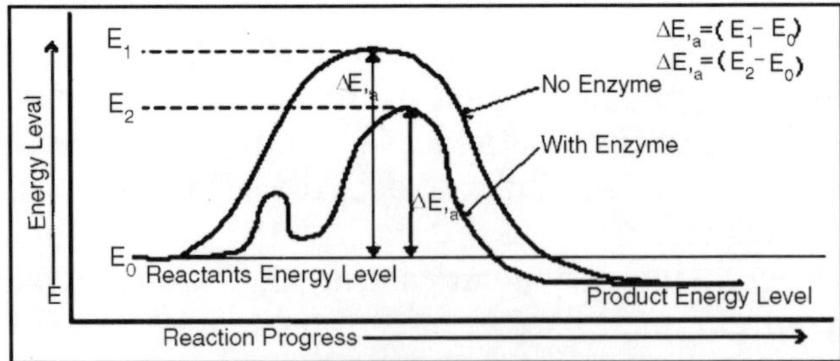

Fig. Energy of Activation ΔE_a is less than ΔE_a due to the Effect of the Enzyme on the Substrate.

Chemists have known for almost a century that for most chemical reactions to proceed, some form of energy is needed. They have termed this quantity of energy, "the energy of activation."

It is the magnitude of the activation energy which determines just how fast the reaction will proceed. It is believed that enzymes lower the activation energy for the reaction they are catalyzing. Figure illustrates this concept.

The enzyme is thought to reduce the "path" of the reaction. This shortened path would require less energy for each molecule of substrate converted to product.

Given a total amount of available energy, more molecules of substrate would be converted when the enzyme is present (the shortened "path") than when it is absent. Hence, the reaction is said to go faster in a given period of time.

ENZYME KINETICS: THE ENZYME SUBSTRATE COMPLEX

A theory to explain the catalytic action of enzymes was proposed by the Swedish chemist Savante Arrhenius in 1888. He proposed that the substrate and enzyme formed some intermediate substance which is known as the enzyme substrate complex. The reaction can be represented as:

$$\underset{\text{substrate}}{S} + \underset{\text{enzyme}}{E} \rightarrow \underset{\text{enzyme substrate complex}}{ES}$$

If this reaction is combined with the original reaction equation [1], the following results:

$$\underset{\text{substrate}}{S} + \underset{\text{enzyme}}{E} \rightarrow \underset{\text{enzyme substrate complex}}{ES} \rightarrow \underset{\text{product}}{P} + \underset{\text{enzyme}}{E}$$

The existence of an intermediate enzyme-substrate complex has been demonstrated in the laboratory, for example, using catalase and a hydrogen peroxide derivative.

At Yale University, Kurt G. Stern observed spectral shifts in catalase as the reaction it catalysed proceeded. This experimental evidence indicates that the enzyme first unites in some way with the substrate and then returns to its original form after the reaction is concluded.

CHEMICAL EQUILIBRIUM

The study of a large number of chemical reactions reveals that most do not go to true completion. This is likewise true of enzymatically-catalysed reactions.

This is due to the reversibility of most reactions. In general:

$$A + B \xrightarrow{K+1} C + D \text{ forward reaction}$$

$$C + D \xrightarrow{K-1} A + B \text{ reverse reaction}$$

where K^{+1} is the forward reaction rate constant and K^{-1} is the rate constant for the reverse reaction.

Combining the two reactions gives:

$$A + B \underset{K-1}{\overset{K+1}{\rightleftarrows}} C + D$$

Applying this general relationship to enzymatic reactions allows the equation:

$$E + S \underset{K-1}{\overset{K+1}{\rightleftarrows}} ES \underset{K-2}{\overset{K+2}{\rightleftarrows}} P + E$$

Equilbrium, a steady state condition, is reached when the forward reaction rates equal the backward rates. This is the basic equation upon which most enzyme activity studies are based.

FACTORS AFFECTING ENZYME ACTIVITY

Knowledge of basic enzyme kinetic theory is important in enzyme analysis in order both to understand the basic enzymatic mechanism and to select a method for enzyme analysis. The conditions selected to measure the activity of an enzyme would not be the same as those selected to measure the concentration of its substrate. Several factors affect the rate at which enzymatic reactions proceed - temperature, pH, enzyme concentration, substrate concentration, and the presence of any inhibitors or activators.

ENZYME CONCENTRATION

In order to study the effect of increasing the enzyme concentration upon the reaction rate, the substrate must be present in an excess amount; *i.e.*, the reaction must be independent of the substrate concentration. Any change in the amount of product formed over a specified period of time will be dependent upon the level of enzyme present. Graphically this can be represented as:

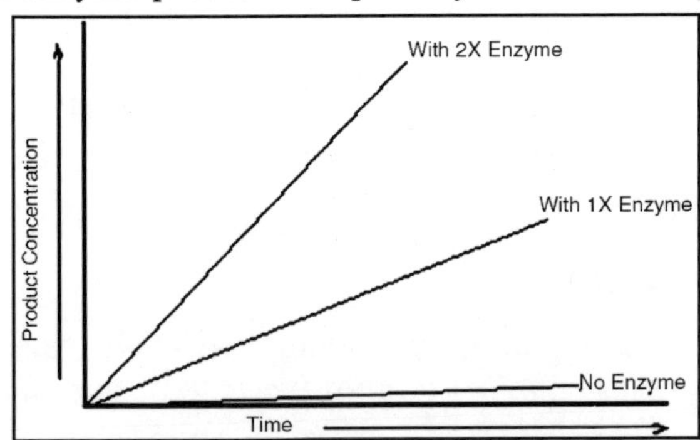

Fig. "Zero order" Reaction rate is Independent of Substrate Concentration.

These reactions are said to be "zero order" because the rates are independent of substrate concentration, and are equal to some constant k. The formation of product proceeds at a rate which is linear with time. The addition of more substrate does not serve to increase the rate. In zero order kinetics, allowing the assay to run for double time results in double the amount of product.

Table. Reaction Orders with Respect to Substrate Concentration.

Order	Rate Equation	Comments
Zero	Rate = k	Rate is independent of substrate concentration
First	Rate = k[S]	Rate is proportional to the first power of substrate concentration
Second	Rate = $k[S][S]=k[S]^2$	Rate is proportional to the square of the substrate concentration
Second	Rate = $k[S_1][S_2]$	Rate is proportional to the first power of each of two reactants

The amount of enzyme present in a reaction is measured by the activity it catalyses. The relationship between activity and concentration is affected by many factors such as temperature, pH, etc. An enzyme assay must be designed so that the observed activity is proportional to the amount of enzyme present in order that the enzyme concentration is the only limiting factor. It is satisfied only when the reaction is zero order. Enzyme activity is generally greatest when substrate concentration is unlimiting.

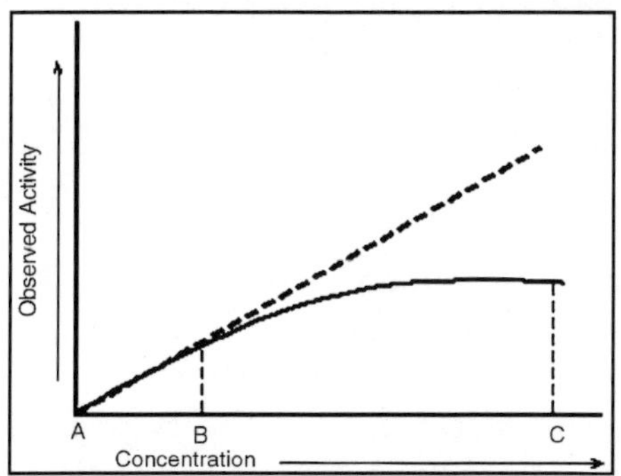

Fig. Activity vs. Concentration.

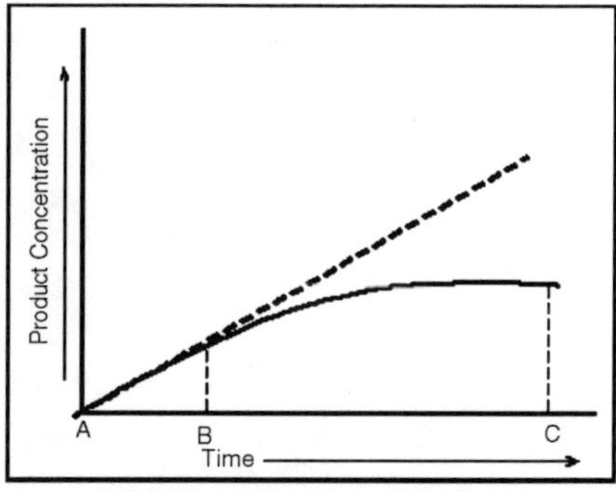

Fig. Reaction Rate Limited by Substrate Concentration.

When the concentration of the product of an enzymatic reaction is plotted against time, a similar curve results, Figure. Between A and B, the curve represents a zero order reaction; that is, one in which the rate is constant with time. As substrate is used up, the enzyme's active sites are no longer saturated, substrate concentration becomes rate limiting, and the reaction becomes first order between B and C. To measure enzyme activity ideally, the measurements must be made in that portion of the curve where the reaction is zero order. A reaction is most likely to be zero order initially since substrate concentration is then highest. To be certain that a reaction is zero order, multiple measurements of product (or substrate) concentration must be made. Figure illustrates three types of reactions which might be encountered in enzyme assays and shows the problems which might be enountered if only single measurements are made.

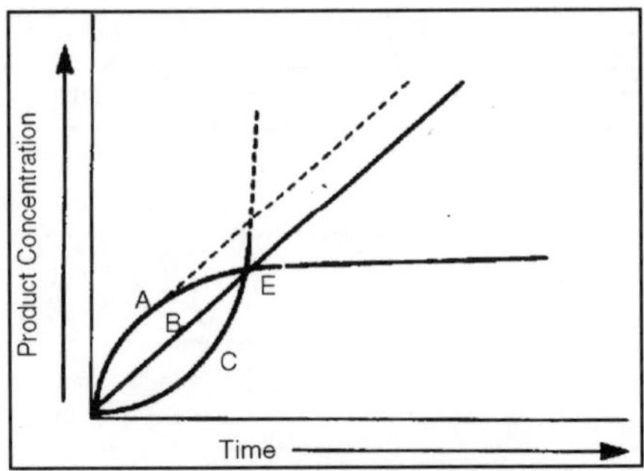

Fig. Leading, lagging, and linear reactions

B is a straight line representing a zero order reaction which permits accurate determination of enzyme activity for part or all of the reaction time. This reaction is zero order initially and then slows, presumably due to substrate exhaustion or product inhibition.

This type of reaction is sometimes referred to as a "leading" reaction. True "potential" activity is represented by the dotted line. Curve C represents a reaction with an initial "lag" phase. Again the dotted line represents the potentially measurable activity. Multiple determinations of product concentration enable each curve to be plotted and true activity determined. A single end point determination at E would lead to the false conclusion that all three samples had identical enzyme concentration.

SUBSTRATE CONCENTRATION

It has been shown experimentally that if the amount of the enzyme is kept constant and the substrate concentration is then gradually increased, the reaction velocity will increase until it reaches a maximum. After this point, increases in substrate concentration will not increase the velocity ($\Delta A/\Delta T$). This is represented graphically as shown.

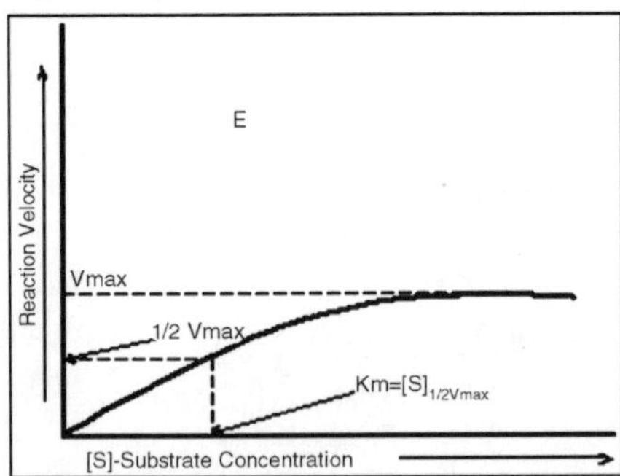

Fig. Effect of Szubstrate Concentration

It is theorized that when this maximum velocity had been reached, all of the available enzyme has been converted to ES, the enzyme substrate complex. This point on the graph is designated Vmax. Using this maximum velocity and equation, Michaelis developed a set of mathematical expressions to calculate enzyme activity in terms of reaction speed from measurable laboratory data.

$$E + S \underset{K-1}{\overset{K+1}{\rightleftarrows}} ES \underset{K-2}{\overset{K+2}{\rightleftarrows}} +E$$

The Michaelis constant Km is defined as the substrate concentration at 1/ 2 the maximum velocity. This is shown in Figure. Using this constant and the fact that Km can also be defined as:

$$Km = K\text{-}1 + K2 / K+1$$

$$K^{+1}, K^{-1} \text{ and } K^{+2}$$

being the rate constants from equation. Michaelis developed the following,

$$V_1 = \frac{V_{mx}[S]}{K_m + [S]}$$

where,

V_t	=	The velocity at any time
[S]	=	The substrate concentration at this time
V_{mx}	=	The highest under this set of experimental conditions (pH,temperature,etc.)
K_m	=	The Michaelis constant for the particular enzyme being inverstigated

Michaelis constants have been determined for many of the commonly used enzymes. The size of Km tells us several things about a particular enzyme.

- A small Km indicates that the enzyme requires only a small amount of substrate to become saturated. Hence, the maximum velocity is reached at relatively low substrate concentrations.
- A large Km indicates the need for high substrate concentrations to achieve maximum reaction velocity.
- The substrate with the lowest Km upon which the enzyme acts as a catalyst is frequently assumed to be enzyme's natural substrate, though this is not true for all enzymes.

EFFECTS OF INHIBITORS ON ENZYME ACTIVITY

Enzyme inhibitors are substances which alter the catalytic action of the enzyme and consequently slow down, or in some cases, stop catalysis. There are three common types of enzyme inhibition - competitive, non-competitive and substrate inhibition.

Most theories concerning inhibition mechanisms are based on the existence of the enzyme-substrate complex ES. As mentioned earlier, the existence of temporary ES structures has been verified in the laboratory.

Competitive inhibition occurs when the substrate and a substance resembling the substrate are both added to the enzyme. A theory called the "lock-key theory" of enzyme catalysts can be used to explain why inhibition occurs.

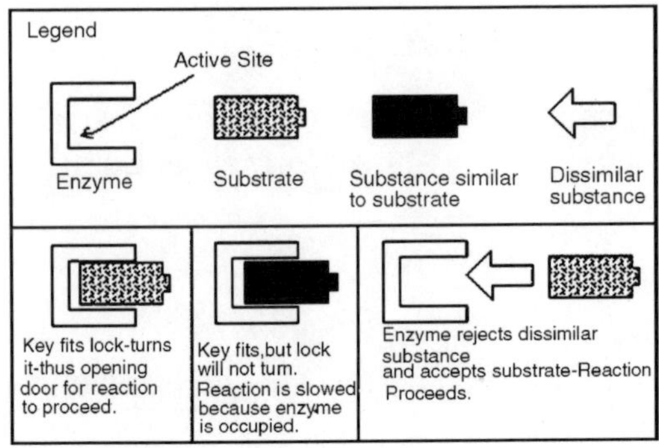

Fig. Lock - Key Theory - Competitive Inhibition

The lock and key theory utilizes the concept of an "active site." The concept holds that one particular portion of the enzyme surface has a strong affinity for the substrate.

The substrate is held in such a way that its conversion to the reaction products is more favourable. If we consider the enzyme as the lock and the substrate the key (Figure) - the key is inserted in the lock, is turned, and the door is opened and the reaction proceeds.

However, when an inhibitor which resembles the substrate is present, it will compete with the substrate for the position in the enzyme lock. When the inhibitor wins, it gains the lock position but is unable to open the lock. Hence, the observed reaction is slowed down because some of the available enzyme sites are occupied by the inhibitor.

If a dissimilar substance which does not fit the site is present, the enzyme rejects it, accepts the substrate, and the reaction proceeds normally.

Non-competitive inhibitors are considered to be substances which when added to the enzyme alter the enzyme in a way that it cannot accept the substrate.

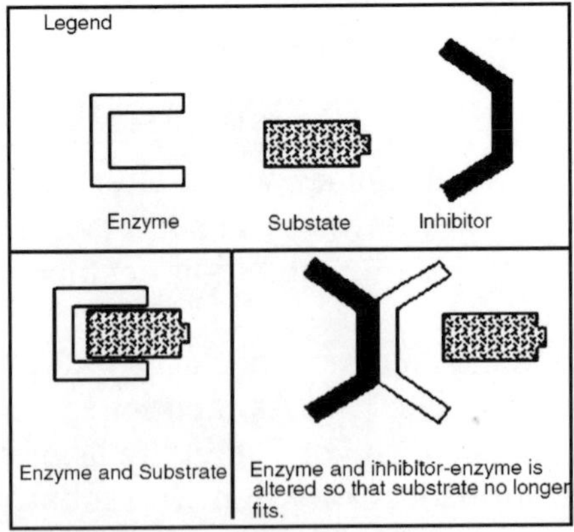

Fig. Non-competitive Inhibition

Substrate inhibition will sometimes occur when excessive amounts of substrate are present. Figure shows the reaction velocity decreasing after the maximum velocity has been reached.

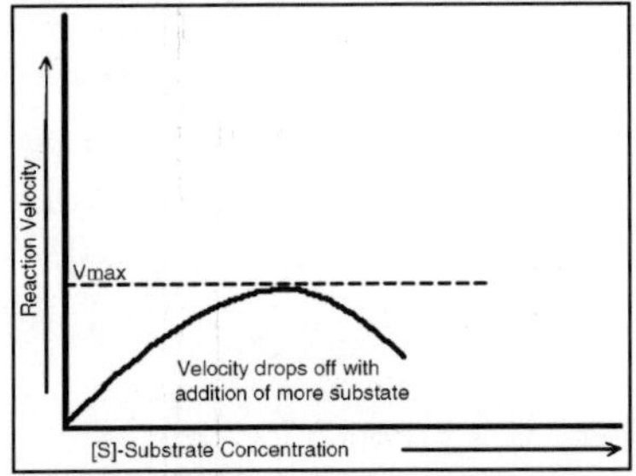

Fig. Substrate Become rate-inhibiting

Additional amounts of substrate added to the reaction mixture after this point actually decrease the reaction rate. This is thought to be due to the fact that there are so many substrate molecules competing for the active sites on the enzyme surfaces that they block the sites and prevent any other substrate molecules from occupying them.

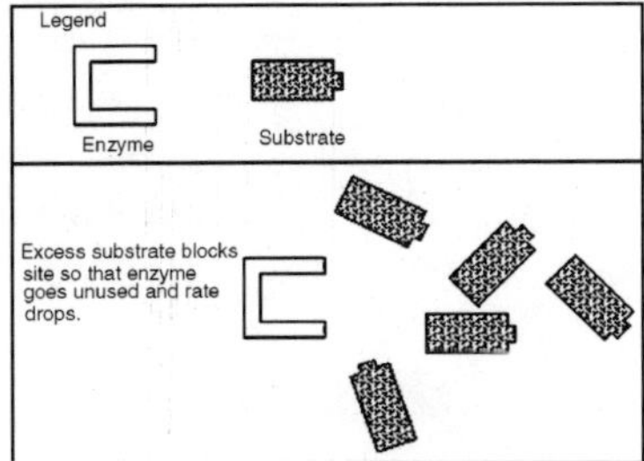

Fig. Substrate Inhibition

This causes the reaction rate to drop since all of the enzyme present is not being used.

TEMPERATURE EFFECTS

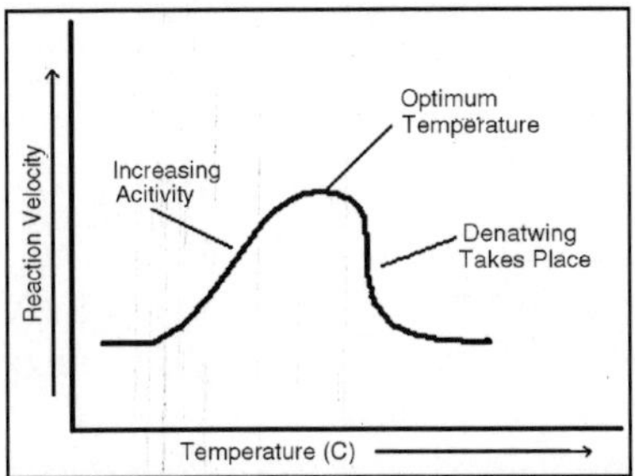

Fig. Effect of Temperature on Reaction rate

Like most chemical reactions, the rate of an enzyme-catalysed reaction increases as the temperature is raised. A ten degree Centigrade rise in temperature will increase the activity of most enzymes by 50 to 100per cent. Variations in reaction temperature as small as 1 or 2 degrees may introduce changes of 10 to 20per cent in the results.

In the case of enzymatic reactions, this is complicated by the fact that many enzymes are adversely affected by high temperatures.

As shown in Figure, the reaction rate increases with temperature to a maximum level, then abruptly declines with further increase of temperature. Because most animal enzymes rapidly become denatured at temperatures above 40°C, most enzyme determinations are carried out somewhat below that temperature.

Over a period of time, enzymes will be deactivated at even moderate temperatures. Storage of enzymes at 5°C or below is generally the most suitable. Some enzymes lose their activity when frozen.

EFFECTS OF pH

Enzymes are affected by changes in pH. The most favourable pH value - the point where the enzyme is most active - is known as the optimum pH. This is graphically illustrated in Figure.

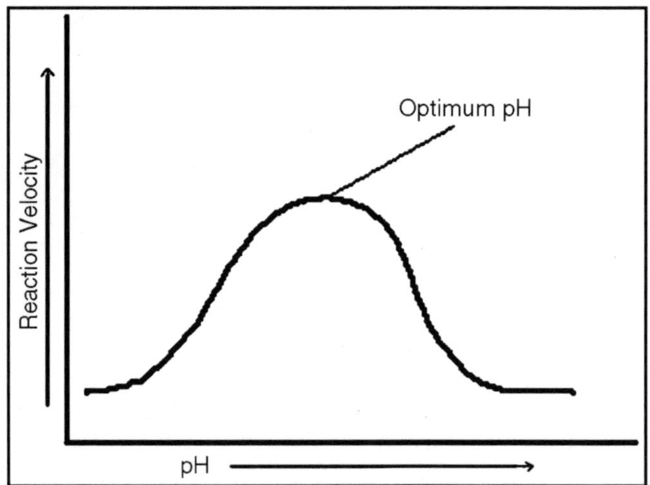

Fig. Effect pH on Reaction Rate

Extremely high or low pH values generally result in complete loss of activity for most enzymes. pH is also a factor in the stability of enzymes. As with activity, for each enzyme there is also a region of pH optimal stability. The optimum pH value will vary greatly from one enzyme to another, as Table shows.

In addition to temperature and pH there are other factors, such as ionic strength, which can affect the enzymatic reaction. Each of these physical and chemical parametres must be considered and optimized in order for an enzymatic reaction to be accurate and reproducible.

Table. pH for Optimum Activity.

Enzyme	pH Optimum
Lipase (pancreas)	8.0
Lipase (stomach)	4.0 – 5.0
Lipase (castor oil)	4.7
Pepsin	1.5 – 1.6
Trypsin	7.8 – 8.7
Urease	7.0
Invertase	4.5
Maltase	6.1 – 6.8
Amylase (pancreas)	6.7 – 7.0
Amylase (malt)	4.6 – 5.2
Catalase	7.0

ENZYMES ARE BIOLOGICAL CATALYSTS

This means that they speed up the chemical reactions in living things. Without enzymes, our guts would take weeks and weeks to digest our food, our muscles, nerves and bones would not work properly and so on - we would not be living! A catalyst is any substance which makes a chemical reaction go faster, without itself being changed. A catalyst can be used over and over again in a chemical reaction: it does not get used up. Enzymes are very much the same except that they are easily denatured (destroyed: but do NOT use this word since the protein molecule is not broken down into amino-acids, it just loses it shape and will not work any more) by heat. Our enzymes work best at body temperature. Our enzymes also have to have the correct pH. All enzymes are made of protein; that is why they are sensitive to heat, pH and heavy metal ions. Unlike ordinary catalysts, they are specific to one chemical reaction. An ordinary catalyst may be used for several different chemical reactions, but an enzyme only works for one specific reaction.

Human saliva contains an enzyme called amylase. This enzyme helps to turn starch into a sugar called maltose. When you swallow a mouthful of food, the amylase stops working because it is much too acid in the stomach pH 2. Amyalse works best in neutral or slightly alkaline conditions, *i.e.* at about pH 7. When your food gets into the small intestine, more amylase is made by the pancreas and this turns the remaining starch into maltose. Another enzyme (maltase) turns all this maltose into glucose. Glucose is then absorbed into the blood.

ENZYMES IN THE HUMAN ALIMENTARY CANAL AND WHAT THEY DIGEST

*All animals, plants, fungi and bacteria produce enzyme*s: so enzymes are not just about digesting food. The enzymes which we use to digest our food are extra-cellular, that means they are found outside cells.

We also have enzymes inside our cells; these are intra-cellular enzymes. Enzymes are used in ALL chemical reactions in living things; this includes respiration, photosynthesis, movement growth, getting rid of toxic chemicals in the liver and so on.

Enzyme	Substrate
Amylase	Starch
Maltase	Maltose
Sucrase	Sucrose
Lipase	Fats
Pepsin	Proteins

Viruses are rather different, but you do not need to know much about them for GCSE, so just make sure that you don't catch any! Enzymes must have the correct shape to do their job.

They are made of proteins, and proteins are very easily affected by heat, pH and heavy metal ions. Some people say that enzymes work like a key in a lock. If the key has been twisted by heat, or dissolved in acid or stuck up with chewing gum it will not work.

Enzymes change their shape if the temperature or pH changes, so they have to have the right conditions. Copper ions are poisonous: if you get copper ions in your blood they will block up some of the important enzymes in red and white blood cells.

Enzymes are catalysts. Most are proteins. (A few rib nucleoprotein enzymes have been discovered and, for some of these, the catalytic activity is in the RNA part rather than the protein part.

Link to discussion of these ribozymes.) Enzymes bind temporarily to one or more of the reactants of the reaction they catalyse. In doing so, they lower the amount of activation energy needed and thus speed up the reaction.

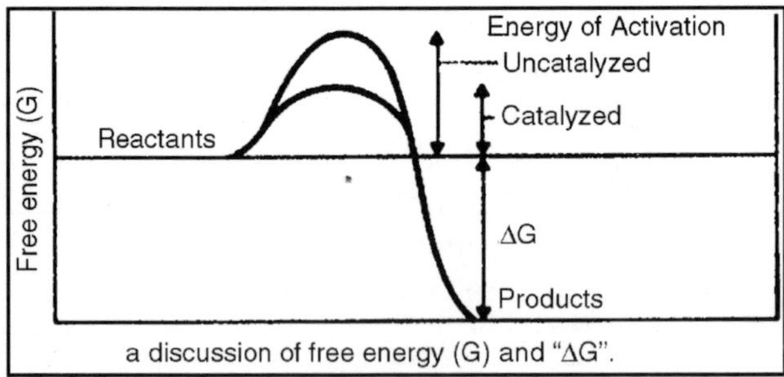

Fig. A Discussion of Free Energy (*G*) and "Δ*G*".

Examples:

- *Catalase*: It catalyses the decomposition of hydrogen peroxide into water and oxygen.

$$2H_2O_2 \rightarrow 2H_2O + O_2$$

One molecule of catalase can break 40 million molecules of hydrogen peroxide each second.

- *Carbonic anhydrase*: It is found in red blood cells where it catalyses the reaction

$$CO_2 + H_2O \leftrightarrow H^+ + HCO_3^-$$

It enables red blood cells to transport carbon dioxide from the tissues to the lungs.

One molecule of carbonic anhydrase can process one million molecules of CO_2 each second.

- *Acetylcholinesterase*: It catalyses the breakdown of the neurotransmitter acetylcholine at several types of synapses as well as at the neuromuscular junction— the specialized synapse that triggers the contraction of skeletal muscle.

One molecule of acetylcholinesterase breaks down 25,000 molecules of acetylcholine each second. This speed makes possible the rapid "resetting" of the synapse for transmission of another nerve impulse. Enzyme activity can be analysed quantitatively. Some of the ways this is done are described in the Enzyme Kinetics.

In order to do its work, an enzyme must unite — even if ever so briefly — with at least one of the reactants. In most cases, the forces that hold the enzyme and its substrate are noncovalent, an assortment of:

HYDROGEN BONDS

If we pass a direct electric current through water containing enough ions to make it a good electrical conductor, it will break down into its constituents: hydrogen and oxygen. Both hydrogen and oxygen gas exist as diatomic molecules so the equation for this chemical reaction is

$$2H_2O \rightarrow 2H_2 + O_2$$

The prefixes tell us that it takes 2 molecules of water to produce one molecule of oxygen and two molecules of hydrogen. If we decompose 36 grams of water (2 moles), we produce 2 moles of hydrogen gas (4 g) and one mole of oxygen gas (32 g). In this reaction, covalent bonds between the hydrogen atoms and oxygen atom in water have been broken and new bonds — between the hydrogen atoms in H_2 and the oxygen atoms in O_2 — have been formed. This reaction requires the input of energy (electrical in this case). This is because:

- It takes energy to break chemical bonds
- Energy is released as chemical bonds form
- But in this case the energy released is less than the energy needed.

Bond Energy

For any particular chemical bond, say the covalent bond between hydrogen and oxygen, the amount of energy it takes to break that bond is exactly the same as the amount of energy released when the bond is formed. This value is called the bond energy. There are many forms of energy:

- Electrical
- Mechanical
- Chemical

but all forms are ultimately converted into heat. So it is convenient for biologists to measure energy in unit of heat. The unit we shall use most often is the kilocalorie(kcal): the amount of heat needed to warm 1 litre of water 1 degree Celsius. The kilocalorie is also the unit used to describe the energy content of foods. It is the "Calorie" used on food labels.

It takes a net of 118 kcal to decompose 2 moles of H_2O into its elements. Actually it takes more than 118 kcal to decompose the water into its atoms, but some of the energy is given back as the atoms immediately bond together to form molecules of hydrogen and oxygen. Let's look at the numbers:

- The bond energy of the H-O bond is 110 kcal.
- The bond energy of H-H bonds is 103 kcal.
- The bond energy of the O=O bonds is 116 kcal.
- The decomposition of 2 molecules of water requires breaking 4 H-O bonds and thus the input of 440 kcal.
- The formation of 2 moles of hydrogen yields 206 kcal (2 x 103).
- The formation of 1 mole of oxygen yields 116 kcal.
- The difference between
  - The energy released (206 + 116 = 322 kcal) and
  - The energy consumed (4 x 110 = 440 kcal)
- Gives the net energy consumed - 118 kcal.

Where has the Energy Gone?

It is now chemical energy stored in the bonds of the hydrogen and oxygen molecules. The energy stored in this reaction is called free energy because it is still available to do work. It is useful to have a symbol for free energy, and we shall use the letter *G* (in honour of Josiah Willard Gibbs who developed the concept of free energy).

What is Free Energy?

It is energy that can be harnessed to do work. The water stored behind a dam has free energy. When allowed to fall through a turbine, it can generate electricity (another form of free energy). But for biologists, the most interesting form of free energy is the energy stored in chemical bonds. It, too, can be harnessed to do work. When you lift a weight, you are using the free energy stored in the bonds of food molecules to run a machine - your skeletal muscles. The conversion of free energy to work is never 100per cent efficient. As you contract your muscles, much of the free energy of your fuel is given off as heat.

It is no longer free; there is no way you can harness the warmth of your muscles to accomplish biologically useful work. A change in free energy is depicted by the letter *G* preceded by the Greek Delta (Δ). By convention, we indicate the storage of free energy with a plus sign. So, our reaction is expressed:

$$2H_2O \rightarrow 2H_2 + O_2, \Delta G = +118 \text{ kcal.}$$

You may have had a chemistry professor ignite a mixture of hydrogen and oxygen. It not, simply accept my word that the result is a dramatic explosion. The equation for this chemical reaction is the reverse of the one we have been studying and is expressed as,

$$2H_2 + O_2 \rightarrow 2H_2O$$

And, as the explosion suggests, this time a release of energy occurs. In fact, the free energy change is once again 118 kcal. This is because it took only 322 kcal to break the H-H and O=O bonds, and 440 kcal were liberated by the 4 moles of H-O bonds that were formed. (The igniting spark provided the initial input of energy; the surplus from the reaction then provided what was needed to get all the other molecules to react.) We express the fact that energy came out of the reacting system by putting a minus sign before Δ *G*.

$$2H_2 + O_2 \rightarrow 2H_2O, \Delta G = -118 \text{ kcal.}$$

These chemical reactions may not seem very "biological" to you, but in fact, they are good models for the reactions at the very heart of life itself.

Cellular Respiration

It turns out that mitochondria exploit a similar reaction to secure free energy. Mitochondria synthesize water using the hydrogen atoms removed from organic molecules, like glucose, and the oxygen atoms they take in as they respire. The process is called cellular respiration. The overall equation is:

$$C_6H_{12}O_6 + 6O_2 \rightarrow 6CO_2 + 6\ H_2O, \Delta G = -686 \text{ kcal.}$$

The same equation describes the burning of glucose, and the same amount of free energy is released. But the energy of burning is released as heat, which is of little value to cells. The achievement of mitochondria is their ability to release the energy of glucose in small, discrete steps so that some of the energy can be trapped in ATP.

Photosynthesis

Similarly, photosynthesis involves the decomposition of water molecules with their hydrogen atoms transferred to carbon atoms to make organic molecules like glucose.

More on Bond Energies

What determines the magnitude of the bond energy for a particular bond? There are several contributing factors but usually the most important is the difference in the electronegativity of the two atoms bonding together. The energies of bonds between atoms of substantially different electronegativities tend to be high, *e.g.*, the 110 kcal of the H-O bond. Another important example is the bonds between oxygen and carbon atoms in carbon dioxide, CO_2. The carbon atom shares two pairs of electrons with each of the oxygen atoms, and each of these double bonds has a bond energy of 187 kcal (or about 93 kcal for each shared pair of electrons). The larger the bond energy, the more energy is needed to break the bond. Thus bonds between atoms of differing electronegativities are apt to be very strong and stable.

On the other hand, the energies of bonds between atoms of similar electronegativity tend to be smaller.

Of course, where the atoms are the same (*e.g.*, O=O, C-C) there is no electronegativity difference and we are not surprised to find lower bond energy values. Each of the shared electron pairs in the oxygen molecule is worth 58 kcal for a total of 116 in each molecule, as we saw above. The bond energy of the C-C bond is 80 kcal.

There is a slight difference in electronegativity between carbon and hydrogen, and a bond energy of 98 kcal. The bonds with smaller bond energies are, by definition, easier to break. Thus these bonds are weaker and less stable.

We should also note that the energy needed to break a particular bond, *e.g.*, between carbon and oxygen, may also be influenced by the nature of the other atoms attached to the ones we are interested in.

Thus the C=O double bond in carbon dioxide (O=C=O) has a bond energy of 187 kcal, whereas when this bond is found as part of a larger molecule, the value is closer to 170 kcal. Because of these variations, we speak of average bond energies. This table gives average bond energies for some of the bonds that are always being broken and formed in biochemical processes.

Average Bond Energies,	**kcal/mole**
C-H	98
O-H	110
C-C	80
C-O	78
H-H	103
C-N	65
O=O	116 (2 × 58)
C=O	187* (2 × 93.5)
C=C	145 (2 × 72.5)

Note:

* As found in CO_2.

IONIC INTERACTIONS

At any given pH, proteins have charged groups that may participate in binding them to each other or to other types of molecules. For example, as the figure shows, negatively-charged carboxyl groups on aspartic acid (Asp) and glutamic acid (Glu) residues may be attracted by the positively-charged free amino groups on lysine(Lys) and arginine (Arg) residues. Ionic interactions are highly sensitive to:

Changes in pH.

- As the pH drops,
  - H^+ bind to the carboxyl groups (COO^-) of aspartic acid (Asp) and glutamic acid (Glu), neutralizing their negative charge, and
  - H^+ bind to the unoccupied pair of electrons on the N atom of the amino (NH_2) groups of lysine (Lys) and arginine (Arg) giving them a positive charge.

The result: Not only does the net charge on the molecule change (it becomes more positive) but many of the opportunities that its R groups have for ionic (electrostatic) interactions with other molecules and ions are altered.

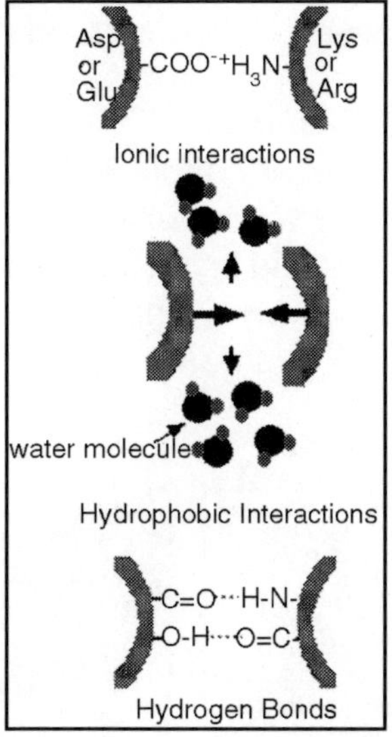

As the pH rises,
  - H^+ are removed from the COOH groups of Asp and Glu, giving them a negative charge (COO^-)
  - H^+ are removed from the NH_3^+ groups of Lys and Arg removing their positive charge.

The result: Again the net charge on the molecule changes (it becomes more negative) and, again, many of the opportunities its R groups have for electrostatic interactions with other molecules or ions are altered.

- Salt concentration. Increasing salt concentration reduces the strength of ionic binding by providing competing ions for the charged residues.

HYDROPHOBIC INTERACTIONS

The side chains (R groups) of such amino acids as phenylalanine and leucine are nonpolar and hence interact poorly with polar molecules like water. For this reason, most of the nonpolar residues in globular proteins are directed towards the interior of the molecule whereas such polar groups as aspartic acid and lysine are on the surface exposed to the solvent. When nonpolar residues are exposed at the surface of two different molecules, it is energetically more favourable for their two "oily" nonpolar surfaces to approach each other closely displacing the polar water molecules from between them.

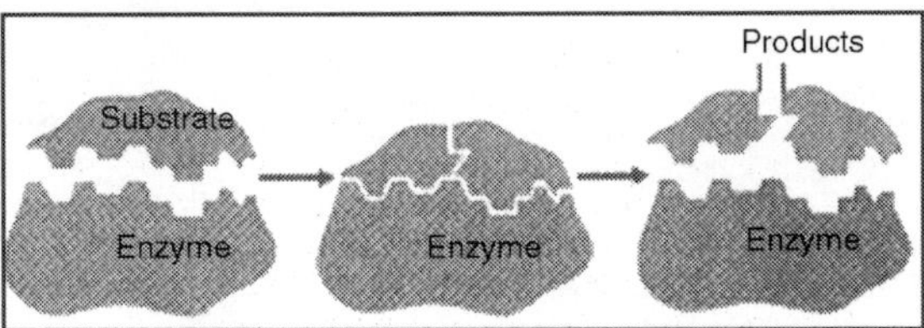

Most of these interactions are weak and especially so if the atoms involved are farther than about one angstromfrom each other. So successful binding of enzyme and substrate requires that the two molecules be able to approach each other closely over a fairly broad surface.

Thus the analogy that a substrate molecule binds its enzyme like a key in a lock. This requirement for complementarity in the configuration of substrate and enzyme explains the remarkable specificity of most enzymes. Generally, a given enzyme is able to catalyse only a single chemical reaction or, at most, a few reactions involving substrates sharing the same general structure.

COMPETITIVE INHIBITION

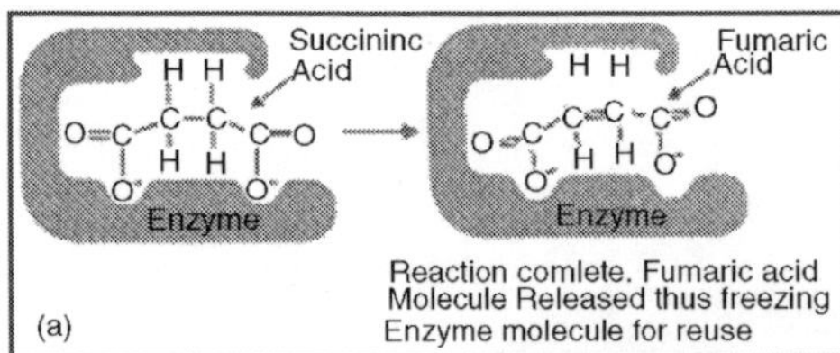

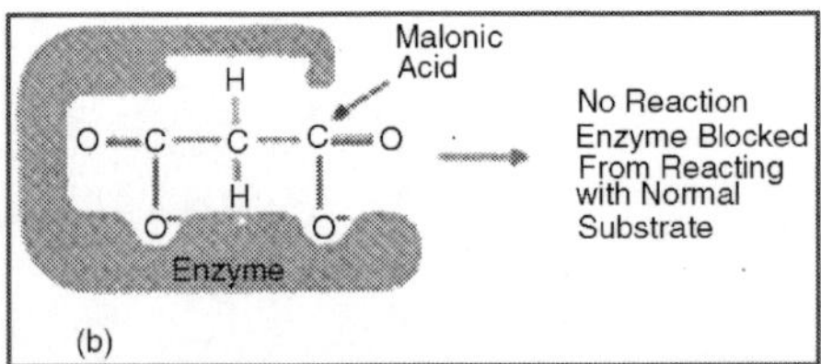

The necessity for a close, if brief, fit between enzyme and substrate explains the phenomenon of competitive inhibition. One of the enzymes needed for the release of energy within the cell is succinic dehydrogenase. It catalyses the oxidation (by the removal of two hydrogen atoms) of succinic acid:

- If one adds malonic acid to cells, or to a test tube mixture of succinic acid and the enzyme, the action of the enzyme is strongly inhibited. This is because the structure of malonic acid allows it to bind to the same site on the enzyme.

- But there is no oxidation so no speedy release of products. The inhibition is called competitive because if you increase the ratio of succinic to malonic acid in the mixture, you will gradually restore the rate of catalysis. At a 50:1 ratio, the two molecules compete on roughly equal terms for the binding (=catalytic) site on the enzyme.

ENZYME COFACTORS

Many enzymes require the presence of an additional, nonprotein, cofactor:

- Some of these are metal ions such as Zn^{2+} (the cofactor for carbonic anhydrase), Cu^{2+}, Mn^{2+}, K^+, and Na^+.
- Some cofactors are small organic molecules called coenzymes. The B vitamins
  - Thiamine (B1)
  - Riboflavin (B2) and
  - Nicotinamide

are precursors of coenzymes. Coenzymes may be covalently bound to the protein part (called the apoenzyme) of enzymes as a prosthetic group. Others bind more loosely and, in fact, may bind only transiently to the enzyme as it performs its catalytic act.

LYSOZYME: A MODEL OF ENZYME ACTION

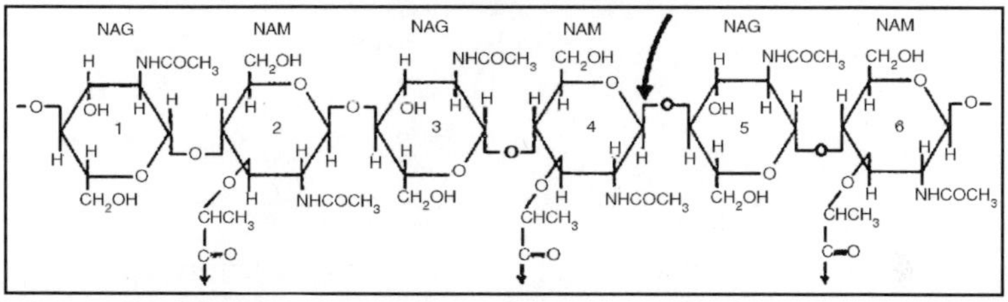

A number of lysozymes are found in nature; in human tears and egg white, for examples. The enzyme is antibacterial because it degrades the polysaccharide that is found in the cell walls of many bacteria. It does this by catalyzing the insertion of a water molecule at the position indicated by the red arrow (a glycosidic bond). This hydrolysis breaks the chain at that point. The bacterial polysaccharide consists of long chains of alternating amino sugars:

- N-acetylglucosamine (NAG)
- N-acetylmuramic acid (NAM)

These hexose units resemble glucose except for the presence of the side chains containing amino groups.

Lysozyme is a globular protein with a deep cleft across part of its surface. Six hexoses of the substrate fit into this cleft:

- With so many oxygen atoms in sugars, as many as 14 hydrogen bonds form between the six amino sugars and certain amino acid R groups such as Arg-114, Asn-37, Asn-44, Trp-62, Trp-63, and Asp-101.

- Some hydrogen bonds also form with the C=O groups of several peptide bonds.
- In addition, hydrophobic interactions may help hold the substrate in position.

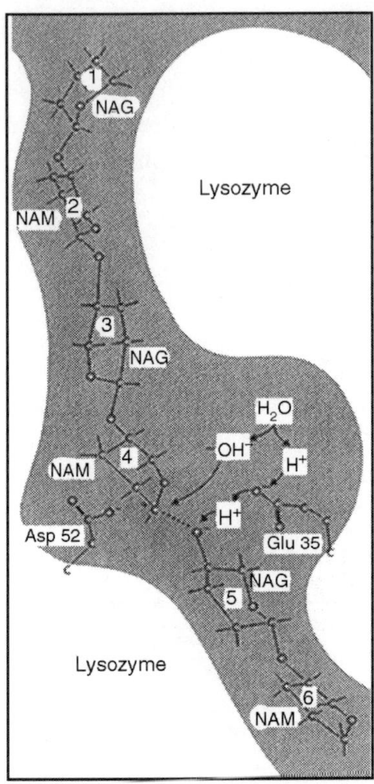

X-ray crystallography has shown that as lysozyme and its substrate unite, each is slightly deformed. The fourth hexose in the chain (ring #4) becomes twisted out of its normal position. This imposes a strain on the C-O bond on the ring-4 side of the oxygen bridge between rings 4 and 5. It is just at this point that the polysaccharide is broken. A molecule of water is inserted between these two hexoses, which breaks the chain. Here, then, is a structural view of what it means to lower activation energy. The energy needed to break this covalent bond is lower now that the atoms connected by the bond have been distorted from their normal position.

As for lysozyme itself, binding of the substrate induces a small (~0.75Å) movement of certain amino acid residues so the cleft closes slightly over its substrate. So the "lock" as well as the "key" changes shape as the two are brought together. (This is sometimes called "induced fit".)

The amino acid residues in the vicinity of rings 4 and 5 provide a plausible mechanism for completing the catalytic act. Residue 35, glutamic acid (Glu-35), is about 3Å from the -O- bridge that is to be broken. The free carboxyl group of glutamic acid is a hydrogen ion donor and available to transfer H^+ to the oxygen atom. This would break the already-strained bond between the oxygen atom and the carbon atom of ring 4.

Now having lost an electron, the carbon atom acquires a positive charge. Ionized carbon is normally very unstable, but the attraction of the negatively-charged carboxyl ion of Asp-52 could stabilize it long enough for an -OH ion (from a spontaneously dissociated water molecule) to unite with the carbon. Even at pH 7, water spontaneously dissociates to produce H^+ and OH^- ions. The hydrogen ion (H^+) left over can replace that lost by Glu-35.

In either case, the chain is broken, the two fragments separate from the enzyme, and the enzyme is free to attach to a new location on the bacterial cell wall and continue its work of digesting it.

FACTORS AFFECTING ENZYME ACTION

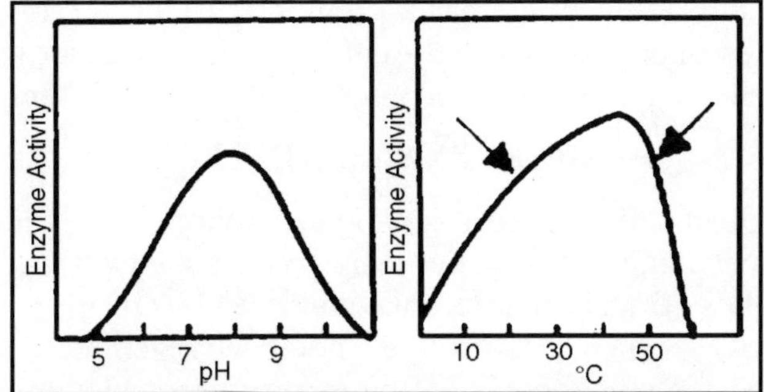

The activity of enzymes is strongly affected by changes in pH and temperature. Each enzyme works best at a certain pH (graph) and temperature (graph), its activity decreasing at values above and below that point.

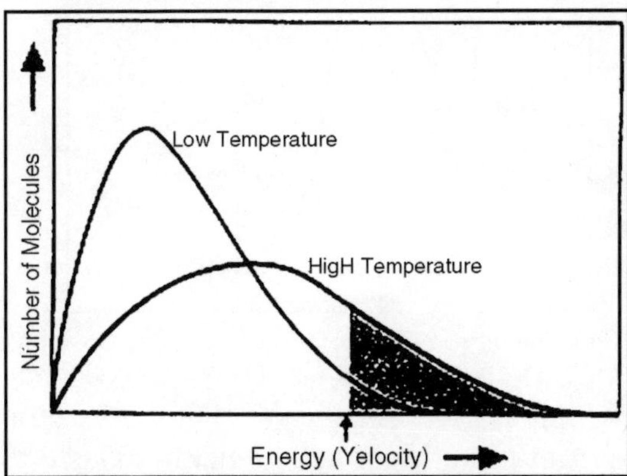

This is not surprising considering the importance of:

- Tertiary structure (*i.e.* shape) in enzyme function and
- Noncovalent forces, *e.g.*, ionic interactions and hydrogen bonds, in determining that shape.

Examples:

- The protease pepsin works best as a pH of 1–2 (found in the stomach) while
- The protease trypsin is inactive at such a low pH but very active at a pH of 8 (found in the small intestine as the bicarbonate of the pancreatic fluid neutralizes the arriving stomach contents).

Changes in pH alter the state of ionization of charged amino acids (*e.g.*, Asp, Lys) that may play a crucial role in substrate binding and/or the catalytic action itself. Without the unionized -COOH group of Glu-35 and the ionized -COO^- of Asp-52, the catalytic action of lysozyme would cease.

Hydrogen bonds are easily disrupted by increasing temperature. This, in turn, may disrupt the shape of the enzyme so that its affinity for its substrate diminishes.

The ascending portion of the temperature curve as shown by arrows reflects the general effect of increasing temperature on the rate of chemical reactions. The descending portion of the curve above reflects the loss of catalytic activity as the enzyme molecules becomedenatured at high temperatures.

BASIC ENZYMES KINETICS

Living organisms seethe with metabolic activity. Thousands of chemical reactions are proceeding very rapidly at any given instant within all living cells. Virtually all of these transformations are mediated by enzymes, proteins (and occasionally RNA) specialized to catalyse metabolic reactions. The substances transformed in these reactions are often organic compounds that show little tendency for reaction outside the cell.

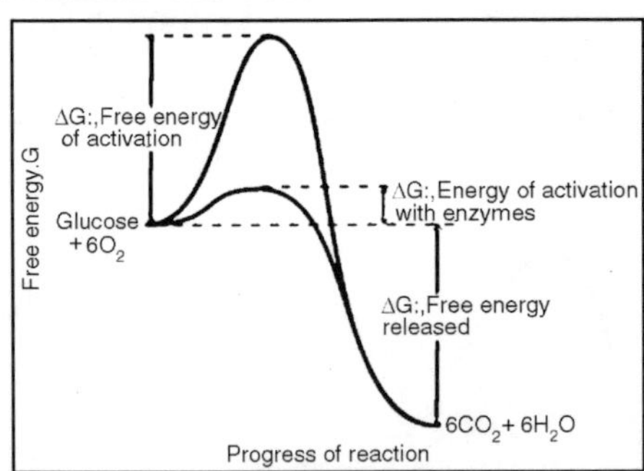

Fig. Reaction Profile Showing large ΔG‡ for Glucose Oxidation, free energy change of -2,870 kJ/mol; Catalysts lower ΔG‡, Thereby Accelerating rate.

An excellent example is glucose, a sugar that can be stored indefinitely on the shelf with no deterioration. Most cells quickly oxidize glucose, producing carbon dioxide and water and releasing lots of energy:

$$C_6H_{12}O_6 + 6\ O_2\ 6\ CO_2 = 6\ H_2O + 2870\ kJ\ \text{of energy}$$

(–2870 kJ/mol is the standard free energy change [ΔG°'] for the oxidation of glucose;. In chemical terms, 2870 kJ is a large amount of energy, and glucose can be viewed as an energy-rich compound even though at ambient temperature it is not readily reactive with oxygen outside of cells.

Stated another way, glucose represents thermodynamic potentiality: its reaction with oxygen is strongly exergonic, but it just doesn't occur under normal conditions. On the other hand, enzymes can catalyse such thermodynamically favourable reactions so that they proceed at extraordinarily rapid rates.

In glucose oxidation and countless other instances, enzymes provide cells with the ability to exert kinetic control over thermodynamic potentiality. That is, living systems use enzymes to accelerate and control the rates of vitally important biochemical reactions.

ENZYMES AS AGENT OF METABOLIC FUNCTION

Acting in sequence, enzymes form metabolic pathways by which nutrient molecules are degraded, energy is released and converted into metabolically useful forms, and precursors are generated and transformed to create the literally thousands of distinctive biomolecules found in any living cell.

Situated at key junctions of metabolic pathways are specialized regulatory enzymes capable of sensing the momentary metabolic needs of the cell and adjusting their catalytic rates accordingly. The responses of these enzymes ensure the harmonious integration of the diverse and often divergent metabolic activities of cells so that the living state is promoted and preserved.

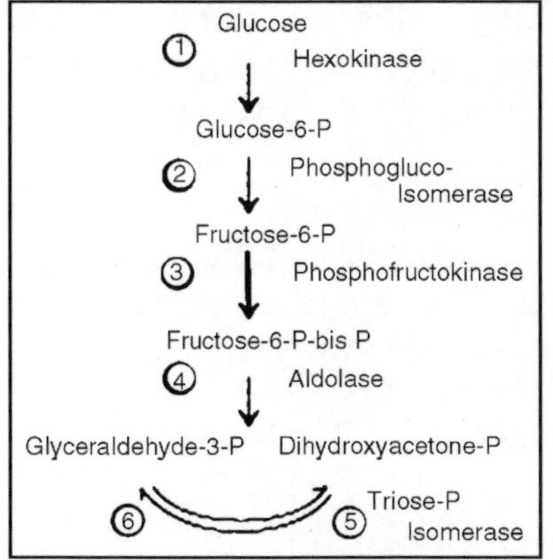

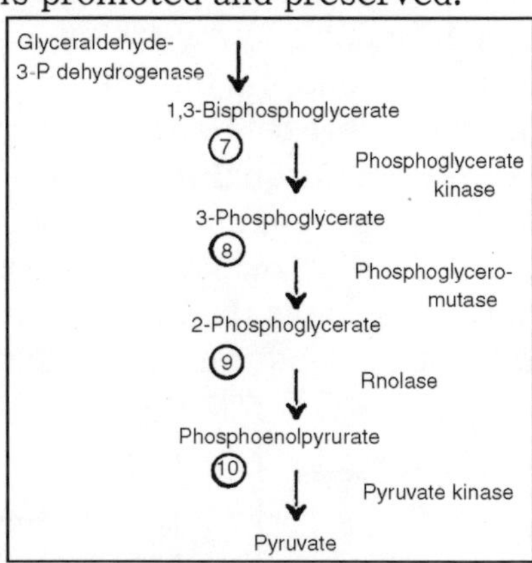

Fig. The Breakdown of Glucose by *Glycolysis* Provides a Prime example of a Metabolic Pathway.

Ten enzymes mediate the reactions of glycolysis. Enzyme 4, *fructose* 1,6, *biphosphate aldolase*, catalyses the C-C bond- breaking reaction in this pathway.

ENZYMES—CATALYTIC POWER, SPECIFICITY, AND REGULATION

Enzymes are characterized by three distinctive features: catalytic power, specificity, and regulation.

CATALYTIC POWER

Enzymes display enormous catalytic power, accelerating reaction rates as much as 10^{16} over uncatalysed levels, which is far greater than any synthetic catalysts can achieve, and enzymes accomplish these astounding feats in dilute aqueous solutions under mild conditions of temperature and pH. For example, the enzyme jack bean*urease* catalyses the hydrolysis of urea:

$$H_2N-\overset{\overset{\displaystyle O}{\|}}{C}-NH_2 + 2H_2O + H^+ \rightarrow 2NH_4^+ + HCO_3^-$$

At 20°C, the rate constant for the enzyme-catalysed reaction is 3 x 10^4/sec; the rate constant for the uncatalysed hydrolysis of urea is 3 x 10^{-10}/sec. Thus, 10^{14} is the ratio of the catalysed rate to the uncatalysed rate of reaction. Such a ratio is defined as the relative catalytic power of an enzyme, so the catalytic power of urease is 10^{14}.

SPECIFICITY

A given enzyme is very selective, both in the substances with which it interacts and in the reaction that it catalyses. The substances upon which an enzyme acts are traditionally called substrates. In an enzyme-catalysed reaction, none of the substrate is diverted into nonproductive side-reactions, so no wasteful by-products are produced. It follows then that the products formed by a given enzyme are also very specific. This situation can be contrasted with your own experiences in the organic chemistry laboratory, where yields of 50per cent or even 30per cent are viewed as substantial accomplishments.

The selective qualities of an enzyme are collectively recognized as itsspecificity. Intimate interaction between an enzyme and its substrates occurs through molecular recognition based on structural complementarity; such mutual recognition is the basis of specificity. The specific site on the enzyme where substrate binds and catalysis occurs is called the active site.

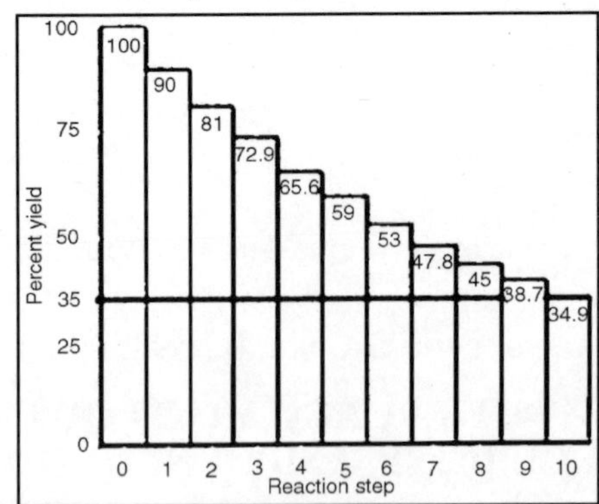

Fig. A 90per cent Yield over 10 steps, for Example, in a Metabolic Pathway, gives an Overall Yield of 35per cent.

Therefore, yields in biological reactions *must be substantially greater*; otherwise, unwanted by-products would accumulate to unacceptable levels.

REGULATION

Regulation of enzyme activity is achieved in a variety of ways, ranging from controls over the amount of enzyme protein produced by the cell to more rapid, reversible interactions of the enzyme with metabolic inhibitors and activators. is devoted to discussions of enzyme regulation. Because most enzymes are proteins, we can anticipate that the functional attributes of enzymes are due to the remarkable versatility found in protein structures.

ENZYME NOMENCLATURE

Traditionally, enzymes often were named by adding the suffix-*ase* to the name of the substrate upon which they acted, as in *urease* for the urea-hydrolyzing enzyme or *phosphatase* for enzymes hydrolyzing phosphoryl groups from organic phosphate compounds. Other enzymes acquired names bearing little resemblance to their activity, such as the peroxide-decomposing enzyme *catalase* or the proteolytic enzymes (*proteases*) of the digestive tract, *trypsin* and *pepsin*. Because of the confusion that arose from these trivial designations, an International Commission on Enzymes was established in 1956 to create a systematic basis for enzyme nomenclature. Although common names for many enzymes remain in use, all enzymes now are classified and formally named according to the reaction they catalyse. Six classes of reactions are recognized.

Within each class are subclasses, and under each subclass are sub-subclasses within which individual enzymes are listed. Classes, subclasses, sub-subclasses, and individual entries are each numbered, so that a series of four numbers serves to specify a particular enzyme. A systematic name, descriptive of the reaction, is also assigned to each entry. To illustrate, consider the enzyme that catalyses this reaction:

$$\text{ATP} + \delta\text{-glucose} \rightarrow \text{ADP} + \delta\text{-glucose-6-phosphate}$$

A phosphate group is transferred from ATP to the C-6-OH group of glucose, so the enzyme is a *transferase*. Subclass 7 of transferases is *enzymes transferring phosphorus-containing groups*, and sub-subclass 1 covers those *phosphotransferases with an alcohol group as an acceptor*. Entry 2 in this sub-subclass is ATP: δ-glucose-6-phosphotransferase, and its classification number is2.7.1.2.

In use, this number is written preceded by the letters E.C., denoting the Enzyme Commission. For example, entry 1 in the same sub-subclass is E.C.2.7.1.1, ATP: δ-hexose-6-phosphotransferase, an ATP-dependent enzyme that transfers a phosphate to the 6-OH of hexoses (that is, it is nonspecific regarding its hexose acceptor). These designations can be cumbersome, so in everyday usage, trivial names are employed frequently.

The glucose-specific enzyme, E.C.2.7.1.2, is called glucokinase and the nonspecific E.C.2.7.1.1 is known as*hexokinase*. *Kinase* is a trivial term for enzymes that are ATP-dependent phosphotransferases.

COENZYMES

Many enzymes carry out their catalytic function relying solely on their protein structure. Many others require nonprotein components, called cofactors. Cofactors may be metal ions or organic molecules referred to as coenzymes. Cofactors, because they are structurally less complex than proteins, tend to be stable to heat (incubation in a boiling water bath). Typically, proteins are denatured under such conditions. Many coenzymes are vitamins or contain vitamins as part of their structure. Usually coenzymes are actively involved in the catalytic reaction of the enzyme, often serving as intermediate carriers of functional groups in the conversion of substrates to products.

In most cases, a coenzyme is firmly associated with its enzyme, perhaps even by covalent bonds, and it is difficult to separate the two. Such tightly bound coenzymes are referred to as prosthetic groups of the enzyme. The catalytically active complex of protein and prosthetic group is called the holoenzyme. The protein without the prosthetic group is called the apoenzyme; it is catalytically inactive.

Table. Enzyme Cofactors: Some Metal Ions and Coenzymes and the Enzymes with Which They Are Associated.

Metal Ions and Some Enzymes That Require Them		**Coenzymes Serving as Transient Carriers of Specific Atoms or Functional Groups**		**Representative Enzymes Using Coenzymes**
Metal Ion	Enzyme	Coenzyme	Entity Transferred	
Fe^{2+} or Fe^{3+}	Cytochrome oxidase Catalase Peroxidase	Thiamine pyrophosphate (TPP) Flavin adenine dinucleotide (FAD) Nicotinamide adenine dinucleotide (NAD)	Aldehydes Hydrogen atoms Hydride ion (H^-)	Pyruvate dehydrogenase Succinate dehydrogenase Alcohol dehydrogenase
Cu^{2+}	Cytochrome oxidase			
Zn^{2+}	DNA polymerase Carbonic anhydrase	Coenzyme A (CoA) Pyridoxal phosphate (PLP)	Acyl groups Amino groups	Acetyl-CoA carboxylase Aspartate aminotransferase
	Alcohol dehydrogenase	5'-Deoxyadenosylcobalamin (vitamin B_{12})	H atoms and alkyl groups	Methylmalonyl-CoA mutase
Mg^{2+}	Hexokinase Glucose-6-phosphatase	Biotin (biocytin)	CO_2	Propionyl-CoA carboxylase
Mn^{2+}	Arginase	Tetrahydrofolate (THF)	Other one-carbon groups	Thymidylate synthase
K^+	Pyruvate kinase (also requires Mg^{2+})			
Ni^{2+}	Urease			
Mo	Nitrate reductase			
Se	Glutathione peroxidase			

CONCEPT OF ENZYME KINETICS

Kinetics is the branch of science concerned with the rates of chemical reactions. The study of enzyme kinetics addresses the biological roles of enzymatic catalysts and how they accomplish their remarkable feats. In enzyme kinetics, we seek to determine the maximum reaction velocity that the enzyme can attain and its binding affinities for substrates and inhibitors. Coupled with studies on the structure and chemistry of the enzyme, analysis of the enzymatic rate under different reaction conditions yields insights regarding the enzyme's mechanism of catalytic action. Such information is essential to an overall understanding of metabolism.

Significantly, it can be exploited to control and manipulate the course of metabolic events.

The science of pharmacology relies on such a strategy. Pharmaceuticals, or drugs, are often special inhibitors specifically targeted at a particular enzyme in order to overcome infection or to alleviate illness. A detailed knowledge of the enzyme's kinetics is indispensable to rational drug design and successful pharmacological intervention.

REVIEW OF CHEMICAL KINETICS

Before beginning a quantitative treatment of enzyme kinetics, it will be fruitful to review briefly some basic principles of chemical kinetics.Chemical kinetics is the study of the rates of chemical reactions. Consider a reaction of overall stoichiometry

$$A \rightarrow P$$

Although we treat this reaction as a simple, one-step conversion of A to P, it more likely occurs through a sequence of elementary reactions, each of which is a simple molecular process, as in,

$$A \rightarrow I \rightarrow J \rightarrow P$$

where I and J represent intermediates in the reaction. Precise description of all of the elementary reactions in a process is necessary to define the overall reaction mechanism for,

$$A \rightarrow P.$$

Let us assume that A → P *is* an elementary reaction and that it is spontaneous and essentially irreversible. Irreversibility is easily assumed if the rate of P conversion to A is very slow *or* the concentration of P (expressed as [P]) is negligible under the conditions chosen. The velocity, *v*, or rate, of the reaction A → P is the amount of P formed or the amount of A consumed per unit time, *t*. That is,

$$v = \frac{d[P]}{dt} \text{ or } v = \frac{-d[A]}{dt}$$

The mathematical relationship between reaction rate and concentration of reactant(s) is the rate law. For this simple case, the rate law is

$$v = \frac{-d[A]}{dt} = k[A]$$

From this expression, it is obvious that the rate is proportional to the concentration of A, and *k* is the proportionality constant, or rate constant. *k* has the units of $(\text{time})^{-1}$, usually $\sec^{-1}$. v is a function of [A] to the first power, or, in the terminology of kinetics, *v* is first-order with respect to A. For an elementary reaction, the order for any reactant is given by its exponent in the rate equation.

The number of molecules that must simultaneously interact is defined as the molecularity of the reaction. Thus, the simple elementary reaction of A $\rightarrow$ P is a first-order reaction.

Figure portrays the course of a first-order reaction as a function of time. The rate of decay of a radioactive isotope, like ^{14}C or ^{32}P, is a first-order reaction, as is an intramolecular rearrangement, such as A $\rightarrow$ P. Both are unimolecular reactions(the molecularity equals 1).

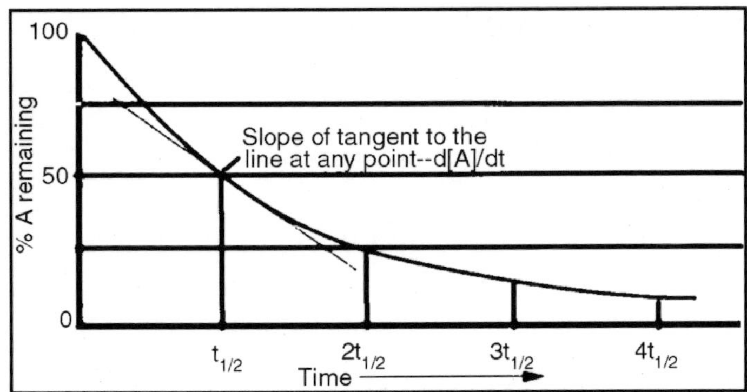

Fig. Plot of the Course of a First-order Reaction. The half-time, $t_{1/2}$, is the time for one-half of the Starting Amount of A to Disappear.

BIOMOLECULAR REACTIONS

Consider the more complex reaction, where two molecules must react to yield products:

$$A + B \rightarrow P + Q$$

Assuming this reaction is an elementary reaction, its molecularity is 2; that is, it is a bimolecular reaction. The velocity of this reaction can be determined from the rate of disappearance of either A or B, or the rate of appearance of P or Q:

$$v = \frac{-d[A]}{dt} = \frac{-d[B]}{dt} = \frac{d[P]}{dt} = \frac{d[Q]}{dt}$$

The rate law is,

$$v = k[A][B]$$

The rate is proportional to the concentrations of both A and B. Because it is proportional to the product of two concentration terms, the reaction is second-order overall, first-order with respect to A and first-order with respect to B. (Were the elementary reaction 2 $\rightarrow$ P + Q, the rate law would be $v = k[A]^2$, second-order overall and Second-order with respect to A.) Second-order rate constants have the units of (concentration)$^{-1}$ (time)$^{-1}$, as in M^{-1} sec^{-1}.

Molecularities greater than two are rarely found (and greater than three, never). When the overall stoichiometry of a reaction is greater than two (for example, as in A+B+Cn or 2A+Bn), the reaction almost always proceeds via uni- or bimolecular elementary steps, and the overall rate obeys a simple first- or Second-order rate law.

At this point, it may be useful to remind ourselves of an important caveat that is the first principle of kinetics: *Kinetics cannot prove a hypothetical mechanism.* Kinetic experiments can only rule out various alternative hypotheses because they don't fit the data. However, through thoughtful kinetic studies, a process of elimination of alternative hypotheses leads ever closer to the reality.

FREE ENERGY OF ACTIVATION AND THE ACTION OF CATALYSTS

In a first-order chemical reaction, the conversion of A to P occurs because, at any given instant, a fraction of the A molecules has the energy necessary to achieve a reactive condition known as the transition state.

In this state, the probability is very high that the particular rearrangement accompanying the A $\rightarrow$ P transition will occur. This transition state sits at the apex of the energy profile in the energy diagram describing the energetic relationship between A and P Figure.

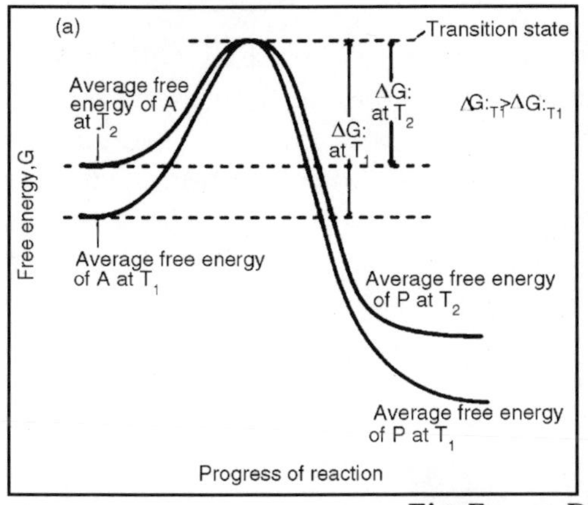

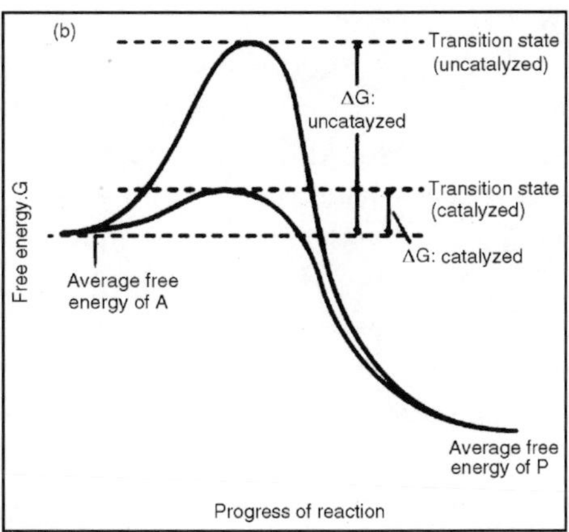

Fig. Energy Diagram for a Chemical reaction (A $\rightarrow$ P) and the Effects

- Raising the Temperature from T_1 to T_2 or
- Adding a Catalyst.

Raising the temperature raises the average energy of A molecules, which increases the population of A molecules having energies equal to the activation energy for the reaction, thereby increasing the reaction rate. In contrast, the average free energy of A molecules remains the same in uncatalysed versus catalysed reactions (conducted at the same temperature). The effect of the catalyst is to lower the free energy of activation for the reaction.

The average free energy of A molecules defines the initial state and the average free energy of P molecules is the final state along the reaction coordinate.

The rate of any chemical reaction is proportional to the concentration of reactant molecules (A in this case) having this transition-state energy. Obviously, the higher this energy is above the average energy, the smaller the fraction of molecules that will have this energy, and the slower the reaction will proceed. The height of this energy barrier is called the free energy of activation, $\Delta G^{\ddagger}$.Specifically, $\Delta G^{\ddagger}$ is the energy required to raise the average energy of one mole of reactant (at a given temperature) to the transition-state energy. The relationship between activation energy and the rate constant of the reaction, *k*, is given by the Arrhenius equation:

$$k = Ae^{-\Delta G^{\ddagger}/RT}$$

where A is a constant for a particular reaction (not to be confused with the reactant species, A, that we're discussing). Another way of writing this is $1/k = (1/A)e^{\Delta G^{\ddagger}/RT}$. That is, *k* is inversely proportional to $e^{\Delta G^{\ddagger}/RT}$. Therefore, if the energy of activation decreases, the reaction rate increases.

DECREASING ΔG‡ INCREASES REACTION RATE

We are familiar with two general ways that rates of chemical reactions may be accelerated. First, the temperature can be raised. This will increase the average energy of reactant molecules, which in effect lowers the energy needed to reach the transition state. The rates of many chemical reactions are doubled by a 10°C rise in temperature. Second, the rates of chemical reactions can also be accelerated by catalysts. Catalysts work by lowering the energy of activation rather than by raising the average energy of the reactants. Catalysts accomplish this remarkable feat by combining transiently with the reactants in a way that promotes their entry into the reactive, transition-state condition.

Two aspects of catalysts are worth noting:

- They are regenerated after each reaction cycle ($A \rightarrow P$), and so can be used over and over again; and
- Catalysts have *no* effect on the overall free energy change in the reaction, the free energy difference between A and P.

KINETICS OF ENZYME-CATALYSED REACTIONS

Examination of the change in reaction velocity as the reactant concentration is varied is one of the primary measurements in kinetic analysis. Returning to A → P, a plot of the reaction rate as a function of the concentration of A yields a straight line whose slope is *k* Figure.

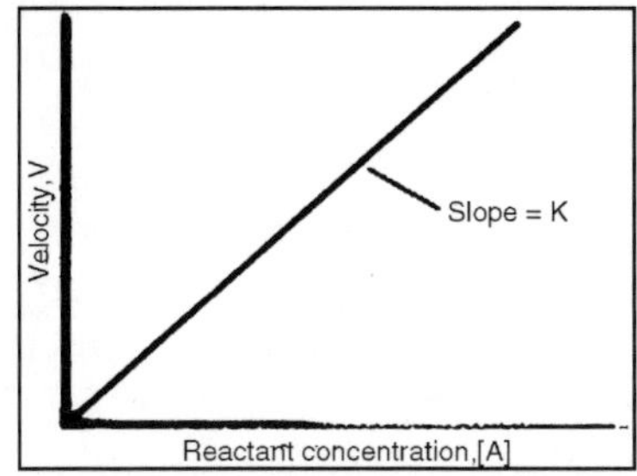

Fig. A plot of v Versus [A] for the Unimolecular Chemical Reaction, A → P, Yields a Straight line having a Slope Equal to k.

The more A that is available, the greater the rate of the reaction, v. Similar analyses of enzyme-catalysed reactions involving only a single substrate yield remarkably different results. At low concentrations of the substrate S, v is proportional to [S], as expected for a first-order reaction. However, v does not increase proportionally as [S] increases, but instead begins to level off. At high [S], v becomes virtually independent of [S] and approaches a maximal limit. The value of v at this limit is written V_{max}. Because rate is no longer dependent on [S] at these high concentrations, the enzyme-catalysed reaction is now obeying zero-order kinetics; that is, the rate is independent of the reactant (substrate) concentration.

This behaviour is a saturation effect: when v shows no increase even though [S] is increased, the system is saturated with substrate. Such plots are called substrate saturation curves. The physical interpretation is that every enzyme molecule in the reaction mixture has its substrate-binding site occupied by S. Indeed, such curves were the initial clue that an enzyme interacts directly with its substrate by binding it.

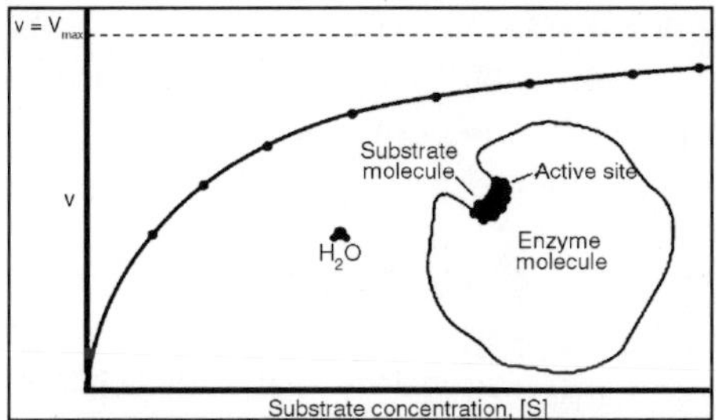

Fig. Substrate Saturation Curve for an Enzyme-catalysed Reaction.

The amount of enzyme is constant, and the velocity of the reaction is determined at various substrate concentrations. The reaction rate, v, as a function of [S] is described by a rectangular hyperbola.

At very high [S], $v = V_{max}$. That is, the velocity is limited only by conditions (temperature, pH, ionic strength) and by the amount of enzyme present; v becomes independent of [S]. Such a condition is termed *zero-order kinetics*. Under zero-order conditions, velocity is directly dependent on [enzyme]. The H_2O molecule provides a rough guide to scale. The substrate is bound at the active site of the enzyme.

THE MICHAELIS - MENTEN EQUATION

Lenore Michaelis and Maud L. Menten proposed a general theory of enzyme action in 1913 consistent with observed enzyme kinetics. Their theory was based on the assumption that the enzyme, E, and its substrate, S, associate reversibly to form an enzyme-substrate complex, ES:

$$E + S \underset{k_{-1}}{\overset{k_1}{\rightleftharpoons}} ES$$

This association/dissociation is assumed to be a rapid equilibrium, and Ks is the *enzyme: substrate dissociation constant.* At equilibrium,

$$k_{-1}[ES] = k_1[E][S]$$

and,

$$K_s = \frac{[E][S]}{[ES]} = \frac{k_{-1}}{k_1}$$

Product, P, is formed in a second step when ES breaks down to yield E + P.

$$E + S \underset{k_{-1}}{\overset{k_1}{\rightleftharpoons}} ES \xrightarrow{k_2} E + P$$

E is then free to interact with another molecule of S.

STEADY-STATE ASSUMPTION

The interpretations of Michaelis and Menten were refined and extended in 1925 by Briggs and Haldane, by assuming the concentration of the enzyme-substrate complex ES quickly reaches a constant value in such a dynamic system.

That is, ES is formed as rapidly from E + S as it disappears by its two possible fates: dissociation to regenerate E + S, and reaction to form E + P. This assumption is termed thesteady-state assumption and is expressed as,

$$\frac{d[ES]}{dt} = 0$$

That is, the change in concentration of ES with time, t, is 0. Figure below illustrates the time course for formation of the ES complex and establishment of the steady-state condition.

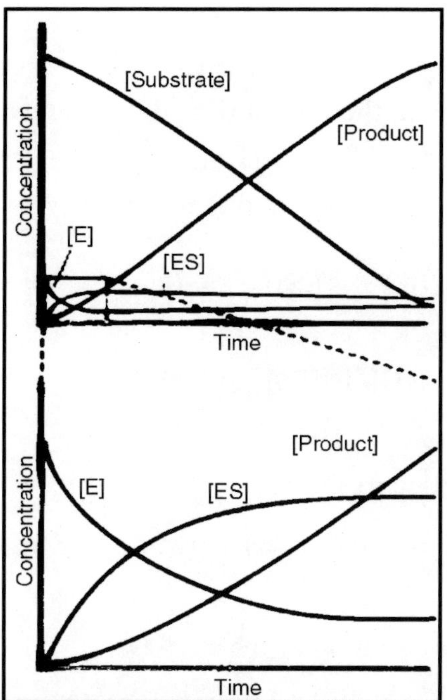

Fig. Time Course for the Consumption of Substrate, the Formation of Product, and the Establishment of a steady-state level of the Enzyme-substrate [ES] complex for a typical Enzyme Obeying the Michaelis-Menten, Briggs-Haldane models for Enzyme Kinetics.

The early stage of the time course is shown in greater magnification in the bottom graph.

INITIAL VELOCITY ASSUMPTION

One other simplification will be advantageous. Because enzymes accelerate the rate of the reverse reaction as well as the forward reaction, it would be helpful to ignore any back reaction by which E1P might form ES. The velocity of this back reaction would be given by $v = k_{-2}$[E][P]. However, if we observe only the *initial velocity* for the reaction immediately after E and S are mixed in the absence of P, the rate of any back reaction is negligible ecause its rate will be proportional to [P], and [P] is essentially 0.

Given such simplification, we now analyse the system described in order to describe the initial velocity v as a function of [S] and amount of enzyme. The total amount of enzyme is fixed and is given by the formula.

Total enzyme,

$$[E_T] = [E] + [ES]$$

where [E] = free enzyme and [ES] = the amount of enzyme in the enzyme-substrate complex. From above Equation, the rate of [ES] formation is

$$v_f = k_1([ET] - [ES])[S]$$

where,

$$[ET] - [ES] = [E]$$

From above Equation, the rate of [ES] disappearance is,

$$v_d = k_{-1}[ES] + k_2[ES] = (k_{-1} + k_2)[ES]$$

At steady state, $d[ES]/dt = 0$, and therefore, $v_f = v_d$.
So,

$$K_1([ET] - [ES])[S] = (k_{-1} + k_2)[ES]$$

Rearranging gives,

$$\frac{([E_T]-[ES])[S]}{[ES]} = \frac{(k_{-1}+k_2)}{k_1}$$

THE MICHAELIS CONSTANT, KM

The ratio of constants $(k_{-1} + k_2)/k_1$ is itself a constant and is defined as the Michaelis constant, K_m

$$K_m = \frac{(k_{-1}+k_2)}{k_1}$$

Note from (14.15) that K_m is given by the ratio of two concentrations (([ET] - [ES]) and [S]) to one ([ES]), so K_m has the units of molarity. From Equation, we can write,

$$\frac{([E_T]-[ES])[S]}{[ES]} = K_m$$

which rearranges to,

$$[ES] = \frac{[E_T]-[S]}{K_m+[S]}$$

Now, the most important parametre in the kinetics of any reaction is the rate of product formation. This rate is given by,

$$v = \frac{d[P]}{dt}$$

and for this reaction,

$$v = k_2[ES]$$

Substituting the expression for [ES] from Equation gives,

$$v = \frac{k_2[E_r][S]}{K_m+[S]}$$

The product k_2[ET] has special meaning. When [S] is high enough to saturate all of the enzyme, the velocity of the reaction, v, is maximal.

At saturation, the amount of [ES] complex is equal to the total enzyme concentration, E_T, its maximum possible value. From Equation, the initial velocity v then equals $k_2[E_T] = V_{max}$. Written symbolically, when [S]

$>> [E_T]$ (and K_m), $[E_T] = [ES]$ and $v = V_{max}$. Therefore,

$$V_{max} = k_2[E_T]$$

Substituting this relationship into the expression for v gives the Michaelis.

MENTEN EQUATION

$$v = \frac{V_{max}[S]}{K_m + [S]}$$

This equation says that the rate of an enzyme-catalysed reaction, v, at any moment is determined by two constants, K_m and V_{max}, and the concentration of substrate at that moment.

WHEN $[S] = K_M$, $V = V_{MAX}/2$

Table. K_m Values for Some Enzymes.

Enzyme	Substrate	K_m(m*M*)
Carbonic anhydrase	CO_2	12
Chymotrypsin	*N*-Benzoyltyrosinamide	2.5
	Acetyl-L -tryptophanamide	5
	N-Formyltyrosinamide	12
	N-Acetyltyrosinamide	32
	Glycyltyrosinamide	122
Hexokinase	Glucose	0.15
	Fructose	1.5
β-Galactosidase	Lactose	4
Glutamate dehydrogenase	NH_4^+	57
	Glutamate	0.12
	α -Ketoglutarate	2
	NAD^+	0.025
	NADH	0.018
Aspartate aminotransferase	Aspartate	0.9
	α -Ketoglutarate	0.1
	Oxaloacetate	0.04
	Glutamate	4
Threonine deaminase	Threonine	5
Arginyl-tRNA synthetase	Argininet	0.003
	RNA^{Arg}	0.0004
	ATP	0.3
Pyruvate carboxylase	HCO_3^-	1.0
	Pyruvate	0.4
	ATP	0.06
Penicillinase	Benzylpenicillin	0.05
Lysozyme	Hex α -*N*-acetylglucosamine	0.006

We can provide an operational definition for the constant K_m by rearranging Equation to give

$$K_m = [S]\left(\frac{V_{max}}{v} - 1\right)$$

Then, at $v = V_{max}/2$, $K_m = [S]$. That is, K_m is defined by the substrate concentration that gives a velocity equal to one-half the maximal velocity gives the K_m values of some enzymes for their substrates.

RELATIONSHIPS BETWEEN V_{max}, K_m, AND LEACTION ORDER

The Michaelis-Menten equation describes a curve known from analytical geometry as a rectangular hyperbola.1 In such curves, as [S] is increased, v approaches the limiting value, V_{max}, in an asymptotic fashion. V_{max} can be approximated experimentally from a substrate saturation curve and K_m can be derived from $V_{max}/2$, so the two constants of the Michaelis-Menten equation can be obtained from plots of v versus [S].

Note, however, that actual estimation of Vmax, and consequently K_m, is only approximate from such graphs. That is, according to Equation, in order to get $v = 0.99\ V_{max}$, [S] must equal 99 K_m, a concentration that may be difficult to achieve in practice.

From Equation, when $[S] >> K_m$, then $v = V_{max}$. That is, v is no longer dependent on [S], so the reaction is obeying zero-order kinetics.

Also, when $[S] < K_m$, then v" $(Vmax/K_m)[S]$. That is, the rate, v, approximately follows a first-order rate equation, $v = k'[A]$, where $k' = V_{max}/K_m$.

K_m and V_{max}, once known explicitly, define the rate of the enzyme-catalysed reaction, provided:

- The reaction involves only one substrate, or if the reaction is multisubstrate, the concentration of only one substrate is varied while the concentration of all other substrates is held constant.
- The reaction $ES \rightarrow E + P$ is irreversible, or the experiment is limited to observing only initial velocities where $[P] = 0$.
- $[S]_0 > [E_T]$ and $[E_T]$ is held constant.
- All other variables that might influence the rate of the reaction (temperature, pH, ionic strength, and so on) are constant.

ENZYME UNITS

In many situations, the actual molar amount of the enzyme is not known. However, its amount can be expressed in terms of the activity observed. The International Commission on Enzymes defines One International Unit of enzyme as the amount that catalyses the formation of one micromole of product in one minute. (Because enzymes are very sensitive to factors such as pH, temperature, and ionic strength, the conditions of assay must be specified.) Another definition for units of enzyme activity is the katal. One katal is that amount of enzyme catalyzing the conversion of one mole of substrate to product in one second. Thus, one katal equals 6 x 10^7 international units.

TURNOVER NUMBER

The turnover number of an enzyme, k_{cat}, is a measure of its maximal catalytic activity. k_{cat} is defined as the number of substrate molecules converted into product per enzyme molecule per unit time when the enzyme is saturated with substrate.

The turnover number is also referred to as the molecular activity of the enzyme. For the simple Michaelis-Menten reaction under conditions of initial velocity measurements, $k_2 = k_{cat}$. Provided the concentration of enzyme, $[E_T]$, in the reaction mixture is known, k_{cat} can be determined from V_{max}. At saturating [S], $v = V_{max} = k_2 [E_T]$. Thus,

$$k_2 = \frac{V_{max}}{[E_T]} = k_{cat}$$

The term k_{cat} represents the kinetic efficiency of the enzyme. Table lists below turnover numbers for some representative enzymes. Catalase has the highest turnover number known; each molecule of this enzyme can degrade 40 million molecules of H_2O_2 in one second! At the other end of the scale, lysozyme requires 2 seconds to cleave a glycosidic bond in its glycan substrate.

Table. Values of k_{cat} (Turnover Number) for Some Enzymes.

Enzyme	k_{cat} (sec^{-1})
Catalase	40,000,000
Carbonic anhydrase	1,000,000
Acetylcholinesterase	14,000
Penicillinase	2,000
Lactate dehydrogenase	1,000
Chymotrypsin	100
DNA polymerase I	15
Lysozyme	0.5

k_{cat}/K_m

Under physiological conditions, [S] is seldom saturating, and kcat itself is not particularly informative. That is, the *in vivo* ratio of $[S]/K_m$ usually falls in the range of 0.01 to 1.0, so active sites often are not filled with substrate. Nevertheless, we can derive a meaningful index of the efficiency of Michaelis-Menten-type enzymes under these conditions by employing the following equations.

As presented in Equation, if,

$$v = \frac{V_{max}[S]}{K_m + [S]}$$

and $V_{max} = k_{cat}$ $[E_T]$, then,

$$v = \frac{K_{cut}[E_T][S]}{K_m + [S]}$$

When [S] << K_m, the concentration of free enzyme, [E], is approximately equal to $[E_T]$, so that

$$v = \left(\frac{K_{cut}}{K_m}\right)[EIS]$$

That is, k_{cat}/K_m is an apparent Second-order rate constant for the reaction of E and S to form product. Because K_m is inversely proportional to the affinity of the enzyme for its substrate and k_{cat} is directly proportional to the kinetic efficiency of the enzyme, k_{cat}/K_mprovides an index of the catalytic efficiency of an enzyme operating at substrate concentrations substantially below saturation amounts.

An interesting point emerges if we restrict ourselves to the simple case where $k_{cat} = k_2$.

Then,

$$\frac{K_{cut}}{K_m} = \frac{K_1K_2}{K_1 + K_2}$$

Table. Enzymes Whose k_{cat}/K_m Approaches the Diffusion-Controlled Rate of Association with Substrate.

Enzyme	Substrate	k_{cat} (sec^{-1})	K_m (*M*)	k_{cat}/K_m (sec^{-1} M^{-1})
Acetylcholinesterase	Acetylcholine	1.4×10^4	9×10^{-5}	1.6×10^8
Carbonic anhydrase	CO_2 HCO_3^-	1×10^6 4×10^5	0.012 0.026	8.3×10^7 1.5×10^7
Catalase	H_2O_2	4×10^7	1.1	4×10^7
Crotonase	Crotonyl-CoA	5.7×10^3	2×10^{-5}	2.8×10^8
Fumarase	Fumarate Malate	800 900	5×10^{-6} 2.5×10^{-5}	1.6×10^8 3.6×10^7
Triosephosphate isomerase	Glyceraldehyde-3-phosphate*	4.3×10^3	1.8×10^{-5}	2.4×10^8
β-Lactamase	Benzylpenicillin	2×10^3	2×10^{-5}	1×10^8

Note:

* K_m for glyceraldehyde-3-phosphate is calculated on the basis that only 3.8per cent of the substrate in solution is unhydrated and therefore reactive with the enzyme.

But k1 must always be greater than or equal to $k_1k_2/(k_{-1} + k_2)$. That is, the reaction can go no faster than the rate at which E and S come together. Thus, k_1 sets the upper limit for k_{cat}/K_m. In other words, *the catalytic efficiency of an enzyme cannot exceed the diffusion-controlled rate of combination of* E *and* S *to form* ES. In H_2O, the rate constant for such diffusion is approximately $10^9/M \times$ sec. Those enzymes that are most efficient in their catalysis have k_{cat}/K_m ratios approaching this value. Their catalytic velocity is limited only by the rate at which they encounter S; enzymes this efficient have achieved so-called catalytic perfection. All E and S encounters lead to reaction because such *"catalytically perfect"* enzymes can channel S to the active site, regardless of where S hits E. Table 14.5 lists the kinetic parametres of several enzymes in this category. Note that k_{cat} and K_m both show a substantial range of variation in this table, even though their ratio falls around $10^8/M \times$ sec.

LINEAR PLOTS CAN BE DERIVED FROM THE MICHAELIS - MENTEN EQUATION

Because of the hyperbolic shape of v versus [S] plots, V_{max} can only be determined from an extrapolation of the asymptotic approach of v to some limiting value as [S] increases indefinitely and K_m is derived from that value of [S] giving $v = V_{max}/2$. However, several rearrangements of the Michaelis-Menten equation transform it into a straight-line equation. The best known of these is theLineweaver-Burk double-reciprocal plot: Taking the reciprocal of both sides of the Michaelis-Menten equation, yields the equality,

$$\frac{1}{v} = \left(\frac{K_m}{V_{max}}\right)\left(\frac{1}{[S]}\right) + \frac{1}{V_{max}}$$

This conforms to y5mx1b (the equation for a straight line), where $y = 1/v$; m, the slope, is K_m/V_{max}; $x = 1/[S]$; and $b = 1/V_{max}$. Plotting $1/v$versus 1/[S] gives a straight line whose x-intercept is $-1/K_m$, whose y-intercept is $1/V_{max}$, and whose slope is K_m/V_{max} (Figure).

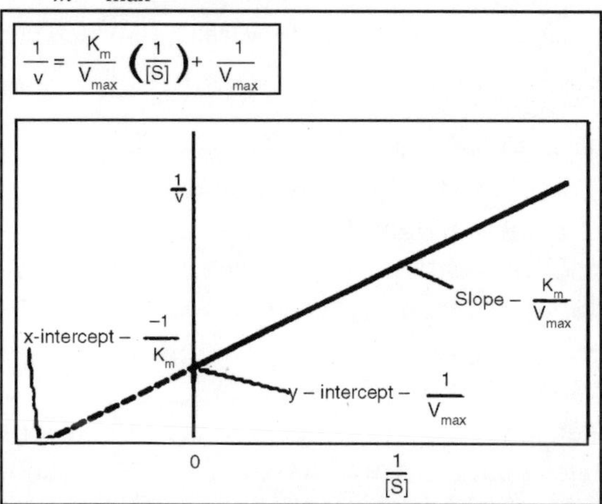

Fig. The Lineweaver-Burk Double-reciprocal plot, Depicting Extrapolations that allow the Determination of the x- and y-Intercepts and slope.

The Hanes-Woolf plot is another rearrangement of the Michaelis-Menten equation that yields a straight line:

Multiplying both sides by [S] gives,

$$\frac{[S]}{v} = [S]\left(\frac{K_m}{V_{max}}\right)\left(\frac{1}{[S]}\right) + \frac{[S]}{V_{max}} = \frac{K_m}{V_{max}} + \frac{[S]}{V_{max}}$$

and,

$$\frac{[S]}{v} = \left(\frac{1}{V_{max}}\right)[S] + \frac{K_m}{V_{max}}$$

Graphing [S]/v versus [S] yields a straight line where the slope is $1/V_{max}$, the y-intercept is K_m/V_{max}, and the x-intercept is $-K_m$, as shown. The common advantage of these plots is that they allow both K_m and V_{max} to be accurately estimated by extrapolation of straight lines rather than asymptotes. Computer fitting of v versus [S] data to the Michaelis-Menten equation is more commonly done than graphical plotting.

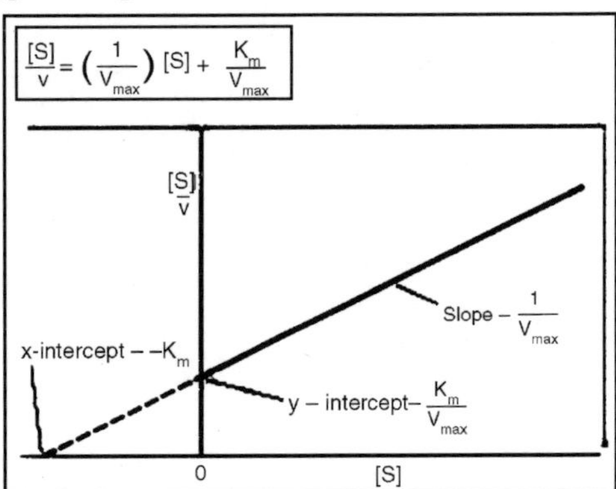

Fig. A Hanes-Wolff plot of [S]/v versus [S], another straight-line Rearrangement of the Michaelis-Menten Equation.

A DEEPER LOOK

An Example of the Effect of Amino Acid Substitutions on K_m and k_{cat}: Wild-Type and Mutant Forms of Human Sulfite Oxidase Mammalian sulfite oxidase is the last enzyme in the pathway for degradation of sulfur-containing amino acids. Sulfite oxidase (SO) catalyses the oxidation of sulfite (SO_3^{2-}) to sulfate (SO_4^{2-}), using the heme-containing protein, cytochrome c, as electron acceptor:

SO_3^{2-} + 2 cytochrome $c_{oxidized}$ + $H_2O \rightleftharpoons SO_4^{2-}$ + 2 cytochrome $c_{reduced}$ + 2 H^+*Isolated sulfite oxidase deficiency* is a rare and often fatal genetic disorder in humans. The disease is characterized by severe neurological abnormalities, revealed as convulsions shortly after birth. R. M. Garrett and K. V. Rajagopalan at Duke UniversityMedical Centre have isolated the human cDNA for sulfite oxidase from the cells of normal (*wild-type*) and SO-deficient individuals.

Expression of these SO cDNAs in transformed *Escherichia coli* cells allowed the isolation and kinetic analysis of wild-type and mutant forms of SO, including one (designated R160Q) in which the Arg at position 160 in the polypeptide chain is replaced by Gln. A genetically engineered version of SO (designated R160K) in whichLys replaces Arg^{160} was also studied.

Table. Kinetic Constants for Wild-type and Mutant Sulfite Oxidase.

Enzyme	$K_m^{sulfite}$(m*M*)	k_{cat}(sec^{-1})	k_{cat}/K_m(10^6 $M^{-1}sec^{-1}$)
Wild-type	17	18	
R160Q	1900	3	0.0016
R160K	360	5.5	0.015

Replacing R^{160} in sulfite oxidase by Q increases K_m, decreases k_{cat}, and markedly diminishes the catalytic efficiency (k_{cat}/K_m) of the enzyme. The R160K mutant enzyme has properties intermediate between wild-type and the R160Q mutant form. The substrate, SO_3^{2-}, is strongly anionic, and R^{160} is one of several Arg residues situated within the SO substrate-binding site. Positively charged side chains in the substrate-binding site facilitate SO_3^{2-} binding and catalysis, with Arg being optimal in this role.

DEPARTURES FROM LINEARITY: A HINT OF REGULATION

If the kinetics of the reaction disobey the Michaelis-Menten equation, the violation is revealed by a departure from linearity in these straight-line graphs. We shall see that deviations from linearity are characteristic of the kinetics of regulatory enzymes known as allosteric enzymes. Such regulatory enzymes are very important in the overall control of metabolic pathways.

EFFECT OF PH ON ENZYMATIC ACTIVITY

Enzyme-substrate recognition and the catalytic events that ensue are greatly dependent on pH. An enzyme possesses an array of ionizable side chains and prosthetic groups that not only determine its secondary and tertiary structure but may also be intimately involved in its active site. Further, the substrate itself often has ionizing groups, and one or another of the ionic forms may preferentially interact with the enzyme. Enzymes in general are active only over a limited pH range and most have a particular pH at which their catalytic activity is optimal. These effects of pH may be due to effects on K_m or V_{max} or both. Figure illustrates the relative activity of four enzymes as a function of pH. Although the pH optimum of an enzyme often reflects the pH of its normal environment, the optimum may not be precisely the same. This difference suggests that the pH-activity response of an enzyme may be a factor in the intracellular regulation of its activity.

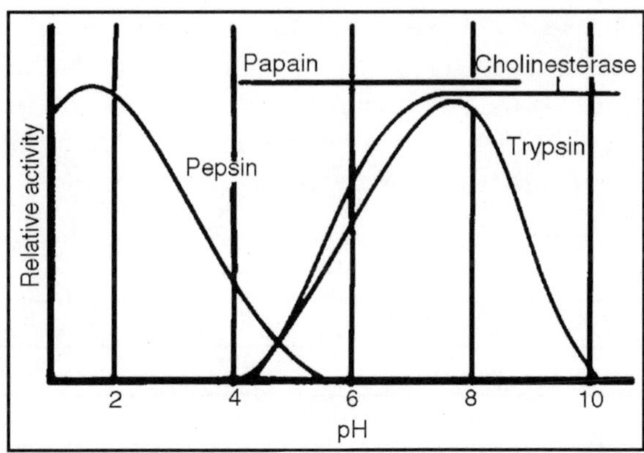

Fig. The pH Activity Profiles of four Different Enzymes.

Trypsin, an intestinal protease, has a slightly alkaline pH optimum, whereas *pepsin*, a gastric protease, acts in the acidic confines of the stomach and has a pH optimum near 2. *Papain*, a protease found in papaya, is relatively insensitive to pHs between 4 and 8.

Cholinesterase activity is pH-sensitive below pH 7 but not between pH 7 and 10. The cholinesterase pH activity profile suggests that an ionizable group with a p*K*' near 6 is essential to its activity. Might it be a histidine residue within the active site?

EFFECT OF TEMPERATURE ON ENZYMATIC ACTIVITY

Like most chemical reactions, the rates of enzyme-catalysed reactions generally increase with increasing temperature. However, at temperatures above 50° to 60°C, enzymes typically show a decline in activity.

Two effects are operating here:

- The characteristic increase in reaction rate with temperature, and
- Thermal denaturation of protein structure at higher temperatures.

Most enzymatic reactions double in rate for every 10°C rise in temperature (that is, $Q_{10} = 2$, where Q_{10} is defined as *the ratio of activities at two temperatures 10° apart*) as long as the enzyme is stable and fully active. Some enzymes, those catalyzing reactions having very high activation energies, show proportionally greater Q_{10} values.

The increasing rate with increasing temperature is ultimately offset by the instability of higher orders of protein structure at elevated temperatures, where the enzyme is inactivated. Not all enzymes are quite so thermally labile. For example, the enzymes of thermophilic bacteria (*thermophilic* = "heat-loving") found in geothermal springs retain full activity at temperatures in excess of 85°C.

The relative activity of an enzymatic reaction as a function of temperature. The decrease in the activity above 50°C is due to thermal denaturation.

Table. The Effect of Temperature on Enzyme Activity.

Optimum pH of Some Enzymes	
Enzyme	Optimum pH
Pepsin	1.5
Catalase	7.6
Trypsin	7.7
Fumarase	7.8
Ribonuclease	7.8
Arginase	9.7

ENZYME INHIBITION

If the velocity of an enzymatic reaction is decreased or inhibited, the kinetics of the reaction obviously have been perturbed. Systematic perturbations are a basic tool of experimental scientists; much can be learned about the normal workings of any system by inducing changes in it and then observing the effects of the change. The study of enzyme inhibition has contributed significantly to our understanding of enzymes.

REVERSIBLE VERSUS IRREVERSIBLE INHIBITION

Enzyme inhibitors are classified in several ways. The inhibitor may interact either reversibly or irreversibly with the enzyme. Reversible inhibitors interact with the enzyme through noncovalent association/dissociation reactions. In contrast, irreversible inhibitors usually cause stable, covalent alterations in the enzyme.

That is, the consequence of irreversible inhibition is a decrease in the concentration of active enzyme. The kinetics observed are consistent with this interpretation, as we shall see later.

REVERSIBLE INHIBITION

Reversible inhibitors fall into two major categories: competitive and noncompetitive (although other more unusual and rare categories are known). Competitive inhibitors are characterized by the fact that the substrate and inhibitor compete for the same binding site on the enzyme, the so-called active site or S-binding site. Thus, increasing the concentration of S favours the likelihood of S binding to the enzyme instead of the inhibitor, I.

That is, high [S] can overcome the effects of I. The other major type, noncompetitive inhibition, cannot be overcome by increasing [S]. The two types can be distinguished by the particular patterns obtained when the kinetic data are analysed in linear plots, such as double-reciprocal (Lineweaver-Burk) plots.

A general formulation for common inhibitor interactions in our simple enzyme kinetic model would include

$$E + I \rightleftharpoons EI \text{ and / or } I + ES \rightleftharpoons IES$$

That is, we consider here reversible combinations of the inhibitor with E and/or ES.

Competitive Inhibition

Consider the following system

$$E + S \underset{k_{-1}}{\overset{k_1}{\rightleftharpoons}} ES \xrightarrow{k_2} E + P \quad E + I \underset{k_{-3}}{\overset{k_3}{\rightleftharpoons}} EI$$

where an inhibitor, I, binds *reversibly* to the enzyme at the same site as S. S-binding and I-binding are mutually exclusive, *competitive*processes. Formation of the ternary complex, EIS, where both S and I are bound, is physically impossible. This condition leads us to anticipate that S and I must share a high degree of structural similarity because they bind at the same site on the enzyme.

Also notice that, in our model, EI does not react to give rise to E + P. That is, I is not changed by interaction with E. The rate of the product-forming reaction is $v = k_2[ES]$. It is revealing to compare the equation for the uninhibited case, the Michaelis-Menten equation for the rate of the enzymatic reaction in the presence of a fixed concentration of the competitive inhibitor, [I]

$$V = \frac{V_{max}[S]}{[S] + K_m}$$

$$V = \frac{V_{max}[S]}{[S] + K_m\left(1 + \frac{[I]}{K_I}\right)}$$

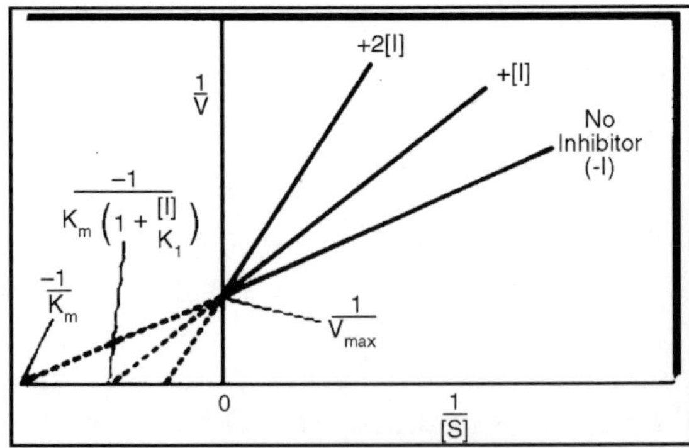

Fig. Lineweaver-Burk plot of Competitive Inhibition, Showing lines for no I, [I], and 2[I].

The K_m term in the denominator in the inhibited case is increased by the factor $(1 + [I]/K_I)$; thus, v is less in the presence of the inhibitor, as expected.

Clearly, in the absence of I, the two equations are identical. Figure shows a Lineweaver-Burk plot of competitive inhibition. Several features of competitive inhibition are evident. First, at a given [I], v decreases ($1/v$ increases). When [S] becomes infinite, $v = V_{max}$ and is unaffected by I because all of the enzyme is in the ES form.

Note that the value of the -x-intercept decreases as [I] increases. This -x-intercept is often termed the *apparent* K_m (or K_{mapp}) because it is the K_m apparent under these conditions.

The diagnostic criterion for competitive inhibition is that V_{max} is unaffected by I; that is, all lines share a common y-intercept. This criterion is also the best experimental indication of binding at the same site by two substances. Competitive inhibitors resemble S structurally.

Note that when [S] is infinitely large (1/[S]50), Vmax is the same, whether I is present or not. In the presence of I, the negative x-intercept521/K_m(11[I]/K_I). *The Equations of Competitive Inhibition:* Given the relationships between E, S, and I described previously and recalling the steady-state assumption that $d[ES]/dt = 0$, from Equations we can write,

$$[ES] = \frac{k_1[E][S]}{(k_2 + k_{-1})} = \frac{[E][S]}{K_m}$$

Assuming that E + I ! EI reaches rapid equilibrium, the rate of EI formation, $v_f' = k_3[E][I]$, and the rate of disappearance of EI, $v_d' = k_{-3}[EI]$, are equal.

So,

$$k_3[E][I] = k_{-3}[EI]$$

Therefore,

$$[EI] = \frac{k_3}{k_{-3}}[E][I]$$

If we define K_I as k_{-3}/k_3, an enzyme-inhibitor dissociation constant, then,

$$[EI] = \frac{[E][I]}{K_I}$$

knowing $[E_T] = [E] + [ES] + [EI]$.

Then,

$$[E_T] = [E] + \frac{[E][S]}{K_m} + \frac{[E][I]}{K_I}$$

Solving for [E] gives,

$$[E] = \frac{K_1 K_m [E_T]}{(K_I K_m + K_I[S] + K_m[I])}$$

Because the rate of product formation is given by $v = k_2[ES]$, from Equation we have,

$$v = \frac{k_2[E][S]}{Km}$$

So,

$$v = \frac{(k_2K_I[E_T][S])}{(K_IKm + K_I[S] + Km[I])}$$

Because $V_{max} = k_2[E_T]$,

$$v = \frac{V_{max}[S]}{Km + [S] + \frac{Km[I]}{K_1}}$$

or

$$v = \frac{V_{max}[S]}{[S] + Km\left(1 + \frac{[I]}{K_I}\right)}$$

Succinate Dehydrogenase—A Classic Example of Competitive Inhibition

The enzyme *succinate dehydrogenase* (SDH) is competitively inhibited by malonate. Figure shows the structures of succinate and malonate. The structural similarity between them is obvious and is the basis of malonate's ability to mimic succinate and bind at the active site of SDH. However, unlike succinate, which is oxidized by SDH to form fumarate, malonate cannot lose two hydrogens; consequently, it is unreactive.

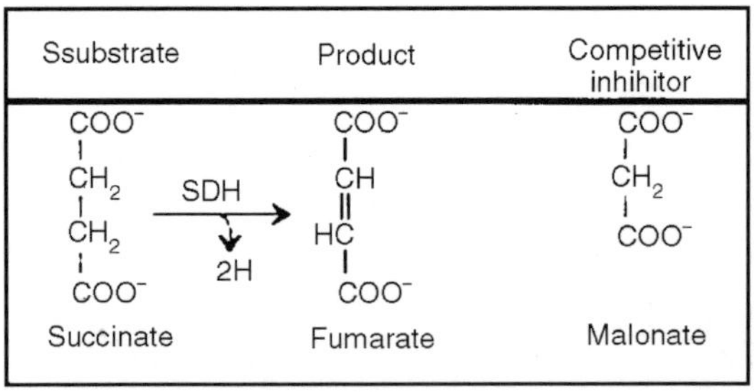

Ssubstrate		Product	Competitive inhihitor
COO^- $\vert$ CH_2 $\vert$ CH_2 $\vert$ COO^-	SDH → ↓ 2H	COO^- $\vert$ CH $\Vert$ HC $\vert$ COO^-	COO^- $\vert$ CH_2 $\vert$ COO^-
Succinate		Fumarate	Malonate

Fig. Structures of Succinate, the Substrate of Succinate Dehydrogenase (SDH), and Malonate, the Competitive Inhibitor.

Fumarate (the product of SDH action on succinate) is also shown.

Noncompetitive Inhibition

Noncompetitive inhibitors interact with both E and ES (or with S and ES, but this is a rare and specialized case). Obviously, then, the inhibitor is not binding to the same site as S, and the inhibition cannot be overcome by raising [S]. There are two types of noncompetitive inhibition: pure and mixed.

Pure Noncompetitive Inhibition

In this situation, the binding of I by E has no effect on the binding of S by E. That is, S and I bind at different sites on E, and binding of I does not affect binding of S. Consider the system

$$E + I \underset{}{\overset{K_I}{\rightleftharpoons}} ES + I \underset{}{\overset{K_I'}{\rightleftharpoons}} IES$$

Pure noncompetitive inhibition occurs if $K_I = K_I'$. This situation is relatively uncommon; the Lineweaver-Burk plot for such an instance is given in Figure below. Note that K_m is unchanged by I (the x-intercept remains the same, with or without I). Note also that V_{max} decreases. A similar pattern is seen if the amount of enzyme in the experiment is decreased. Thus, it is as if I lowered [E].

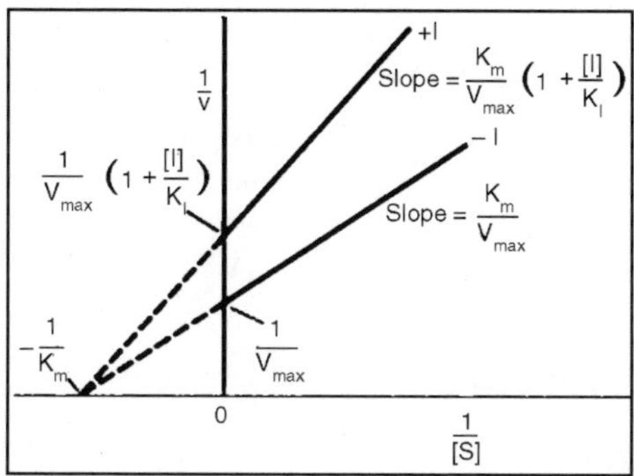

Fig. Lineweaver-Burk Plot of Pure Noncompetitive Inhibition. Note that I does not alter K_m but that it decreases V_{max}. In the presence of I, the y-intercept is equal to $(1/V_{max})(1 + I/K_I)$.

MIXED NONCOMPETITIVE INHIBITION

In this situation, the binding of I by E influences the binding of S by E. Either the binding sites for I and S are near one another or conformational changes in E caused by I affect S binding. In this case, K_I and K_I', as defined previously, are not equal. Both K_m and V_{max} are altered by the presence of I, and K_m/V_{max} is not constant.

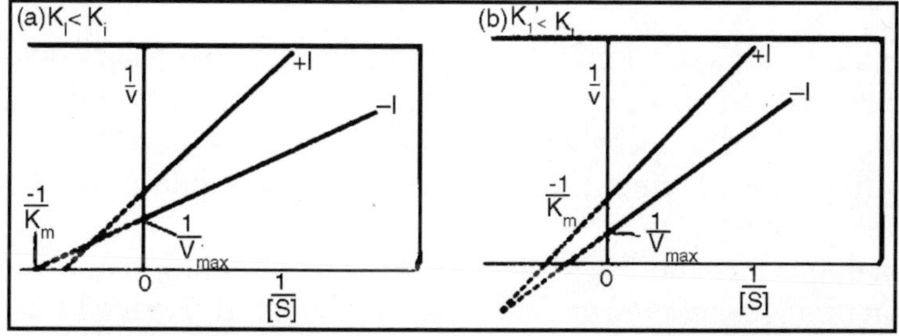

Fig. Lineweaver-Burk plot of mixed noncompetitive inhibition. Note that both intercepts and the slope change in the presence of I.

- When K_I is less than K_I';
- When K_I is greater than K_I'.

This inhibitory pattern is commonly encountered. A reasonable explanation is that the inhibitor is binding at a site distinct from the active site, yet is influencing the binding of S at the active site. Presumably, these effects are transmitted via alterations in the protein's conformation. Table below includes the rate equations and apparent K_m and V_{max} values for both types of noncompetitive inhibition.

Table. The Effect of Various Types of Inhibitors on the Michaelis–Menten RateEquation and on Apparent K_m and Apparent Vmax

Inhibition Type	Rate Equation	Apparent K_m	Apparent Vmax
None	$v = V_{max}[S]/(K_m + [S])$	K_m	V_{max}
Competitive	$v = V_{max}[S]/([S] + K_m(1 + [I]/K_I))$	$K_m(1 + [I]/K_I)$	V_{max}
Noncompetitive	$v = (V_{max}[S]/(1 + [I]/K_I))/(K_m + [S])$	K_m	$V_{max}/(1 + [I]/K_I)$
Mixed	$v = V_{max}[S]/((1 + [I]/K_I) K_m 1(1 + [I]/K_I' [S]))$	$K_m(1 + [I]/K_I)/(1 + [I]/K_I')$	$V_{max}/(1 + [I]/K_I')$

K_I is defined as the enzyme:inhibitor dissociation constant K_I = [E][I]/[EI]; K_I' is defined as the enzyme substrate complex: inhibitor dissociation constant K_I' = [ES][I]/[ESI]

IRREVERSIBLE INHIBITION

If the inhibitor combines irreversibly with the enzyme—for example, by covalent attachment—the kinetic pattern seen is like that of noncompetitive inhibition, because the net effect is a loss of active enzyme. Usually, this type of inhibition can be distinguished from the noncompetitive, reversible inhibition case since the reaction of I with E (and/or ES) is not instantaneous. Instead, there is a *time-dependent decrease in enzymatic activity* as $E + I \rightarrow EI$ proceeds, and the rate of this inactivation can be followed. Also, unlike reversible inhibitions, dilution or dialysis of the enzyme: inhibitor solution does not dissociate the EI complex and restore enzyme activity.

Suicide Substrates—Mechanism-Based Enzyme Inactivators

Suicide substrates are inhibitory substrate analogs designed so that, via normal catalytic action of the enzyme, a very reactive group is generated. This reactive group then forms a covalent bond with a nearby functional group within the active site of the enzyme, thereby causing irreversible inhibition. Suicide substrates, also called *Trojan horse substrates*, are a type of affinity label. As substrate analogs, they bind with specificity and high affinity to the enzyme active site; in their reactive form, they become covalently bound to the enzyme. This covalent link effectively labels a particular functional group within the active site, identifying the group as a key player in the enzyme's catalytic cycle.

Penicillin—A Suicide Substrate

Several drugs in current medical use are mechanism-based enzyme inactivators. For example, the antibiotic penicillin exerts its effects by covalently reacting with an essential serine residue in the active site of *glycoprotein peptidase*, an enzyme that acts to cross-link the peptidoglycan chains during synthesis of bacterial cell walls. Once cell wall synthesis is blocked, the bacterial cells are very susceptible to rupture by osmotic lysis, and bacterial growth is halted.

Variable group
Thiazolidine ring
Reactive peptide bond of β-lactam ring
Penicillin
Glycopeptide Transpeptidase
Active enzyme
Glycopeptide Transpeptidase
Penicilloyl-enzyme complex (enzymatically inactive)

Fig. Penicillin is an Irreversible Inhibitor of the Enzyme *Glycoprotein Peptidase,* which Catalyses an Essential step in Bacterial cell wall Synthesis.

Penicillin consists of a thiazolidine ring fused to a b-lactam ring to which a variable group R is attached. A reactive peptide bond in the b-lactam ring covalently attaches to a serine residue in the active site of the glycopeptide transpeptidase. (The conformation of penicillin around its reactive peptide bond resembles the transition state of the normal glycoprotein peptidase substrate.) The penicilloyl-enzyme complex is catalytically inactive. The bond between the enzyme and penicillin is indefinitely stable; that is, penicillin binding is irreversible.

INVOLVING TWO OR MORE SUBSTRATES

Thus far, we have considered only the simple case of enzymes that act upon a single substrate, S. This situation is not common. Usually, enzymes catalyse reactions in which two (or even more) substrates take part. Consider the case of an enzyme catalyzing a reaction involving two substrates, A and B, and yielding the products P and Q:

$$A + B \xrightarrow{\text{enzyme}} P + Q$$

Such a reaction is termed a bisubstrate reaction. In general, bisubstrate reactions proceed by one of two possible routes:

- *Both A and B are bound to the enzyme and then reaction occurs to give P1Q*:

$$E + A + B \rightarrow AEB \rightarrow PEQ \rightarrow E + P + Q$$

  Reactions of this type are defined as sequential or single-displacement reactions. They can be either of two distinct classes:
  - Random, where either A or B may bind to the enzyme first, followed by the other substrate, or
  - Ordered, where A, designated the *leading substrate*, must bind to E first before B can be bound.

Double-reciprocal plots of the rates observed with different fixed concentrations of one substrate (B here) are graphed versus a series of concentrations of A. Note that, in these Lineweaver-Burk plots for single-displacement bisubstrate mechanisms, the lines intersect to the left of the $1/v$ axis.

- The other general possibility is that one substrate, A, binds to the enzyme and reacts with it to yield a chemically modified form of the enzyme (E') plus the product, P. The second substrate, B, then reacts with E', regenerating E and forming the other product, Q.

$$E + A \longrightarrow EA \longrightarrow E'P \longrightarrow E' \longrightarrow E'B \longrightarrow EQ \longrightarrow E + Q$$
(P released from E'P; B enters at E')

Reactions that fit this model are called ping-pong or double-displacement reactions. Two distinctive features of this mechanism are the obligatory formation of a modified enzyme intermediate, E', and the pattern of parallel lines obtained in double-reciprocal plots. Figure Double-displacement (ping-pong) bisubstrate mechanisms are characterized by Lineweaver-Burk plots of parallel lines when double-reciprocal plots of the rates observed with different fixed concentrations of the second substrate, B, are graphed versus a series of concentrations of A.

RANDOM, SINGLE-DISPLACEMENT REACTIONS

In this type of sequential reaction, all possible binary enzyme: substrate complexes (AE, EB, QE, EP) are formed rapidly and reversibly when the enzyme is added to a reaction mixture containing A, B, P, and Q:

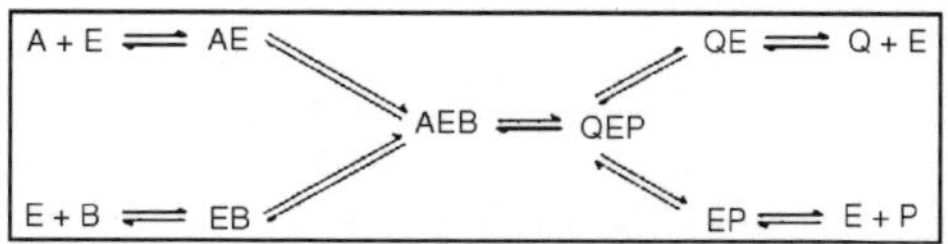

The rate-limiting step is the reaction AEB → QEP. It doesn't matter whether A or B binds first to E, or whether Q or P is released first from QEP. Sometimes, reactions that follow this random order of addition of substrates to E can be distinguished mechanistically from reactions obeying an ordered, single-displacement mechanism, *if* A has *no* influence on the binding constant for B (and vice versa); that is, the mechanism is purely random. Then, the lines in a Lineweaver-Burk plot intersect at the 1/[A] axis.

Note that the lines intersect at the 1/[A] axis. (If [B] were varied in an experiment with several fixed concentrations of A, the lines would intersect at the 1/[B] axis in a $1/v$ versus 1/[B] plot.)

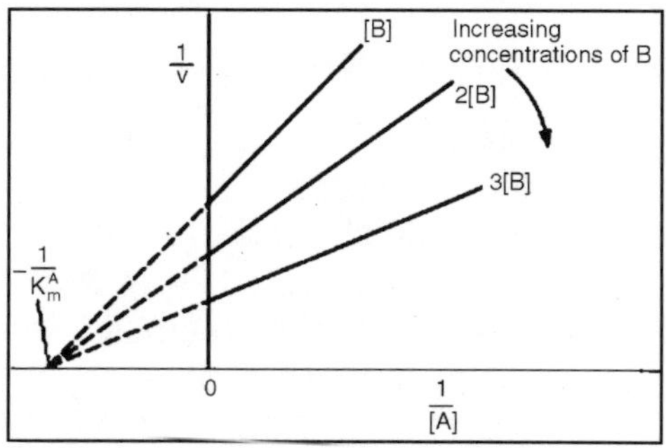

Fig. Random, single-displacement Bisubstrate Mechanism where A does not affect B Binding, and Vice Versa.

Creatine Kinase Acts by a Random, Single-Displacement Mechanism

An example of a random, single-displacement mechanism is seen in the enzyme creatine kinase, a phosphoryl-transfer enzyme that uses ATP as a phosphoryl donor to form creatine phosphate (CrP) from creatine (Cr). Creatine-P is an important reservoir of phosphate-bond energy in muscle cells.

The overall direction of the reaction will be determined by the relative concentrations of ATP, ADP, Cr, and CrP and the equilibrium constant for the reaction.

The enzyme can be considered to have two sites for substrate (or product) binding: an adenine nucleotide site, where ATP or ADP binds, and a creatine site, where Cr or CrP is bound. In such a mechanism, ATP and ADP compete for binding at their unique site, while Cr and CrP compete at the specific Cr-, CrP-binding site. Note that no modified enzyme form (E'), such as an E-PO_4intermediate, appears here.

The reaction is characterized by rapid and reversible binary ES complex formation, followed by addition of the remaining substrate, and the rate-determining reaction taking place within the ternary complex.

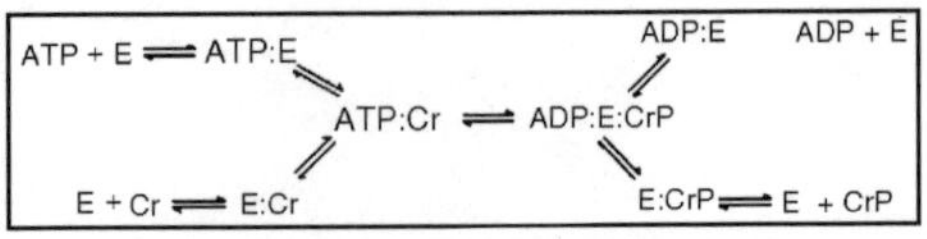

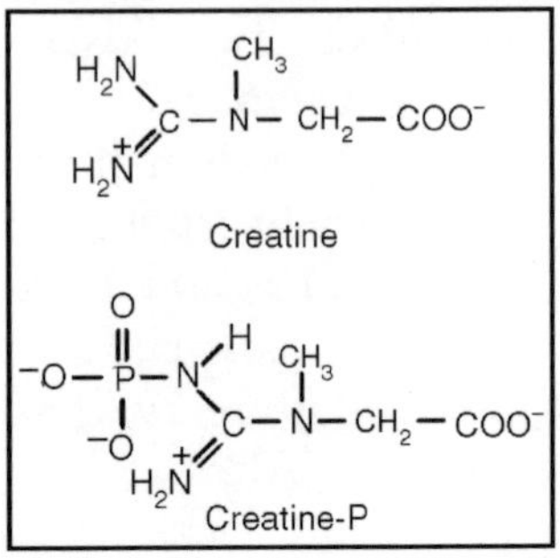

Fig. The Structures of Creatine and Creatine Phosphate, Guanidinium Compounds that are Important in Muscle Energy Metabolism.

ORDERED, SINGLE-DISPLACEMENT REACTIONS

In this case, the leading substrate, A (also called The obligatory or compulsory substrate), must bind first. Then the second substrate, B, binds. Strictly speaking, B cannot bind to free enzyme in the absence of A. Reaction between A and B occurs in the ternary complex, and is usually followed by an ordered release of the products of the reaction, P and Q. In the schemes below, Q is the product of A and is released last. One representation, suggested by W. W. Cleland, follows:

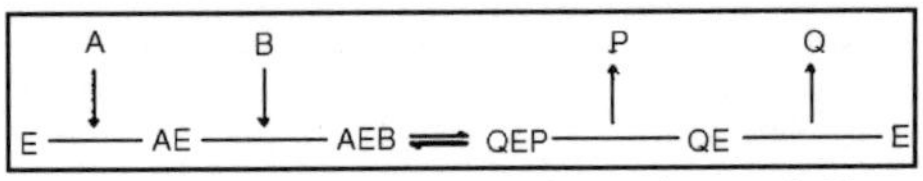

Another way of portraying this mechanism is as follows:

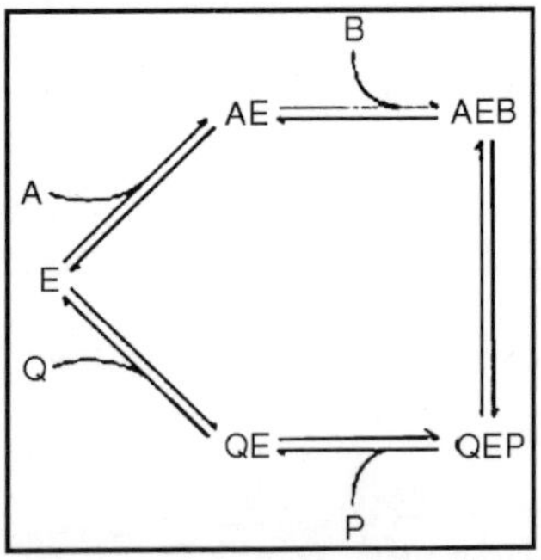

Note that A and Q are competitive for binding to the free enzyme, E, but not A and B (or Q and B).

NAD$^+$-Dependent Dehydrogenases Show Ordered

Single-Displacement Mechanisms

Nicotinamide adenine dinucleotide (NAD$^+$)-dependent dehydrogenases are enzymes that typically behave according to the kinetic pattern just described.

A general reaction of these dehydrogenases is,

$$NAD^+ + BH_2 \rightleftharpoons NADH + H^+ + B$$

The leading substrate (A) is nicotinamide adenine dinucleotide (NAD^+), and NAD^+ and NADH (product Q) compete for a common site on E. A specific example is offered by alcohol dehydrogenase (ADH):

$$NAD^+ + CH_3CH_2OH \rightleftharpoons NADH + H^+ + CH_3CHO$$

DOUBLE-DISPLACEMENT (PING-PONG) REACTIONS

Reactions conforming to this kinetic pattern are characterized by the fact that the product of the enzyme's reaction with A (called P in the following schemes) is released *prior* to reaction of the enzyme with the second substrate, B. As a result of this process, the enzyme, E, is converted to a modified form, E9, which then reacts with B to give the second product, Q, and regenerate the unmodified enzyme form, E:

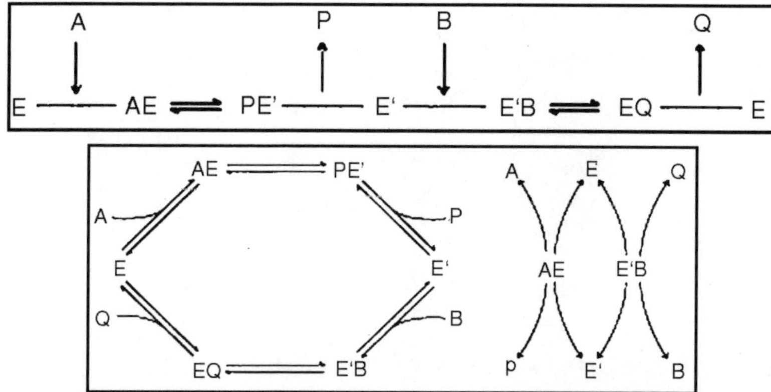

Note that these schemes predict that A and Q compete for the free enzyme form, E, while B and P compete for the modified enzyme form, E'. A and Q do not bind to E', nor do B and P combine with E.

Aminotransferases Show Double-Displacement Catalytic Mechanisms

One class of enzymes that follow a ping-pong-type mechanism are *aminotransferases* (previously known as transaminases). These enzymes catalyse the transfer of an amino group from an amino acid to an a-keto acid. The products are a new amino acid and the keto acid corresponding to the carbon skeleton of the amino donor:

amino acidl + keto acid2 → keto acidl + amino acid2

A specific example would be glutamate: *aspartate aminotransferase*. Figure depicts the scheme for this mechanism. Note that glutamate and aspartate are competitive for E, and that oxaloacetate and a-ketoglutarate compete for E'. In glutamate: aspartate aminotransferase, an enzyme-bound coenzyme, *pyridoxal phosphate* (a vitamin B_6 derivative), serves as the amino group acceptor/donor in the enzymatic reaction. The unmodified enzyme form, E, has the coenzyme in the aldehydic pyridoxal form, whereas the modified enzyme form, E9, is actually pyridoxamine phosphate. Not all enzymes displaying ping-pong-type mechanisms require coenzymes as carriers for the chemical substituent transferred in the reaction.

Figure Glutamate: aspartate aminotransferase, an enzyme conforming to a double-displacement bisubstrate mechanism. Glutamate: aspartate aminotransferase is a pyridoxal phosphate-dependent enzyme. The pyridoxal serves as the $-NH_2$ acceptor from glutamate to form pyridoxamine. Pyridoxamine is then the amino donor to oxaloacetate to form asparate and regenerate the pyridoxal coenzyme form. (The pyridoxamine: enzyme is the E' form.)

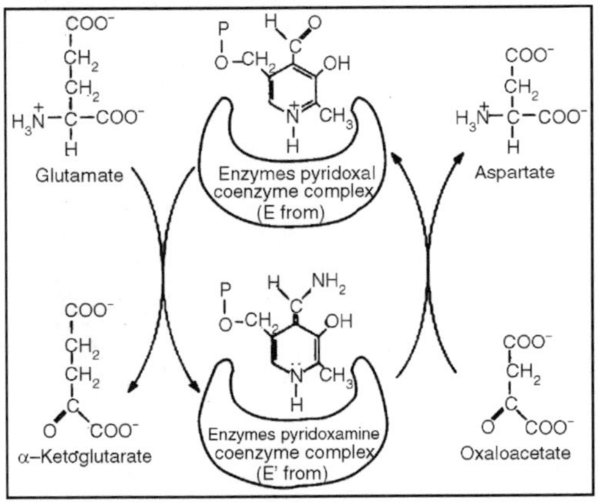

DIAGNOSIS OF BISUBSTRATE MECHANISMS

Kineticists rely on a number of diagnostic tests for the assignment of a reaction mechanism to a specific enzyme. One is the graphic analysis of the kinetic patterns observed. It is usually easy to distinguish between single- and double-displacement reactions in this manner, and examining competitive effects between substrates aids in assigning reactions to random versus ordered patterns of S-binding. A second diagnostic test is to determine whether the enzyme catalyses an exchange reaction.

Consider as an example the two enzymes *sucrose phosphorylase* and *maltose phosphorylase*. Both catalyse the phosphorolysis of a disaccharide and both yield glucose-1-phosphate and a free hexose:

$$\text{Sucrose} + P_i \rightleftharpoons \text{glucose} - 1 - \text{phosphate} + \text{fructose}$$

$$\text{Maltose} + P_i \rightleftharpoons \text{glucose} - 1 - \text{phosphate} + \text{glucose}$$

Interestingly, in the absence of sucrose and fructose, sucrose phosphorylase will catalyse the exchange of inorganic phosphate, Pi, into glucose-1-phosphate. This reaction can be followed by using $^{32}P_i$ as a radioactive tracer and observing the appearance of ^{32}P into glucose-1-phosphate:

$$^{32}P_i + G-1-P \rightleftharpoons P_i + G-1-^{32}P$$

Maltose phosphorylase cannot carry out a similar reaction. The ^{32}P exchange reaction of sucrose phosphorylase is accounted for by a double-displacement mechanism where E' = E-glucose:

$$\text{Sucrose} + E \rightleftharpoons E - \text{glucose} + \text{fructose}$$

$$E - \text{glucose} + P_i \rightleftharpoons E + \text{glucose} - 1 - \text{phosphate}$$

Thus, in the presence of just $^{32}P_i$ and glucose-1-phosphate, sucrose phosphory-lase still catalyses the second reaction and radioactive P_i is incorporated into glucose-1-phosphate over time. Maltose phosphorylase proceeds via a single-displacement reaction that necessarily requires the formation of a ternary maltose: E: P_i (or glucose: E: glucose-1-phosphate) complex for any reaction to occur. Exchange reactions are a characteristic of enzymes that obey double-displacement mechanisms at some point in their catalysis.

MULTISUBSTRATE REACTIONS

Thus far, we have considered enzyme-catalysed reactions involving one or two substrates. How are the kinetics described in those cases in which more than two substrates participate in the reaction? An example might be the glycolytic enzyme *glyceraldehyde-3-phosphate dehydrogenase*:

$$NAD^+ + \text{glyceraldehyde-3-P} + Pi \rightarrow NADH + H^+ + \text{1,3-bisphosphoglycerate}$$

Many other multisubstrate examples abound in metabolism. In effect, these situations are managed by realizing that the interaction of the enzyme with its many substrates can be treated as a series of uni- or bisubstrate steps in a multi-step reaction pathway. Thus, the complex mechanism of a multisubstrate reaction is resolved into a sequence of steps, each of which obeys the single- and double-displacement patterns just discussed.

RNA AND ANTIBODY MOLECULES AS ENZYMES: RIBOZYMES AND ABZYMES

CATALYTIC RNA MOLECULES: RIBOZYMES

It was long assumed that all enzymes are proteins. However, in recent years, more and more instances of biological catalysis by RNA molecules have been discovered. These catalytic RNAs, or ribozymes, satisfy several enzymatic criteria: They are substrate-specific, they enhance the reaction rate, and they emerge from the reaction unchanged. For example, RNase P, an enzyme responsible for the formation of mature tRNA molecules from tRNA precursors, requires an RNA component as well as a protein subunit for its activity in the cell.

In vitro, the protein alone is incapable of catalyzing the maturation reaction, but the RNA component by itself can carry out the reaction under appropriate conditions. In another case, in the ciliated protozoan *Tetrahymena*, formation of mature ribosomal RNA from a pre-rRNA precursor involves the removal of an internal RNA segment and the joining of the two ends in a process known as splicing out. The excision of this intervening internal sequence of RNA and ligation of the ends is, remarkably, catalysed by the intervening sequence of RNA itself, in the presence of Mg^{2+} and a free molecule of guanosine nucleoside or nucleotide (Figure). *In vivo*, the intervening sequence RNA probably acts only in splicing itself out; *in vitro*, however, it can act many times, turning over like a true enzyme.

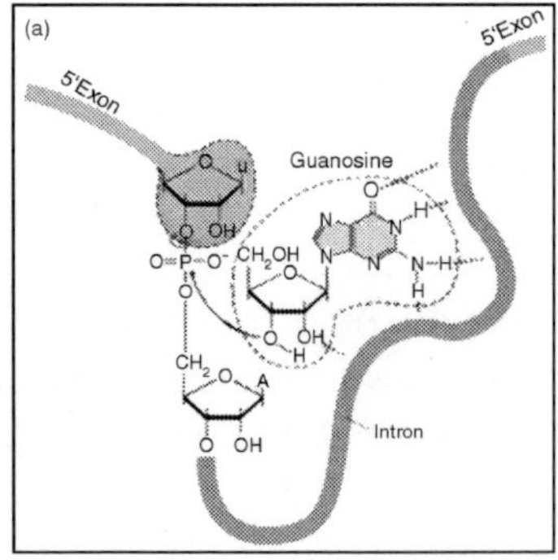

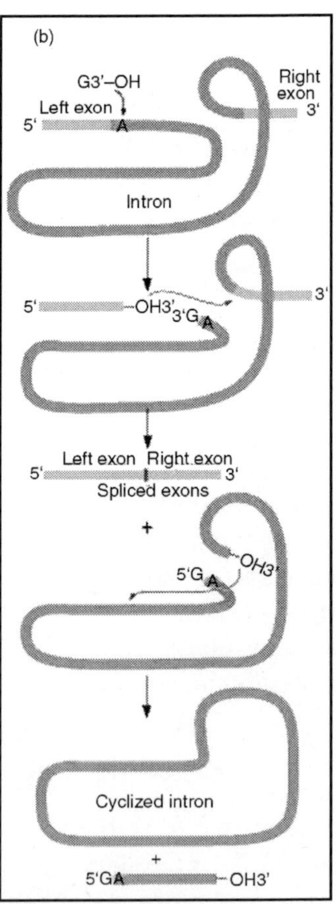

Fig. RNA splicing in *Tetrahymena* rRNA Maturation:

- The guanosine-mediated reaction involved in the autocatalytic excision of the *Tetrahymena* rRNA intron, and
- The overall splicing process. The cyclized intron is formed via nucleophilic attack of the 3'-OH on the phosphodiester bond that is 15 nucleotides from the 5'-GA end of the spliced-out intron. Cyclization frees a linear 15-mer with a 5'-GA end.

Protein-Free 50S Ribosomal Subunits Catalyse Peptide Bond Formation In Vitro

Perhaps the most significant case of catalysis by RNA occurs in protein synthesis. Harry F. Noller and his colleagues have found that the peptidyl transferase reaction, which is the reaction of peptide bond formation during protein synthesis, can be catalysed by 50S ribosomal subunits from which virtually all of the protein has been removed. These experiments imply that just the 23S rRNA by itself is capable of catalyzing peptide bond formation.

Also, the laboratory of Thomas Cech has created a synthetic 196-nucleotide-long ribozyme capable of performing the peptidyl transferase reaction.

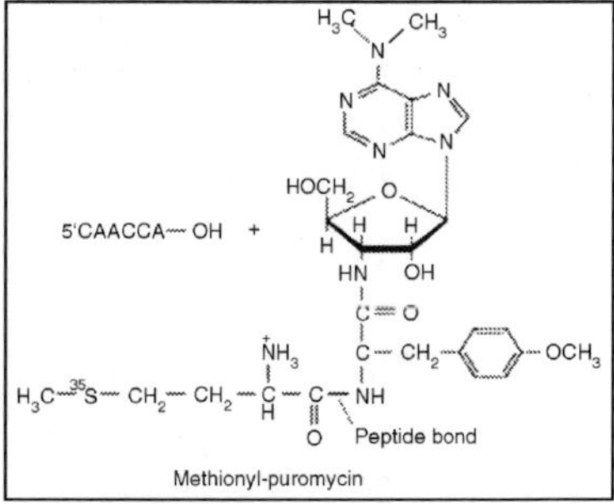

Fig. Protein-free 50S Ribosomal Subunits have Peptidyl Transferase Activity.

Peptidyl transferase is the name of the enzymatic function that catalyses peptide bond formation. The presence of this activity in protein-free 50S ribosomal subunits was demonstrated using a model assay for peptide bond formation in which an aminoacyl-tRNA analog (a short RNA oligonucleotide of sequence CAACCA carrying S-labeled methionine attached at its 3'-OH end) served as the peptidyl donor and puromycin (another amino-acyl-tRNA analog) served as the peptidyl acceptor. Activity was measured by monitoring the formation of S-labeled methioninyl-puromycin.

Several features of these "RNA enzymes," or ribozymes, lead to the realization that their biological efficiency does not challenge that achieved by proteins. First, RNA enzymes often do not fulfill the criterion of catalysis *in vivo* because they act only once in intramolecular events such as self-splicing. Second, the catalytic rates achieved by RNA enzymes *in vivo* and *in vitro* are significantly enhanced by the participation of protein subunits. Nevertheless, the fact that RNA can catalyse certain reactions is experimental support for the idea that a primordial world dominated by RNA molecules existed before the evolution of DNA and proteins.

CATALYTIC ANTIBODIES: ABZYMES

Antibodies are *immunoglobulins*, which, of course, are proteins. Like other antibodies,catalytic antibodies, so-called abzymes, are elicited in an organism in response to immunological challenge by a foreign molecule called an antigen for discussions on the molecular basis of immunology). In this case, however, the antigen is purposefully engineered to be *an analog of the transition-state intermediate in a reaction*. The rationale is that a protein specific for binding the transition-state intermediate of a reaction will promote entry of the normal reactant into the reactive, transition-state conformation.

Thus, a catalytic antibody facilitates, or catalyses, a reaction by forcing the conformation of its substrate in the direction of its transition state. (A prominent explanation for the remarkable catalytic power of conventional enzymes is their great affinity for the transition-state intermediates in the reactions they catalyse;

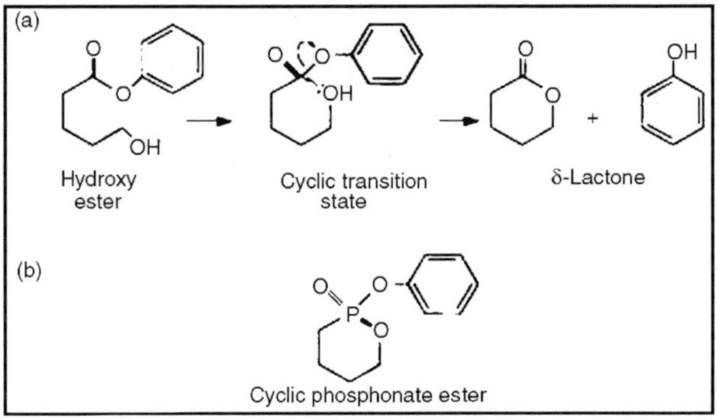

Fig. Catalytic Antibodies are Designed to Specifically Bind the Transition-state Intermediate in a Chemical Reaction.

(a) The intramolecular hydrolysis of a hydroxy ester to yield as products a d-lactone and the alcohol phenol. Note the cyclic transition state.

(b) The cyclic phosphonate ester analog of the cyclic transition state. Antibodies raised against this phosphonate ester act as *enzymes*: they are catalysts that markedly accelerate the rate of ester hydrolysis.

One strategy has been to prepare ester analogs by substituting a phosphorus atom for the carbon in the ester group. The phospho-compound mimics the natural transition state of ester hydrolysis, and antibodies elicited against these analogs act like enzymes in accelerating the rate of ester hydrolysis as much as 1000-fold. Abzymes have been developed for a number of other classes of reactions, including COC bond formation via aldol condensation (the reverse of the aldolase reaction and the pyridoxal 5'-P-dependent aminotransferase reaction. In this latter instance, N_a-(5'-

phosphopyridoxyl)-lysine (Figure a) coupled to a carrier protein served as the antigen. An antibody raised against this antigen catalysed the conversion of d-alanine and pyridoxal 5'-P to pyruvate and pyridoxamine 5'-P. This biotechnology offers the real possibility of creating "designer enzymes," specially tailored enzymes designed to carry out specific catalytic processes.

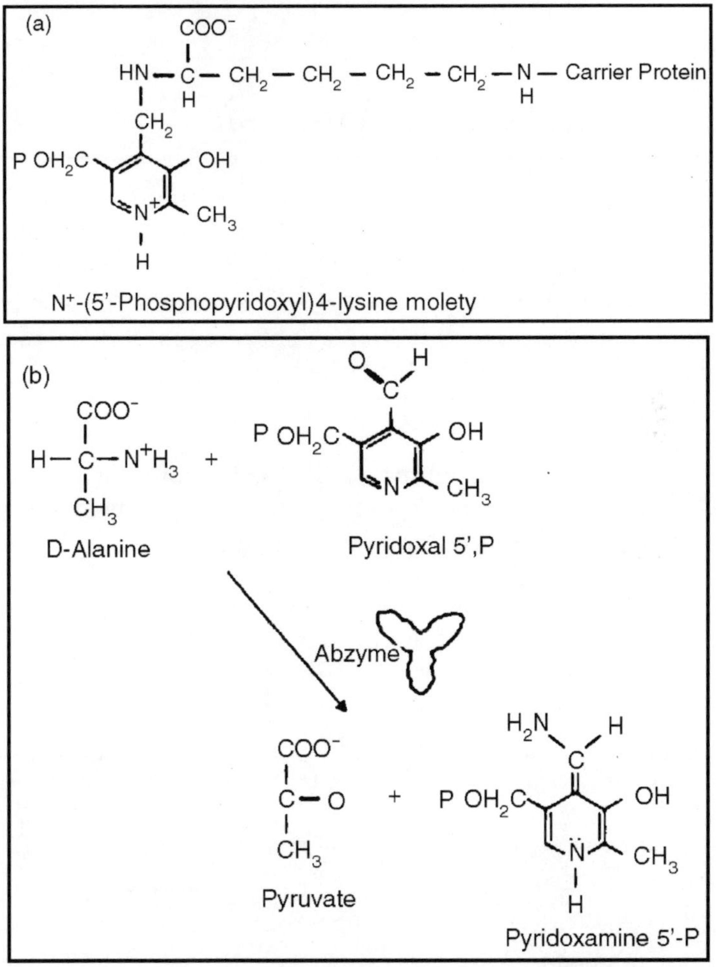

(a) N^+-(5'-Phosphopyridoxyl)4-lysine molety

(b) D-Alanine + Pyridoxal 5',P → (Abzyme) → Pyruvate + Pyridoxamine 5'-P

Fig. (a) Antigen used to Create an Abzyme with Aminotransferase Activity. (b) Aminotransferase Reaction Catalysed by the Abzyme.

4

Protein Structure and Analysis

CONCEPT

It is assumed that students will be already familiar with basic concepts of protein and nucleic acid structure, as well as enzyme kinetics and mechanisms, before using the Biochemistry of Metabolism.

PROTEIN PRIMARY STRUCTURE

Proteins are polymers of amino acids. Each amino acid has the same fundamental structure, differing only in the side-chain, designated the R-group. The carbon atom to which the amino group, carboxyl group, and side chain (R-group) are attached is the alpha carbon (C^{α}).

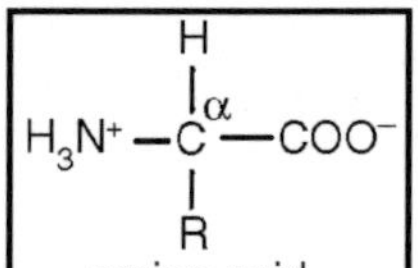

$H_3N^+-C^{\alpha}(H)(R)-COO^-$

amino acid

Alanine(Ala, A) Isoleucinen (Ile, I) Leucine (Leu,L) Valine (Val,V) Glycine (Gly, G)

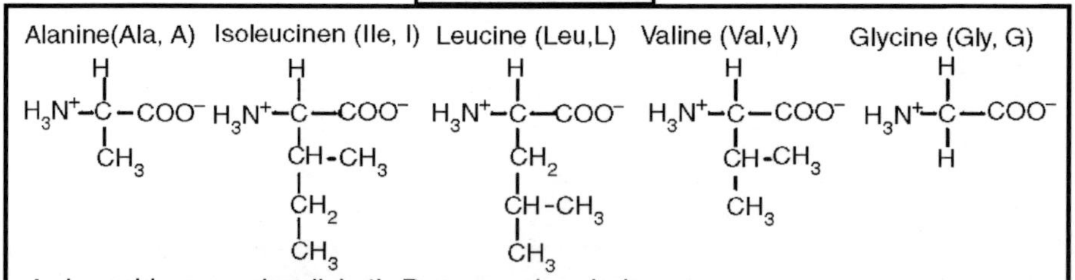

Amino acids: non-polar aliphatic R-groups; plus glycine

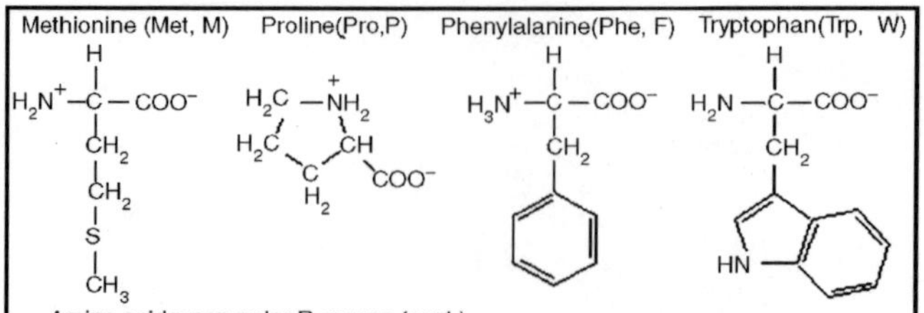

Methionine (Met, M) Proline(Pro,P) Phenylalanine(Phe, F) Tryptophan(Trp, W)

Amino acids: non-polar R-groups (cont.)

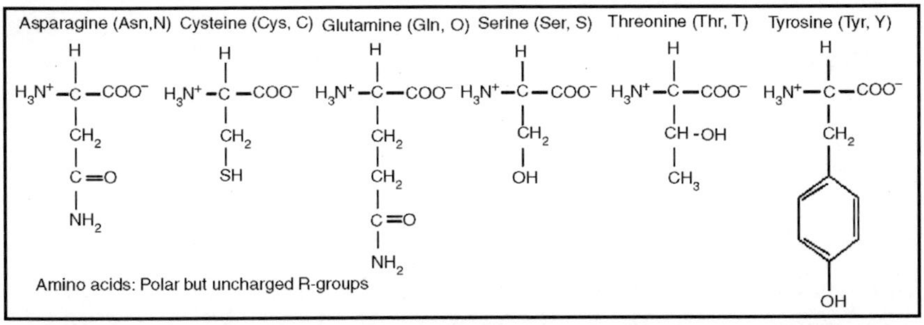

Asparagine (Asn,N) Cysteine (Cys, C) Glutamine (Gln, Q) Serine (Ser, S) Threonine (Thr, T) Tyrosine (Tyr, Y)

Amino acids: Polar but uncharged R-groups

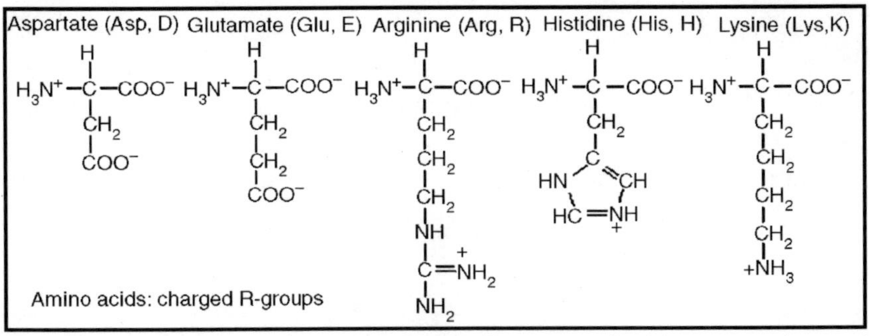

Aspartate (Asp, D) Glutamate (Glu, E) Arginine (Arg, R) Histidine (His, H) Lysine (Lys,K)

Amino acids: charged R-groups

Structures of amino acids, with their R-groups in blue, are shown below with their three-letter and one-letter abbreviated names. Glycine has just a hydrogen atom in place of an R-group. At physiological pH, some amino acid R-groups are charged, because of dissociation or association of a proton by, *e.g.,* a carboxyl or amino group.

Note that histidine is shown charged, but its pK is close to the physiological range. Some side-chain groups that are uncharged at the near-neutral pH of the cytosol or extracellular space, may dissociate or gain a proton in the microenvironment of an enzyme active site.

Peptide bonds link amino acid residues within proteins. The sequence of covalently linked amino acids is known as theprimary structure of a protein. The reaction by which two amino acids are joined in a peptide bond, with elimination of H_2O, is represented at right.

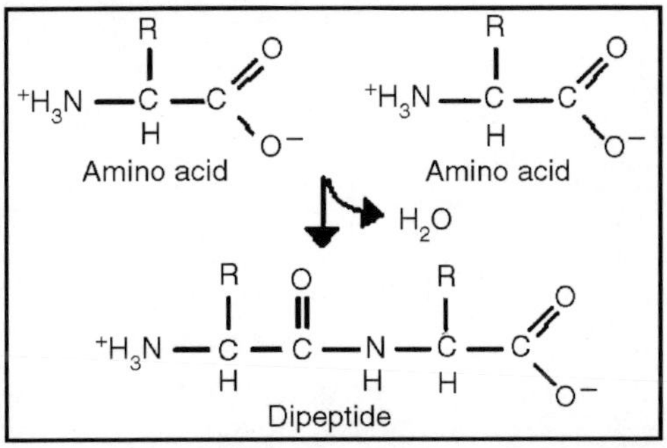

Amino acid Amino acid

H_2O

Dipeptide

A protein is a polypeptide, a linear polymer of many amino acids, linked by peptide bonds. The peptide linkages, along with the α-carbon atoms to which

R-groups are attached, form the protein backbone, with sequence NCCNCCNCCNCC...

Polypeptide

Protein Secondary Structure

Segments of polypeptides often fold locally into stable structures that include α-helices and β-pleated sheets.

α-Helix

In an α-helix (alpha helix), the polypeptide backbone follows a helical path. There are 3.6 amino acid residues per turn of the helix. Some protein domains assume other helical structures, but the α-helix is most common.

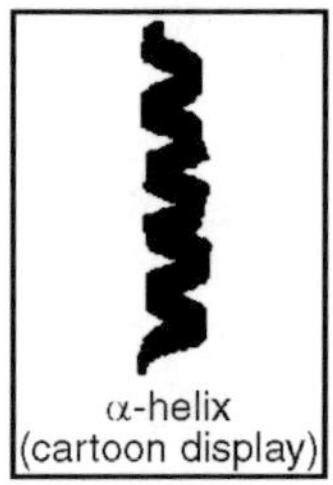
α-helix
(cartoon display)

An α-helix is stabilized by hydrogen bonds between backbone amino and carbonyl groups and those in the next turn of the helix, represented as N-H····O=C.

The hydrogen and oxygen atoms are attracted to one another because the H atom carries a partial positive charge and the O atom carries a partial negative charge, due to unequal sharing of electrons in N-H and O=C bonds.

Peptide backbone H-bond
(H & R-group on α-Comitted)

In an α-helix, the amino acid R-groups protrude out from the helically coiled polypeptide backbone. The surface of an α-helix largely consists of the R-groups of amino acid residues. At right, an α-helix is shown end-on and from the side. In this image, H atoms are not visible. Colours: C N O R-group

Some amino acids have a greater tendency to be found within an α-helix. The amino acid proline tends to interrupt an α-helix. Its fused ring, which includes the α-carbon and the peptide-forming amino N, prevents the polypeptide backbone from assuming a conformation compatible with an a-helix in the vicinity of a proline.

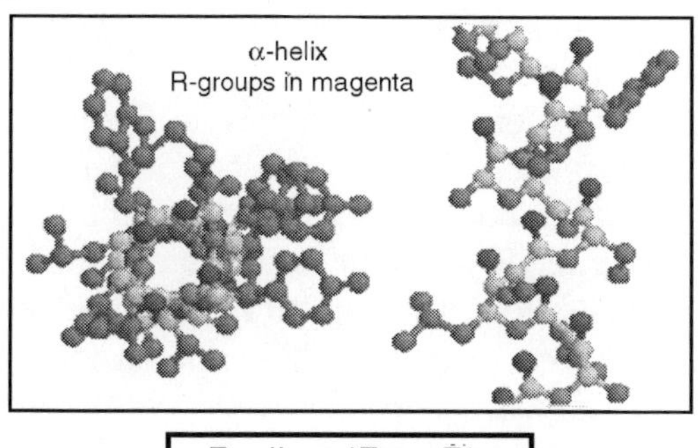

Proline (Pro, P)

$H_2C-\overset{+}{N}H_2$, H_2C, CH, C, H_2, COO^-

Explore below the structure of an α-helix, using MDL's software plug-in Chime.

- With Chime, usually one selects something, and then alters its display, colour, etc.
- Use the left mouse button to drag the image to view the a-helix from different perspectives.

Using the right mouse button, choose display backbone. Drag to view the spiraling backbone from the side as well as down its axis. Now choose display ball and stick with colour CPK (a colour convention in which C is grey, O is red, N is blue, etc.) To distinguish the R-groups, select protein-sidechain, and then display as sticks.

Question: Structures of individual amino acids are given above. Based on the R-group structures, identify each amino acid residue and specify the sequence of amino acids in this peptide. Now select protein - sidechain; then select - change colour to and pick a colour. This will give the R-groups a colour distinct from the CPK-coloured backbone atoms. Select protein - protein. Try other display options including spacefill-Van der Waals, and ribbons.

Questions: What part of the polypeptide is mainly exposed to the surrounding medium. Is an α-helix a hollow structure?

Beta Pleated Sheets

Another common secondary structure is the β sheet (beta sheet). In a β sheet, strands of protein lie adjacent to one another, interacting laterally via H bonds between backbone carbonyl oxygen and amino H atoms. The strands may be parallel (N-termini of both strands at the same end) or antiparallel. Because of the tetrahedral nature of carbon bonds, a β-sheet is puckered, leading to the designation pleated sheet. R groups of amino acids in a β-strand alternately point to one side or the other of a β-strand. Hence every other amino acid is exposed on one side or the other of ab-sheet. Explore at right two strands of a β-sheet. Recommended displays: Display as cartoon.

Question: Are the two β-strands parallel or antiparallel? Now change the display to ball and stick, with colour CPK. Then select protein-sidechain, and select-change colour to. Specify a colour not already visible, such as green.

View the 2-stranded β-sheet from the side. Note the "pleated" appearance of each β-strand. Note how the protein side-chains (R-groups) alternate in extending above and below the β-sheet. Note how, within the plane of the sheet, backbone carbonyl oxygen atoms point towards backbone amino N atoms of the adjacent strand. (H atoms involved in interchain H-bonds are not visible in this structure, which is based on X-ray crystallo graphic analysis.)

These two β-strands are actually part of a larger protein that you will explore below. C O N S. A common structural motif, the β-barrel, is equivalent to a β-sheet that is rolled up to form a cylinder. An example of a protein that consists mainly of a b-barrel is the bacterial channel porin. In some cases, a β-barrel may be partly flattened, to form what is called a β-clam structure.

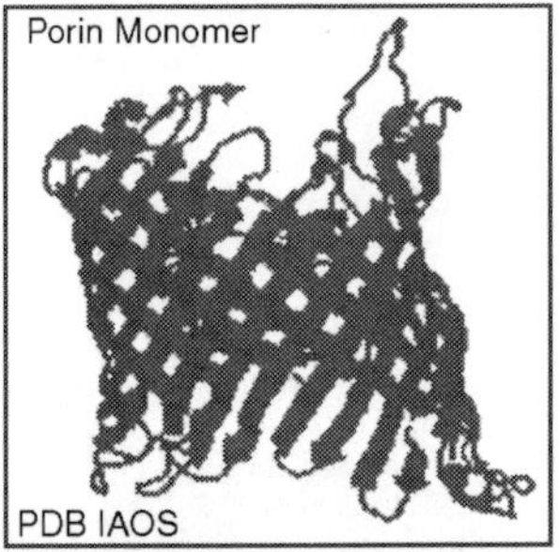

Other common folding motifs involve combinations of α-helices and β-strands. One example is the α,β-barrel, explored elsewhere in an exercise on Triose Phosphate Isomerase (TIM).

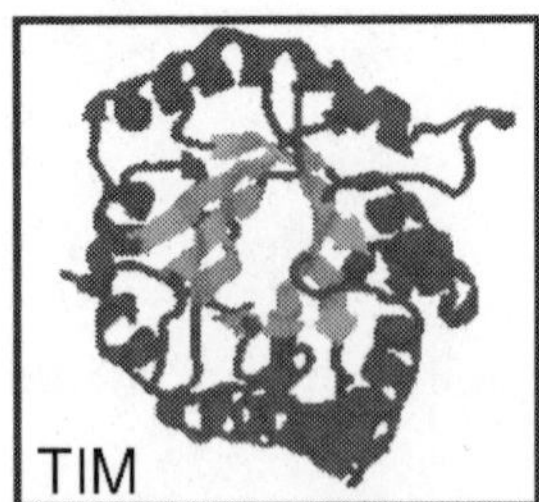

Explore at right an intestinal fatty acid binding protein. Recommended displays: Display as cartoon, and colour structure. Different colours distinguish the β-strands, α-helices and sharp turns called hairpin loops.

Question: Would you describe the predominant structure as a β-sheet, β-barrel, or β-clam? To view the fatty acid, select hetero-ligand and display as spacefill with colour CPK. Now select protein-protein and display as spacefill with colour chain. Is the fatty acid well enclosed by its binding protein?

Tertiary protein structure refers to the complete three dimensional folding of a protein. Stabilization of a protein's tertiary structure may involve interactions between amino acids located far apart along the primary sequence. These may include:

- Weak interactions such as hydrogen bonds and Van der Waals interactions.
- Ionic bonds involving negatively charged and positively charged amino acid side-chain groups.
- Disulfide bonds, covalent linkages that may form as the thiol groups of two cysteine residues are oxidized to a disulfide: 2 R-SH → R-S-S-R.

Interactions with the aqueous solvent, known as the hydrophobic effect results in residues with non-polar side-chains typically being buried in the interior of a protein. Conversely, polar amino acid side-chains tend to on the surface of a protein where they are exposed to the aqueous milieu.

There are, however, many exceptions in which polar residues are buried or non-polar residues exposed on the surface of a protein. Such atypical locations might be stabilized, *e.g.,* by interaction of amino acid side-chains with enzyme prosthetic groups or other ligands, by interactions between amino acid side-chains, or by association of proteins with lipid membranes.

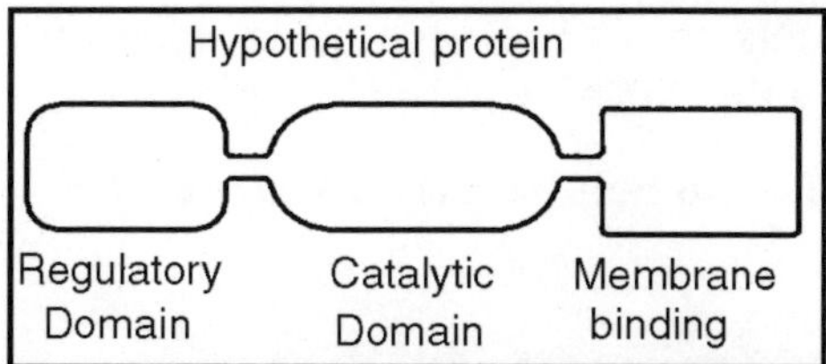

Many proteins have a modular design with multiple distinct domains resulting from gene fusion events during evolution. A domain with a particular structure and function may be part of the structure of several otherwise distinct proteins. For example, an enzyme's primary structure may include a segment that folds to produce an active site with particular catalytic activity, plus other segments that may mediate regulation of the enzyme or binding of the enzyme to a membrane.

Quaternary protein structure refers to the regular association of two or more polypeptide chains to form a complex. A multi-subunit protein may be composed of two or more identical polypeptides, or it may include different polypeptides. Quaternary structure tends to be stabilized mainly by weak interactions between residues exposed on surfaces polypeptides within a complex.

A multimeric complex may be important to enzyme activity, *e.g.*, in cases in which an active site is formed by residues from more than one polypeptide subunit, or when adjacent active sites may be involved sequentially in catalysis of a complex reaction.

Regulation of functional activity may involve cooperative interactions among protein subunits in a complex. Examples of these are included throughout.

PROTEIN STRUCTURE

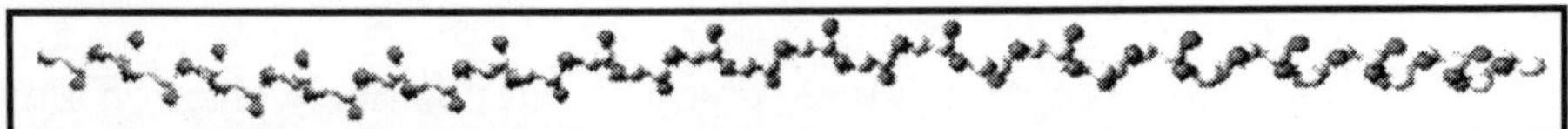

Low-Tech (but very Instructive) Preliminary Exercises

- Use your organic-chemistry model kit to build a model of hexa-alanine, ala_6. Restrict the peptides bonds to the planar, trans, conformation by making the peptide bond a double bond.
- By rotation about single bonds involving the alpha carbons, adjust the conformation of your model to form an alpha helix.
- Identify hydrogen bonds that would stabilize this helix.
- Break the model into two models of tri-alanine, ala_3. By rotation about single bonds involving the alpha carbons, adjust the conformations of both models to form extended, or beta, structure.
- Align the models antiparallel to each other. Identify hydrogen bonds that would stabilize this little two-stranded pleated sheet.
- Align the models parallel to each other. Identify hydrogen bonds that would stabilize this little two-stranded pleated sheet.

Some Simple Structures (to help you read your text)

Collagen

Study 1bkv.pdb and explore it with Deep as you read the description of collagen in your textbook.

Silk Fibroin

Study SilkFib.pdb and explore it with Deep as you read the description of beta keratins in your textbook.

Fun With Polypeptide Conformation

First, read the material in your text about conformational angles in polypeptides (look up Ramachandran diagram). This exercise will reward you with a better understanding of backbone conformation, and the meaning of the phi and psi conformational angles. If you have not already completed the graphics exercises for the topic Amino Acids, do so now before continuing.

Build:Remove Hydrogens (all)). In the Control Panel, all residues should be selected (red). If not, select them. Then Wind:Ramachandran Plot. Move and resize the plot so that you can see the graphics and the Control Panel.

Each dot on the Rama plot represents one residue in oxytocin. They dot lies at values of phi (horizontal axis) and psi (vertical axis) that correspond to the conformational angles on either side of the alpha carbon of that residue.

Touch the cursor to a dot the name and number of the residue appears in the upper left corner of the window. Now select residues 7, 8, and 9 only, and press the return key. Only three residues remain on the screen, and only three dots remain on the plot. On the Rama plot, find the dot for LEU8. You can restrict changes to phi only by holding down"9" while you drag. Holding down"0" (zero) restricts the movement to changing psi.

Now use these tools to explore the following questions:

- What three bonds and four atoms are involved in the dihedral angle phi for LEU8?
- What three bonds and four atoms are involved in psi?
- Get a sense of what"postive and negative conformation angles" means, as follows:

If you look down the middle bond of phi (LEU8-N in front, LEU8-C-alpha behind), and increase phi (move dot to right), do the atoms on the far end of the bond rotate clockwise or counterclockwise?

- If you look down the middle bond of psi (LEU8-C-alpha in front LEU8-CO behind), and increase psi (move dot up), do the atoms on the far end of the bond rotate clockwise or counterclockwise?

Now for some conformational fun. Select: All and press return to display the whole model. It's probably a mess now after your previous tweaking. Turn off all side chains by removing their checkmarks in the Control Panel. Now all dots are on the Rama plot. Find the dot for ILE3 in the lower right corner of the yellow region at the lower left of the plot (phi ~ -30, psi ~ -30). Drag all the other dots onto this one.

Now centre and look at your model:

- The backbone of you model now forms a helix. Is this helix right- or left-handed? Consult your text on the subject of alpha helices.
- Study all the dots into the smallest region (right side of plot, phi ~ +30, psi ~ +60). Again you have a helix. Is it right- or left-handed?
- Study all the dots to phi ~ 180, psi ~ 180. What secondary structure has this conformation?

Guided Tour of Cytochrome b_5 (PDB 1cyo)

Our classroom introduction to the three-dimensional structure of proteins begins with a guided tour of the cytoplasmic domain of cytochrome b_5. You can take this tour again, and move off its path at any time to explore in your own way, by downloading the file provided below.

The cytochrome-b_5 model presented here is an 87-residue, water-soluble fragment that was proteolytically cleaved from an approximately 50-residue domain that anchors the protein in the membrane of the endoplasmic reticulum of mammalian liver cells. This cleavage was necessary in order to crystllize the protein and determine its structure by x-ray crystallography.

Intact cytochrome b_5 takes part in liver fatty-acid metabolism. By way of its heme-iron prosthetic group, cytochrome b_5 accepts electrons from an NADPH-containing enzyme, and then passes them to a second enzyme (a desaturase) that removes double bonds from fatty acids by reduction.

The 87-residue fragment that you will explore contains the heme-iron prosthetic group, and despite its separation from its membrane anchor, is fully functional.

Although very small, this protein illustrates many of fundamental concepts of protein structure. This tour treats aspects of primary, secondary, and tertiary structure. I will discuss quaternary structure in the views concerning protein function.

Exploring

A Swiss-PdbViewer project file containing 8 different views of the cytoplasmic domain of cytochrome b_5. Each view (or layer) is the starting point for exploring a different aspect of protein structure.

Swiss-PdbViewer 3.5 or later is Required for Viewing this File

After the file opens in Swiss-PdbViewer, press the"=" key to centre the view. Display the Layer Infos window (Wind: Layer Infos) and move the window to a convenient location.

Hold down the control key and press tab repeatedly until the first layer, labeled 3B5C, is highlighted in the Layer Infos window. Then begin exploring the structure.

To move to the next view, press control - tab. Do not change the selected residues at each layer until you have carried out the excercises for that layer. If you accidently do so, quit Swiss-PdbViewer, restart it, and reopen the file. After carrying out the exercises at a layer, explore at will!

Layer 1cyo: Plain PDB File

- Rotate, translate, and zoom the structure to get a feeling for its overall shape.
- Turn off all side chains. Rotate the model and see if you can make out elements of secondary structure: helices or sheets of extended backbone.
- Find the heme group; turn side chains back on and try to identify the side chains that bind the iron ion in the centre of the heme.
- Identify residue represented by dots outside of “allowed” regions.

Layer 1cyo01: Ribbon Model

- Rotate the structure and count the number of helices and beta strands in the structure.
- Use Colour:Ribbon:Secondary Structure to confirm your count. This command colours helices red and beta strands yellow.
- Describe how the heme is contained within the elements of secondary structure.

Layer 1cyo02: Detail of Alpha Helix

- Remove the ribbon from the display and add hydrogen bonds. Confirm by counting or labeling that most of the H-bonds connect the backbone carbonyl oxygen of residue n with the amide hydrogen of residue n+4.
- Add side chains to the helix. Look at the helix end-on. Can you tell, in the absence of the rest of the structure, which side of the helix is in contact with the interior of the protein?
- Add van der Waals surface dots to the helix. Note that the helix is quite compact and dense, with no empty space in its interior.
- The dots on the diagram represent the backbone conformational angles (phi and psi) for the selected residues only. Notice that all dots are within the yellow polygon at the left of centre, at conformational angles near (phi, psi) = (-60, -60). Why are all the dots in this region?

Layer 1cyo03: Detail of Beta Strands

- Remove the ribbons from the display and add hydrogen bonds. Measure the distance between Ns and Os that are sharing a hydrogen (not shown). Find a way to display all H-bond distances in one step. Notice that alternating carbonyl oxygens point in opposite directions.
- Use labels to determine whether adjacent strands are parallel or antiparallel.
- Beta sheets are twisted. Imagine yourself walking down the centre strand of this sheet, holding out your arms to point at the adjacent strands. As you walk, will you have to move your arms clockwise or counterclockwise in order to keep pointing at adjacent strands. If your answer is clockwise, then we say that the twist is righthanded.
- Display side chains. Notice that alternating side chains face opposite side of the sheet. Is this sheet amphipathic?
- Display the Ramachandran Plot. Most (but not all) of the dots are within the yellow polygon at the upper left, at conformational angles near (phi, psi) = (-120, +120). Why are most of the dots in this region?

- Slide the cursor onto a dot that does not lie in this region, and you will see the residue number of the dot in the upper left corner of the Rama Plot.

Layer 1cyo04: Locations of Hydrophobic Side Chains

- This view presents backbone atoms in white, and heme in CPK. Only hydrophobic side chains are on display. Are most of the hydrophobic side chains located on the exterior or in the interior of the protein?
- Predict the answer to this question for the membrane fragment of cytochrome b_5, which is soluble in nonpolar solvents but not water.

Layer 1cyo05: Locations of Polar Side Chains

- In this view, only polar and charged side chains are on display. What can you say about their locations?
- Can you see any patterns or clusters of positive charge (basic side chains) or negative charge (acidic side chains)?

Layer 1cyo06: Heme Environment Overview

- This view shows includes those sidechains that have an atom within 4.5 angstroms of the heme group.
- Identify and characterize the side chains that make contact with the heme.
- Add H-bonds to the view. Swiss-PdbViewer draws some funny H-bonds within the heme group. Ignore them, and look for H-bonds between heme and side chains.

Layer 1cyo07: Heme Environment in Cross-Section

- Colour in this view is green for heme, CPK for all other. Only the heme and its neighbours (within 4.5 anstroms) are on display.
- *Choose Display*: Slab (or press command -/). Now you see only those residues that have an atom within a 7-angstrom-thick slab at the centre of the view. You can move the atoms through this slab by holding down the command key while translating the model forward and back. This way of looking at the model makes it easier to see van der Waals contacts. Study the contacts between the heme and the protein.
- The heme periphery is mostly nonpolar. What forces hold it in its pocket?
- Can you imagine any other amino acid that could fit into position 41? In a comparison of cytochrome b_5 from various mammals, would you expect to find that position 41 is conserved, conservatively substituted, or hypervariable?

Take time to study with the contents of this file to deepen your understanding of basic concepts of protein structure. Quaternary Structure, Domains, Folds, and Motifs in Malate Dehydrogenase (PDB 1BMD)

A Swiss-PdbViewer project file containing 4 different views of the enzyme malate dehydrogenase (MDH). Each view (or layer) is the starting point for exploring a different aspect of protein structure.

Swiss-PdbViewer 3.5 or later is Required for Viewing this file

After the file opens in Swiss-PdbViewer, press the "=" key to centre the view. Display the Layer Infos window (Wind: Layer Infos) and move the window to a convenient location. Hold down the control key and press tab repeatedly until the first layer, labeled 1BMD.01, is highlighted in the Layer Infos window. Then begin exploring the structure. To move to the next view, press control - tab.

First, cycle the view through views 01-04 repeatedly. Each successive layer displays a smaller unit of the protein structure. In the first layer, the two subunits (separate chains) of this dimeric enzyme appear in different colours. In the next layer, you see only the A chain, divided by colour to show its two domains. Third, you see the first domain of the A chain, divided by colour to show its two similar subdomains, which are examples of folding motifs. Finally, the fourth layer shows a common motif that is part of the first subdomain. To help you keep your orientation, the cofactor NAD appears in all layers.

Layer 1bmd01

- Rotate the model until you have a clear view of the NAD in subunit A. Subunits A and B are identical protein chains. How many residues are in each?
- Simplify the view by eliminating side chains and see if you can find a two-fold axis that interchanges the two chains. Use the two molecules of NAD to guide you. When you have found the axis, align it with the Z-axis (pointing towards you) and rotate while holding down the command key, which limits rotation to the Z-axis. This rotation should interchange the subunits.
- In what sense is a description of MDH incomplete if it refers only to the primary, secondary, and tertiary structure of the enzyme?

Layer 1bmd02

- Rotate the model until you can see the residue at which the chain colour changes. This is the approximate boundary between the two domains. Can you see any other strands that cross this boundary? If so, speculate about the role of any such strands in maintaining the structural integrity of one MDH subunit.
- Which of the two domains shown is the N-terminal domain?

- Use labels to determine whether neighbouring strands are parallel or antiparallel. Do the two domains differ in their content of parallel and antiparallel strands?
- Would you say that the two domains are similar or dissimilar in overall fold?

Layer 1bmd03

- The N-terminal domain of the A subunit is shown divided by colours into its two subdomains (each a $\beta\alpha\beta\alpha\beta$ motif). The fold of this full domain is found in many proteins that bind nucleotides. In fact, it is often called the nucleotide-binding fold (or the Rossmann fold, for Michael Rossmann of Purdue University, who first recognized it as a feature common to several different enzymes).
- Notice the alpha helix that points directly at the pyrophosphate group of NAD. This is a common feature of the nucleotide-binding fold. Common structural features are usually stable ones. What stabilizes this feature?
- Would you say that the two subdomains of the Rossmann fold are similar or dissimilar in their overall fold?
- Find a rough two-fold axis that interchanges the two subdomains.

Layer 1bmd04

- This small portion of malate dehydrogenase is a beta-alpha-beta motif. Are the two beta strands parallel or antiparallel?
- The alpha helix crosses from one end of this two-strand sheet to the other. Crossovers between successive strands of parallel pleated sheet are usually right-handed. Try to view the entire backbone of this little fold as about one and one-half turns of a very irregular helix. Is this crude helix right- or left-handed? Stereo viewing will help a lot!

Do not change the selected residues at each layer until you have carried out the excercises for that layer.

If you accidently do so, quit Swiss-PdbViewer, restart it, and reopen the file.

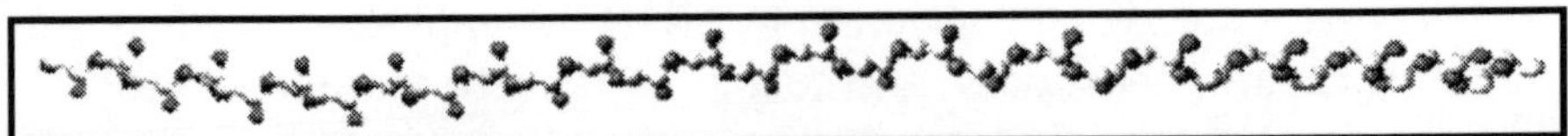

At pH 7, so-called "acidic" side chains like those of glu and asp are unprotonated and negatively charged (pH is higher than their pKa values, so they have already given up their protons as good acids do). So they are actually weak bases. So-called "basic" side chains are protonated and positively charged, so they are actually weak acids at pH 7. Confusing, huh? In most cases, a group is called "acidic" if its neutral form is an acid (for example, R-COOH), and "basic" if its neutral form is a base. It's more important to know the ionization state, including the charge, of the side chain at the pH in question. Then you can infer whether it will act as an acid or base.

PROTEIN/PEPTIDE SEPARATION TECHNIQUES

PROTEIN SEPARATION

While mass spectrometry has become the method of choice for the identification of proteins, several alternative appropraches are being employed for the separation of complex mixtures that precedes their MS analysis. Traditionally, the most fequently applied protein separation strategy has been on two-dimensional polyacrylamide gel electrophoresis, a technique that has the ability to separate up to 10,000 components. While the independent manual digestion of multiple gel spots is time-consuming, robotic digestion can imporve this limitation.

In the last few years, enzymatic digestion of useparated protein mixtures followed by spearation of peptides by multidimentional liquid chormatography (LC) has been used as an alterative. Among other beneifts, this LC-based approach lends itself to automated peptide separation together with the acquisition and analysis of MS data.

Despite concerns regarding the perils of factionation to proteins, fractionating proteomes for analysis has an overriding advantage in that it simplies them. One's ability detect multiple protein species in a sample depends on one's ability to resolve many peptides from the sample and obtain MS data on as many of them as possible.

Selection of a subcellular fraction (*e.g.,* the mitochondria) for analysis reduces the task from analysis of perhaps 25k proteins in a human cell sample to about 1000-2000. There is a better chance of identifying less abundant proteins when they are present in a mixture of 1000 proteins then when they are in a mixture of 14K.

ELECTROPHORESIS

Electrophoresis is used to separate complex mixtures of proteins (*e.g.,* from cells) to investigate subunit compositions and to purify the protein for subsequent applications. In polyacrylamide gel electrophoresis, proteins migrate due to an electrical field through pores in the gel matrix. Pore size decreases with higher acrylamide concentrations. The migrations of the protein is determined by the gel pore size and protein charges, size and shape.

One dimensional gel (1-D) electrophoresis under denaturing conditions (*i.e.,* in the presence of 0.1per cent SDS) separates proteins based on molecular size. Most proteins bind SDS in a constant weight ratio, leading to identical charge densities for the denatured proteins. Thus the SDS protein complexes migrate in the polyacrylamide gel according to size, not charge. Most proteins are resolved on polyacrylamide gels containing from 5per cent to 15per cent acrylamide. The relationship between the relative mobility and log molecular weight is linear over these ranges. After the proteins are solubilized by boiling in the presence of SDS, an aliquot of the protein solution is applied to a gel lane, and the individual proteins are separated electrophoretically. 2-mercaptoethanol is added during solubilization to reduce disulfide bonds. Comparison of reducing and nonreducing gels can provide valuable information about the number of disulfide cross linked subunits in a protein complex. If the subunits are held together by disulfide linkages, the protein will separate in denaturing gels as smaller sized subunits as compared to nonreducing conditions where the protein will separate as a complex.

The polyacrylamide gel is cast as a separating gel topped by a stacking gel and secured in an electrophoresis apparatus. After leaving the stacking gel, the protein enters the separating gel which has a smaller pore size, a higher salt concentration and higher pH compared to the stacking gel. The proteins are separated according to either molecular size in a denaturing gel (containing SDS) or molecular shape, size, and charge in a nondenaturing gel.

Two-dimensional (2-D) gel electrophoresis separates proteins in the first dimension by isoelectric focusing and in the second dimension by electrophoresis in the presence of SDS. Thus information is obtained not only about size as in one-dimensional gels but also about the charge of the protein. In isoelectric focusing a pH gradient is established using ampholines. Proteins migrate to their isoelectric point (pH) at which there is no net charge.

The protein spots can be visualized by staining. An imaging system is used to record an image of the stained gel to provide a record of the protein distribution in the sample. These images can be analysed, compared, and archived with software packages.

A concern with 2D gels is that despite their resolving power, 2D gels do not completely resolve all proteins into single spots. Many spots contain 2-5 proteins. Another concern is that even with the most sensitive stains, there is a limited dynamic range for protein detection. Cellular expression levels of different proteins can differ by as much as a million-fold whereas the dynamic range for protein staining is about 100-2000 fold. Thus, 2D gels typically detect only the most abundantly expressed proteins.

In a powerful technique, 2D-SDS-PAGE is combined with a high-throuput MS analytical method (MALDI-TOF MS). In gel digestion is used to cleave the proteins to peptides which are then analysed by MALDI-TOF MS. The MS data is then analysed with a peptide mass fingerprinting algorithm and software which identifies the proteins present. A second approach is to use peptide sequence identification by tandem MS. Here, one digests the proteins in the mixture to peptides which are then resolved (at least partially) by chromatography and then electrospray tandem MS. These spectra are mapped to protein sequences from databases with the aid of Sequest or similar search tools. The 2 distingushing characteristics of this approach are 1) the analysis primarily involves working with peptides rather than with proteins and the protein identification is based on the MS-MS fragmentation spectra, rather than on peptide mass fingerprinting.

Western blotting is used to identify a specific protein in a complex mixture of proteins. The technique exploits both the efficiency of SDS-PAGE to separate a mixture of proteins into distinct protein bands, adn the ability of immunochemical reagents to interact specifically with a given protein antigen.

A typical Western-blotting protocol incluces the following steps:

- The mixture is first electrophoretically separated on a polyacrylamide slab gel in the presence of SDS.
- The protein bands are then transferred to a nitrocellulose membrane by electrophoresis.
- The membrane contianing the protein bands is serially incubated with
  - A suitable blocking reagent to prevent non-specific protein binding,
  - A wash solution to rinse any unbound blocking reagent
  - A probing antibody (anti-protein-of interest antibody) that forms a specific immune complex with Protein-of interst,
  - Additional wash solution to remove any unbound antibody,
  - An enzyme-linked antibody that binds specifically to the Fc region of the anti-protein-of interest antibody,
  - additional wash solution to remoe any unbound enzyme-lined anntibody and finally,
  - A substrate solution, which int he presence of the enzyme, yields an insoluble, coloured product that precipitates at the site of the immune complex, thereby rending the Protein of interest band visible.

CHROMATOGRAPHY

Column Chromatography can be used to fractionate proteins. The mixture of proteins in solution is passed through a column containing a porous solid matrix.

The 3 types of matrices used are:

- Ion-exchange chromatography,
- Gel-filtration chromatography
- Affinity chromatography
  - Ion-exchange chromatography uses an insoluble matrix that carries ionic charges that retard the movement of molecules of opposite charge. There are 2 types. anion and cation. Protein purification using ion-exchange chromatography usually employs positively charged anion exchangers because the majority of

proteins are negative charged at neutral pH (*i.e.,* have a low isoelectric point).
- Gel-Filtration Chromatography uses a porous matrix. Molecules that are small enough to penetrate into the matrix are delayed and travel more slowly through the column.
- Affinity Chromatography can be used to isolate and identify proteins that interact physically. The method takes advantage of a protein's binding site and its ligand. The ligand, when immobilized, attracts the protein from a mixture, while other molecules are washed away. Most proteins have specific ligands; For example, enzymes have subtrates and cofactors.

Beads Coated with Avidin

One often used method of affinity chromatography is to use a column containing avidin-coated beads. A sample is incubated with an antibody that is conjugated to biotin. When the sample is passed through the column the biotin binds to the avidin. This has been used to isolate hematopoietic stem cells by conjugating CD34 to biotin and passing them through the column.

High Pressure Liquid Chromatography (HPLC)

- A sample is dissolved in mobile phage
- *Column*: the sample is pumped under high pressure onto a column. Need to consider the mode of separation here (ie., adsorption, reversed phase, ion exchange).
- *Elution*: the sample is eluted through the column
- *Detection*: the eluant is monitored with a detector. Detector possibilities include UV, radiochemical, fluorescent, Mass Spec.
  A new method is evaporative light scattering where there is:
  - Nebulization (the column effluent passes through a needle, mixes with nitrogen gas and forms a dispersion of droplets,
  - Mobile phage evaporation (the droplets pass through a heated drift tube where the mobile phase evaporates, leaving a fine mist of dried sample particles
  - Detection (these sample particles pass through a flow cell where they intercept a laser light beam which scatters the light generating an electrical signal).
- *Analysis*: Data from the detectors is fed into a computer.

Multidimensional Liquid Chromatography

A sample is fed through a HPLC using a particular type of separation method, and peaks are selected and fed into a second column using a different mode of separation.

To capture interacting proteins, a target protein is attached to polymer beads that are packed into a column. Cellular proteins are washed through the column and those proteins that interact with the target adhere to the affinity matrix. These proteins can then be eluted and their identity determined by mass spectrometry or another method.

PROTEIN/PEPTIDE SEPARATION TECHNIQUES

Waters Peptide Separation Technology consists of a new unique family of columns that meet the demanding requirements of peptide separations from proteomics to peptide mapping to isolation and offer an improved chromatography of peptides and generate narrow, symmetrical peaks for best resolution.

Peptide Separation Technology provides a consistent set of chromatographic tools usable across all research and development applications that require isolation and analysis of peptides.

Peptide mapping continues to be the preferred technique for the comprehensive characterization of biopharmaceutical products. Its applications include: the identification of proteins based on the elution pattern of peptide fragments, the determination of post-translational modifications, the confirmation of genetic stability, and the analysis of protein sequences when interfaced to a mass spectrometer. In a peptide map, it is necessary to resolve each peptide fragment into a single peak.

Therefore, peptide mapping represents a significant chromatographic challenge, due to the inherent complexity of protein digests.

In addition to the large number of peptide fragments that are generated from the enzymatic digestion of a protein, the number of alternative peptide structures (*e.g.,* post-translational modifications, oxidations, etc.) can be significant..

PEPTIDE SEPARATION TECHNOLOGY COLUMNS

Peptide Separation Technology columns are based on the C18 BEH Technology™ particles and are available from size 1.7 μm to 10 μm. The range of column dimensions spans from I.D. of 75 μm to 30 mm and lengths from 50 to 250 mm. There are over 100 standard columns and others can be custom prepared. There is no need for compromise in matching the column to the application.

These columns not only meet the demanding specifications for the BEH Technology particles, but also are specifically QC certified with a peptide map. These controls ensure the stability of well-developed peptide separation methods used in biotechnology development as well as predictable Behaviour with the many different samples encountered in proteomics, protein characterization and in peptide synthesis.

The surface chemistry of all particle sizes, in either 130Å or 300Å pore sizes, gives sharp symmetrical peaks over a wide range of peptide properties and application requirements. Peptide Separation Technology columns are integral elements of Waters Assured Performance Solutions, combinations of instrumentation, chemistry and software optimized for particular applications.

Peptide mapping for protein characterization requires the best possible chromatographic resolution. In addition to the large number of fragments that are generated from the enzymatic digestion of a protein, the number of alternative structures (*e.g.* post-translational modifications, deamidation, etc.) can be sizeable. Since these maps are often used to measure small amounts of modifications, a wide linear dynamic range must be preserved with the highest possible resolution. Optimized mapping methods are often used for QC of biopharmaceuticals so stability of the analytical method requires long term column-to-column and batch-to-batch reproducibility.

HIGH RESOLUTION FOR SUPERIOR ANALYSES

The surface chemistry of Peptide Separation Technology columns minimizes secondary interactions with peptides. Narrow symmetrical peaks are observed across a wide range of peptide properties. This results in the highest resolution across the entire peptide map.

USE UV OR MS DETECTION WITHOUT COMPROMISE IN PERFORMANCE

Historically, the best peptide separations have been obtained with TFA as a mobile phase additive because it combines ion-pairing and ion-suppression for symmetrical peak shape and good resolution. TFA may, however, cause significant signal suppression in ESI/MS so formic acid may be preferred for LC/MS methods. Specialized "no TFA" columns are often required to preserve chromatographic performance. Peptide Separation Technology columns show minimal differences in performance between TFA and formic acid.

The expected changes in selectivity from mobile phase changes will still be easily recognized. UV or MS detection can be used; there is no need to compromise performance or change columns.

Improved quantitation of modified peptides Peptide mapping is used to quantitate the amount of modified protein in a sample. This application requires that variant peptides be separated from the normal peptides.

The higher resolution and increased sensitivity delivered by the Peptide Separation Technology columns allow modified peptides to be seen at lower levels because they are more easily separated from the unmodified peptides.

IMPROVED SEPARATIONS OF GLYCOPEPTIDES

Glycoproteins show significant microheterogeneity at a single glycosylation site. Analyzing this population of glycans is challenging because glycopeptides often elute as broad, overlapping peaks. The surface chemistry of Peptide Separation Technology columns yield sharper and more symmetrical peaks to simplify the analysis.

UNMATCHED REPRODUCIBILITY FOR INCREASED DATA CONFIDENCE

All Peptide Separation columns are QC-tested and certified using a protein digest. This level of testing ensures that a peptide mapping method developed today can be performed with the same results with a column purchased years from now.

SIGNIFICANT IMPROVEMENTS FOR PEPTIDE MAPPING WITH UPLC

Peptide Separation Technology ACQUITY UPLC columns are part of the UPLC Peptide Analysis Solution. This total system solution combines instrumentation, software, and chemistry for unmatched performance in separating complex peptide samples.

The unique surface chemistry of the Peptide Separation Technology columns yields even sharper peaks and better resolution when used as sub 2-μm particles on instruments that are fully optimized for Ultra Performance LC™. Scientists can be confident of high-quality performance in protein characterization when using this full system application solution.

PROTEIN PURIFICATION

Isolating a protein of interest in sufficiently pure form is an essential step prior to any structural and functional characterization of any proteins of interest. Low or high pressure liquid chromatography is the preferred method for protein purification.

This can be a simple one-step procedure exploiting the binding affinity of or for a protein of interest, or a laborious multistep process that takes advantage of differences in protein size and physico-chemical properties. Protein separations can range from nano, capillary, micro, analytical to preparative scale and often involves fraction collection for subsequent work.

Dionex offers next generation protein purification HPLC systems and an outstanding array of column innovations that addresses every facet of protein purifications; the high resolution that is mandated in nano scale separation for biomarker discovery to high capacity required at preparative scale; for the research scientists that demand highest application flexibility, to highly specialized and regulated purification of recombinant protein and monoclonal antibody therapeutics where robustness, reliability,and throughput is considered absolutely necessary.

PROTEIN MASS SPECTROMETRY

New mass spectrometric methods developed over the last several years have led to the establishment of mass spectrometry as a powerful technique for protein structure determination. Key to this development was the introduction of fast atom bombardment (FAB) ionization which permitted production of intact molecular ions from peptides and small proteins as well as from other labile biological molecules. Other ionization methods (electrospray ionization [ESI], matrix assisted laser desorption ionization [MALDI]) have subsequently been developed which have been demonstrated to permit measurement of protein molecular weights in excess of several hundred thousand daltons.

In combination with these new ionization methods, tandem mass spectrometry permits amino acid sequencing of peptide fragments of proteins as well as characterization of posttranslational modifications. Mass spectrometry therefore provides a means of determining the complete primary structure of a protein. Use of chemical modifications in conjunction with mass spectrometric analysis provides a means of gaining information on the three dimensional structure as well. The use of mass spectrometry in the study of the various aspects of protein structure is discussed in more detail on subsequent pages.

MOLECULAR WEIGHT DETERMINATION

All three of the major approaches to mass spectrometric determination of the molecular weights of intact proteins are available in the Medical University of South Carolina Mass Spectrometry Laboratory. These include FAB (the term as used here also includes cesium ion bombardment), electrospray ionization (ESI), and matrix assisted laser desorption ionization (MALDI). The JEOL HX110/HX110 tandem mass spectrometer is equipped with a high voltage (35 kV.) cesium gun and has a mass range of 14,500. Molecular weights of proteins in excess of 10,000 daltons have been successfully determined on this magnetic sector type instrument using FAB ionization. The resolution and mass accuracy of the JEOL instrument is such that the molecular weights can be determined to better than a single mass unit. In practice the protein is applied as a solution (on the order of 1 microliter) to the tip of a sample probe and mixed with a matrix liquid (*e.g.* glycerol, thioglycerol or nitrobenzyl alcohol). The probe is then inserted into the mass spectrometer and the sample bombarded with high energy cesium ions to sputter off intact (usually protonated) molecular ions of the protein in the sample. The ions are then accelerated into the mass spectrometer and the mass to charge ratio determined. Since one is usually observing singly charged ions, the result is a direct measurement of molecular weight. A pure sample is not necessary, and it is possible to measure molecular weights of multiple components of a mixture although competition effects can cause some components to be observed more easily than others. Buffer salts and detergents can impede the observation of sample components; optimal samples are those collected from a reversed phase HPLC separation.

Electrospray ionization permits measurement of much larger molecular weights by virtue of the fact that it produces multiply charged ions. Since mass spectrometers normally measure mass to charge ratio, increasing the number of charges on the ion effectively multiplies the mass range of the instrument. Mass measurement accuracy on the order of 0.01per cent is possible with this technique. In practice the sample is introduced into the ion source in a liquid stream containing an organic modifier and an acid delivered from a pump driven microliter syringe or as an HPLC effluent. A variety of acids and concentrations are used in ESI; a typical solvent system for discrete samples is 50per cent methanol in water containing 5per cent acetic acid. Buffer salts and ionic detergents must be avoided since they can dominate the ion current and prevent observation of the protein. Since electrospray ionization gives multiple peaks for each protein, mixtures can give very complex spectra. Algorithms have been developed to resolve the complex mixtures of multiply charged ion peaks into a spectrum with a true mass scale and one peak per component, but the technique works best with relatively pure samples.

Matrix assisted laser desorption (MALDI) mass spectrometry permits measurement of still larger molecular weights. In this technique, the sample is mixed with a UV absorbing matrix compound (commonly sinapinic acid) typically in a 30per cent aqueous acetonitrile solution, and 1-3 microliters of the solution is dried on the end of a sample probe or as a spot on a sample plate. The dried sample is then inserted into the mass spectrometer and the sample mixture exposed to the focussed beam from a pulsed UV laser.

Absorption of the laser energy by the matrix results in ejection of intact molecular ions of the protein. The ions produced are typically singly charged, therefore the mass analyser must be of a different type to measure very large masses. A time-of-flight analyser is used to measure mass by measuring the time it takes for an ion, after electrostatic acceleration, to travel from the ion source to the detector.

Heavier ions travel slower, hence, by measuring long times, the mass range of this type of analyser is theoretically unlimited. Molecular weights as high as 160,000 have been measured on our home built instrument with mass measurement errors less than 1per cent (less than 0.1per cent for masses under 20,000). The newly installed (11/96) commercial instrument will provide higher performance. The MALDI technique is applicable to mixture analysis and is less affected than ESI by the presence of salts or ionic detergents.

DETERMINATION OF PRIMARY STRUCTURE

The first step is to determine the molecular weight of the intact protein. This can be done using either FAB, electrospray, or matrix assisted laser desorption mass spectrometry. Knowledge of the molecular weight of the intact protein is necessary to be sure that the entire protein is accounted for in analyzing fragments of the protein.

The next step is to cleave the protein into smaller fragments and determine the amino acid sequence of each fragment. If the protein contains cysteine residues, it is normally subjected to reduction and carboxymethylation of the cysteine sulfhydryl groups prior to cleavage (alternatively carboxamidomethyl or pyridylethyl derivatives may be prepared). Cleavage is then performed either chemically or enzymatically.

Large proteins are usually cleaved in two stages: a first cleavage is performed at relatively low abundance sites (step 2a, *e.g.* cyanogen bromide cleavage at methionine residues) to yield large fragments which are separated and then cleaved at more abundant sites (step 2b, *e.g.* trypsin cleavage at lysines and arginines).

Smaller proteins can be initially cleaved at higher abundance sites. The cleavage mixtures are then separated into simpler mixtures by HPLC (step 2c). Unlike with Edman degradation where it is necessary to individually purify each degradation product, the mass spectrometric approach can be carried out with mixtures of cleavage fragments.

The fractionation into simpler mixtures is done to overcome potential competitive effects in the ionization process to increase the probability of observing all of the fragments in the mass spectrometer. The fragment mixtures are first subjected to single stage mass spectrometry to determine the molecular weights of the fragments (step 2d) and then analysed by tandem mass spectrometry (step 2e) to determine the amino acid sequence of each fragment.

LENS AQUAPORIN 0 STRUCTURE IN AGING AND CATARACTOGENESIS

We examine the posttranslational modifications to the most abundant lens membrane protein, Aquaporin 0 (also known as the lens major intrinsic protein, MIP). Numerous modifications have been identified by mass spectrometry.

A goal of this research is to determine those modifications which lead to lens opacification through structural studies of human lenses and through functional assays of recombinant modified protein. Additional areas of interest involve protein-protein interactions of lens proteins with Aquaporin 0, changes in the lens membrane proteome with age and cataractogenesis, and lens protein oxidation.

MEMBRANE PROTEINS

As stated above, integral membrane proteins present greater challenges not only for the mass spectrometry, but also for the preceding peptide chemistry. The MUSC laboratory has a particular interest in membrane receptor proteins. Work is underway to develop improved procedures for protein cleavage and sample preparation for mass spectrometry of integral membrane proteins and their peptide cleavage products. Recent developments in HPLC separations of cyanogen bromide cleavage products promise to greatly expedite our work on membrane proteins.

SAMPLE REQUIREMENTS

The molecular weight of a protein can usually be obtained with a few picomoles by electrospray or laser desorption techniques if the protein has favourable solubility properties. Sample quantity requirements in these cases are usually dictated more by sample manipulation requirements than by the low femptomole actual sample consumption in the measurement. Hydrophobic proteins, particularly integral membrane proteins, present greater difficulty; however, we have developed methodology which permits analysis of intact integral membrane proteins by MALDI. Molecular weight measurement of smaller proteins and peptides (under ca. 2000 mass units) by FAB ionization can often be obtained with low picomole amounts of material. Larger species usually require larger amounts due to the greater difficulty of producing ions from larger molecules. Extremely hydrophobic or extremely hydrophilic molecules tend to be difficult to ionize by FAB, but the problem can often be overcome by forming a more favourable chemical derivative.

ESI and MALDI generally require less sample. Tandem mass spectrometry requires significantly more sample than that required for molecular weight measurement. Present collision dissociation technology limits the ability to obtain complete sequences of peptides by tandem mass spectrometry to peptides under molecular weight of about 2500-3000 (approximately 25-30 amino acids). Partial sequence information can often be obtained, however, for larger peptides. With a peptide of molecular weight 2000 for which the molecular ion could be measured with picomole amounts, as much as two orders of magnitude more sample could be needed to obtain a good tandem mass spectrum.

Use of the array detector on the four sector instrument and use of the new ion trap instrument should significantly reduce these sample requirements. Since the current technology for tandem mass spectrometric sequencing requires peptide fragments of 25-30 amino acids or less, sequencing of a protein requires that it be cleaved into smaller fragments. The sample size requirement for sequencing a protein is therefore dictated not only by the mass spectrometry but also by the preceding peptide chemistry.

Due to the practical aspects of sample manipulations in cleaving and isolating peptide fragments one should expect to require as much as nanomole to tens of nanomole amounts for small proteins in the 10-15,000 molecular weight range (tens to hundreds of micrograms). In theory a larger protein should not require any more sample on a molar basis, but the increasing complexity of the problem with larger proteins can lead to need for more sample.

It should be emphasized that while state of the art Edman sequencing can claim smaller sample requirements, the mass spectrometric methods do not require individual purification of each peptide fragment (which leads to a practical requirement for more sample). Furthermore, most Edman sequencing facilities do not operate at state of the art sensitivity for real samples. The above discussion of sample quantity requirements for tandem mass spectrometry relates primarily to sector type tandem instruments employing a point detector.

The new scanning array detector on the MUSC four sector instrument is expected to be fully operational soon (11/96). Use of an array detector can increase sensitivity by as much as two orders of magnitude. The new (11/96) LCQ instrument is also expected to require significanly less sample. Two orders of magnitude improvement in instrument sensitivity does not necessarily directly translate to two orders of magnitude lower sample requirement, however, since sample manipulation limitations become more significant with extremely small samples.

The answer to the question of how much sample is required is therefore not a firm figure. Every sample is a different molecular species with different properties, and the technology is constantly evolving. It can safely be said, however, that even with the current state of the art in protein and peptide mass spectrometry, the limitations lie more in the practical aspects of sample handling and peptide chemistry than with the mass spectrometry itself.

Another issue with respect to sample size requirement is that of the question being approached. For example, if the objective is to obtain some partial sequences for DNA probe construction, the sample requirement can be far less than would be required for full sequencing.

INTRODUCTION

WHAT IS MASS SPECTROMETRY

Mass spectrometry is an analytical tool used for measuring the molecular mass of a sample.

For large samples such as biomolecules, molecular masses can be measured to within an accuracy of 0.01per cent of the total molecular mass of the sample *i.e.* within a 4 Daltons (Da) or atomic mass units (amu) error for a sample of 40,000 Da. This is sufficient to allow minor mass changes to be detected, *e.g.* the substitution of one amino acid for another, or a post-translational modification.

For small organic molecules the molecular mass can be measured to within an accuracy of 5 ppm or less, which is often sufficient to confirm the molecular formula of a compound, and is also a standard requirement for publication in a chemical journal.

Structural information can be generated using certain types of mass spectrometers, usually those with multiple analysers which are known as tandem mass spectrometers.

This is achieved by fragmenting the sample inside the instrument and analysing the products generated. This procedure is useful for the structural elucidation of organic compounds and for peptide or oligonucleotide sequencing.

WHERE ARE MASS SPECTROMETERS USED

Mass spectrometers are used in industry and academia for both routine and research purposes. The following list is just a brief summary of the major mass spectrometric applications:

- *Biotechnology*: The analysis of proteins, peptides, oligonucleotides
- *Pharmaceutical*: Drug discovery, combinatorial chemistry, pharmacokinetics, drug metabolism
- *Clinical*: Neonatal screening, haemoglobin analysis, drug testing
- *Environmental*: PAHs, PCBs, water quality, food contamination
- *Geological*: Oil composition

HOW CAN MASS SPECTROMETRY HELP BIOCHEMISTS

- *Accurate molecular weight measurements*: sample confirmation, to determine the purity of a sample, to verify amino acid substitutions, to detect post-translational modifications, to calculate the number of disulphide bridges
- *Reaction monitoring*: to monitor enzyme reactions, chemical modification, protein digestion
- *Amino acid sequencing*: sequence confirmation, de novo characterisation of peptides, identification of proteins by database searching with a sequence "tag" from a proteolytic fragment
- *Oligonucleotide sequencing*: the characterisation or quality control of oligonucleotides
- *Protein structure*: protein folding monitored by H/D exchange, protein-ligand complex formation under physiological conditions, macromolecular structure determination

HOW DOES A MASS SPECTROMETER WORK

INTRODUCTION

Mass spectrometers can be divided into three fundamental parts, namely the ionisation source, the analyser, and the detector.

The sample has to be introduced into the ionisation source of the instrument. Once inside the ionisation source, the sample molecules are ionised, because ions are easier to manipulate than neutral molecules.

These ions are extracted into the analyser region of the mass spectrometer where they are separated according to theirmass (m) -to-charge (z) ratios (m/z). The separated ions are detected and this signal sent to a data system where the m/z ratios are stored together with their relative abundance for presentation in the format of a m/z spectrum.

The analyser and detector of the mass spectrometer, and often the ionisation source too, are maintained under high vacuum to give the ions a reasonable chance of travelling from one end of the instrument to the other without any hindrance from air molecules. The entire operation of the mass spectrometer, and often the sample introduction process also, is under complete data system control on modern mass spectrometers.

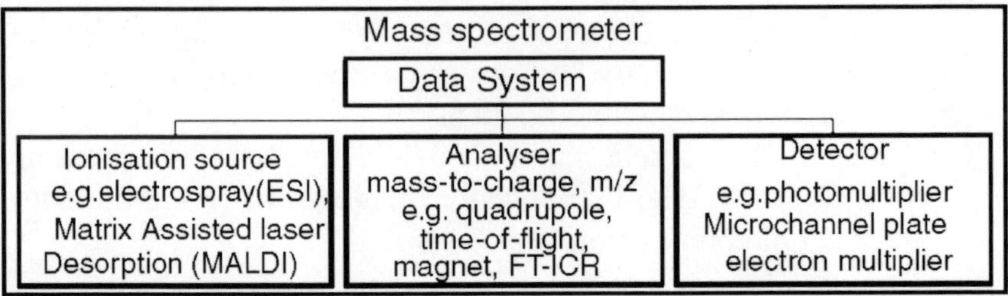

SIMPLIFIED SCHEMATIC OF A MASS SPECTROMETER

The method of sample introduction to the ionisation source often depends on the ionisation method being used, as well as the type and complexity of the sample. The sample can be inserted directly into the ionisation source, or can undergo some type of chromatography en route to the ionisation source.

This latter method of sample introduction usually involves the mass spectrometer being coupled directly to a high pressure liquid chromatography (HPLC), gas chromatography (GC) or capillary electrophoresis (CE) separation column, and hence the sample is separated into a series of components which then enter the mass spectrometer sequentially for individual analysis.

METHODS OF SAMPLE IONISATION

Many ionisation methods are available and each has its own advantages and disadvantages ("Ionization Methods in Organic Mass Spectrometry")

The ionisation method to be used should depend on the type of sample under investigation and the mass spectrometer available. Ionisation methods include the following:

- Atmospheric Pressure Chemical Ionisation (APCI)
- Chemical Ionisation (CI)
- Electron Impact (EI)
- Electrospray Ionisation (ESI)
- Fast Atom Bombardment (FAB)
- Field Desorption/Field Ionisation (FD/FI)
- Matrix Assisted Laser Desorption Ionisation (MALDI)
- Thermospray Ionisation (TSP)

The ionisation methods used for the majority of biochemical analyses are Electrospray Ionisation (ESI) and Matrix Assisted Laser Desorption Ionisation (MALDI).

With most ionisation methods there is the possibility of creating both positively and negatively charged sample ions, depending on the proton affinity of the sample. Before embarking on an analysis, the user must decide whether to detect the positively or negatively charged ions.

ANALYSIS AND SEPARATION OF SAMPLE IONS

The main function of the mass analyser is to separate, or resolve, the ions formed in the ionisation source of the mass spectrometer according to their mass-to-charge (m/z) ratios. There are a number of mass analysers currently available, the better known of which include quadrupoles, time-of-flight (TOF) analysers,magnetic sectors, and both Fourier transform and quadrupole ion traps.

These mass analysers have different features, including the m/z range that can be covered, the mass accuracy, and the achievable resolution. The compatibility of different analysers with different ionisation methods varies. For example, all of the analysers listed above can be used in conjunction with electrospray ionisation, whereas MALDI is not usually coupled to a quadrupole analyser.

Tandem (MS-MS) mass spectrometers are instruments that have more than one analyser and so can be used for structural and sequencing studies. Two, three and four analysers have all been incorporated into commercially available tandem instruments, and the analysers do not necessarily have to be of the same type, in which case the instrument is a hybrid one. More popular tandem mass spectrometers include those of the quadrupole-quadrupole, magnetic sector-quadrupole, and more recently, the quadrupole-time-of-flight geometries.

DETECTION AND RECORDING OF SAMPLE IONS

The detector monitors the ion current, amplifies it and the signal is then transmitted to the data system where it is recorded in the form of mass spectra. The m/z values of the ions are plotted against their intensities to show the number of components in the sample, the molecular mass of each component, and the relative abundance of the various components in the sample.

The type of detector is supplied to suit the type of analyser; the more common ones are the photomultiplier, the electron multiplier and the micro-channel platedetectors.

ELECTROSPRAY IONIZATION

ELECTROSPRAY IONIZATION

Electrospray Ionisation (ESI) is one of the Atmospheric Pressure Ionisation (API) techniques and is well-suited to the analysis of polar molecules ranging from less than 100 Da to more than 1,000,000 Da in molecular mass.

During standard electrospray ionisation (J. Fenn, J. Phys. Chem., 1984, 88, 4451), the sample is dissolved in a polar, volatile solvent and pumped through a narrow,stainless steel capillary (75 - 150 micrometers i.d.) at a flow rate of between 1 L/min and 1 mL/min.

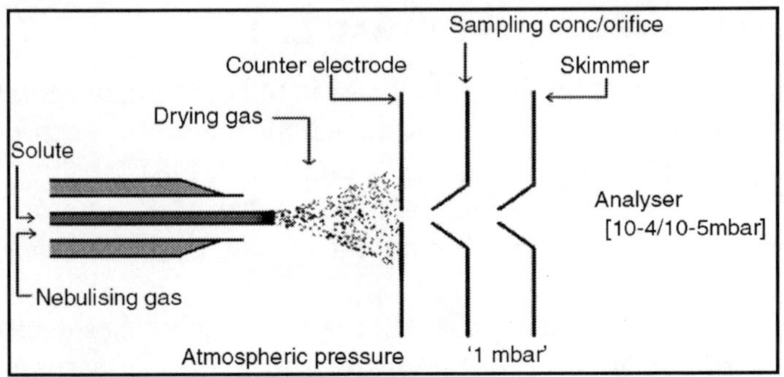

Fig. Standard Electrospray Ionisation Source (Platform II)

A high voltage of 3 or 4 kV is applied to the tip of the capillary, which is situated within the ionisation source of the mass spectrometer, and as a consequence of this strong electric field, the sample emerging from the tip is dispersed into an aerosol of highly charged droplets, a process that is aided by a co-axially introduced nebulising gas flowing around the outside of the capillary.

This gas, usually nitrogen, helps to direct the spray emerging from the capillary tip towards the mass spectrometer. The charged droplets diminish in size by solvent evaporation, assisted by a warm flow of nitrogen known as the drying gas which passes across the front of the ionisation source.

Eventually charged sample ions, free from solvent, are released from the droplets, some of which pass through a sampling cone or orifice into an intermediate vacuum region, and from there through a small aperture into the analyser of the mass spectrometer, which is held under high vacuum. The lens voltages are optimised individually for each sample.

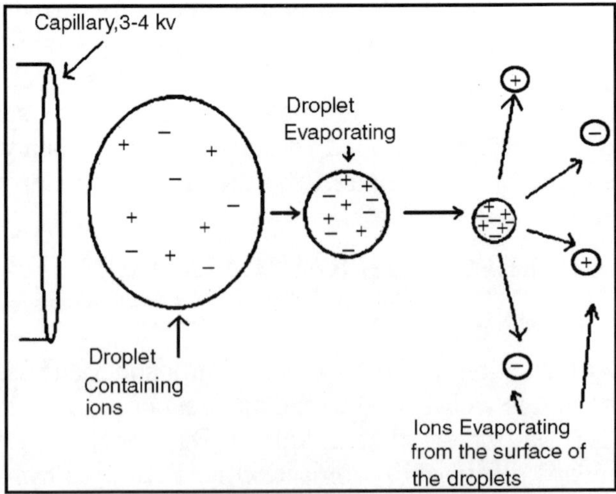

Fig. The Electrospray Ionisation Process

NANOSPRAY IONIZATION

Nanospray ionisation (M. Wilm, M. Mann, Anal. Chem., 1996, 68, 1) is a low flow rate version of electrospray ionisation. A small volume (1-4 microL) of the sample dissolved in a suitable volatile solvent, at a concentration of ca. 1 - 10 pmol/microL, is transferred into a miniature sample vial. A reasonably high voltage(ca. 700 - 2000 V) is applied to the specially manufactured gold-plated vial resulting in sample ionisation and spraying.

The flow rate of solute and solvent using this procedure is very low, 30 - 1000 nL/min, and so not only is far less sample consumed than with the standard electrospray ionisation technique, but also a small volume of sample lasts for several minutes, thus enabling multiple experiments to be performed. A common application of this technique is for a protein digestmixture to be analysed to generate a list of molecular masses for the components present, and then each component to be analysed further by tandem mass spectrometric (MS-MS) amino acid sequencing techniques.

ESI and nanospray ionisation are very sensitive analytical techniques but the sensitivity deteriorates with the presence of non-volatile buffers and other additives, which should be avoided as far as possible. In positive ionisation mode, a trace of formic acid is often added to aid protonation of the sample molecules; in negative ionisation mode a trace of ammonia solution or a volatile amine is added to aid deprotonation of the sample molecules. Proteins and peptides are usually analysed under positive ionisation conditions and saccharides and oligonucleotides under negative ionisation conditions. In all cases, the m/z scale must be calibrated by analysing a standard sample of a similar type to the sample being analysed (*e.g.* a protein calibrant for a protein sample), and then applying a mass correction.

DATA PROCESSING

ESI and nanospray ionisation generate the same type of spectral data for samples, and so the data processing procedures are identical. In ESI, samples (M) with molecular masses up to ca. 1200 Da give rise to singly charged molecular-related ions, usually protonated molecular ions of the formula $(M+H)^+$ in positive ionisation mode, and deprotonated molecular ions of the formula $(M-H)^-$ in negative ionisation mode. An example of this type of sample analysis is shown in the m/z spectrum of the pentapeptide leucine enkephalin, YGGFL. The molecular formula for this compound is $C_{28}H_{37}N_5O_7$ and the calculated monoisotopic molecular weight is 555.2692 Da.

The m/z spectrum shows dominant ions at m/z 556.1, which are consistent with the expected protonated molecular ions, $(M+H^+)$. Protonated molecular ions are expected because the sample was analysed under positive ionisation conditions. These m/z ions are singly charged, and so the m/z value is consistent with the molecular mass, as the value of z (number of charges) equals 1. Hence the measured molecular weight is deduced to be 555.1 Da, in good agreement with the theoretical value.

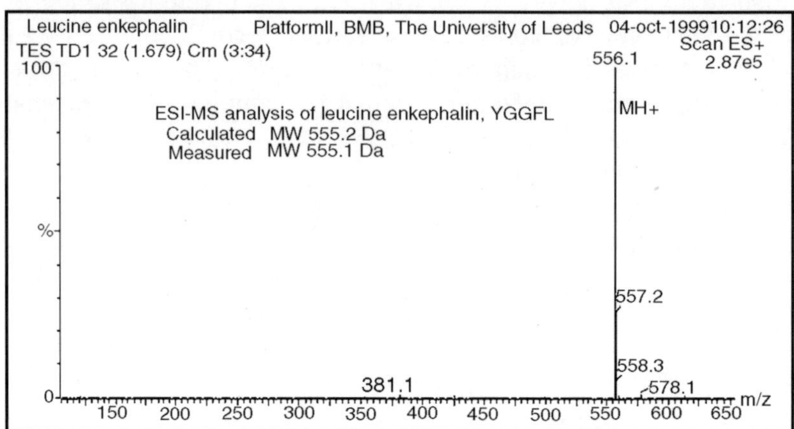

Fig. Positive ESI-MS m/z Spectrum of Leucine Enkaphalin, YGGFL.

The m/z spectrum also shows other ions of lower intensity (ca. 25per cent of the m/z 556.1 ions) at m/z 557.2. These represent the molecule in which one ^{12}C atom has been replaced by a ^{13}C atom, because carbon has a naturally occurring isotope one atomic mass unit (Da) higher. The intensity of these isotopic ions relates to the relative abundance of the naturally occurring isotope multiplied by the total number of carbon atoms in the molecule. Additionally the fact that the ^{13}C ions are one Da higher on the m/z scale than the ^{12}C ions is an indication that $z = 1$, and hence the sample ions are singly charged. If the sample ions had been doubly charged, then the m/z values would only differ by 0.5 Da as z, the number of charges, would then be equal to 2.

The m/z spectrum also contains ions at m/z 578.1, some 23 Da higher than the expected molecular mass. These can be identified as the sodium adduct ions, $(M+Na)^+$, and are quite common in electrospray ionisation. Instead of the sample molecules being ionised by the addition of a proton H^+, some molecules have been ionised by the addition of a sodium cation Na^+. Other common adduct ions include K^+ (+39) and NH_4^+ (+18) in positive ionisation mode and Cl^- (+35) in negative ionisation mode. Electrospray ionisation is known as a "soft" ionisation method as the sample is ionised by the addition or removal of a proton, with very little extra energy remaining to cause fragmentation of the sample ions.

Samples (M) with molecular weights greater than ca. 1200 Da give rise to multiply charged molecular-related ions such as $(M+nH)^{n+}$ in positive ionisation modeand $(M\text{-}nH)^{n-}$ in negative ionisation mode. Proteins have many suitable sites for protonation as all of the backbone amide nitrogen atoms could be protonated theoretically, as well as certain amino acid side chains such as lysine and arginine which contain primary amine functionalities. An example of multiple charging, which is practically unique to electrospray ionisation, is presented in the positive ionisation m/z spectrum of the protein hen egg white lysozyme.

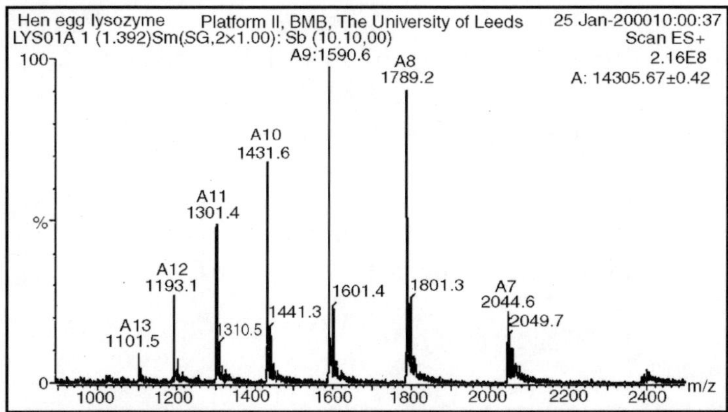

Fig. Positive ESI-MS m/z Spectrum of the Protien hen Egg white Lysozyme.

The sample was analysed in a solution of 1:1 (v/v) acetonitrile: 0.1per cent aqueous formic acid and the m/z spectrum shows a Gaussian-type distribution of multiply charged ions ranging from m/z 1101.5 to 2044.6. Each peak represents the intact protein molecule carrying a different number of charges (protons).

The peak width is greater than that of the singly charged ions seen in the leucine enkephalin spectrum, as the isotopes associated with these multiply charged ions are not clearly resolved as they were in the case of the singly charged ions. The individual peaks in the multiply charged series become closer together at lower m/z values and, because the molecular weight is the same for all of the peaks, those with more charges appear at lower m/z values than do those with fewer. The m/z values can be expressed as follows:

$$m/z = (MW + nH^+) / n$$

where,

m/z: The mass-to-charge ratio marked on the abscissa of the spectrum;

MW: The molecular mass of the sample

n: The integer number of charges on the ions

H: The mass of a proton = 1.008 Da.

If the number of charges on an ion is known, then it is simply a matter of reading the m/z value from the spectrum and solving the above equation to determine the molecular weight of the sample.

Usually the number of charges is not known, but can be calculated if the assumption is made that any two adjacent members in the series of multiply charged ions differ by one charge.

For example, if the ions appearing at m/z 1431.6 in the lysozyme spectrum have "n" charges, then the ions at m/z 1301.4 will have "n+1" charges, and the above equation can be written again for these two ions:

$$1431.6 = (MW + nH^+)/n \text{ and } 1301.4 = [MW + (n+1)H^+]/(n+1)$$

These simultaneous equations can be rearranged to exclude the MW term:

- n(1431.6) - nH^+ = (n+1)1301.4 - (n+1)H^+ and so:
- n(1431.6) = n(1301.4) +1301.4 - H^+ therefore:
- n(1431.6 - 1301.4) = 1301.4 - H^+ and so:
- n = (1301.4 - H^+)/(1431.6 - 1301.4)

hence the number of charges on the ions at m/z 1431.6 = 1300.4/130.2 = 10.

Putting the value of n back into the equation:

- 1431.6 = (MW + nH^+) n gives 1431.6 × 10
- = MW + (10 × 1.008) and so MW
- = 14,316–10.08 therefore MW
- = 14,305.9 Da

The observed molecular mass is in good agreement with the theoretical molecular mass of hen egg lysozyme (based on average atomic masses) of 14305.14 Da. The individual isotopes cannot be resolved when the ions have a large number of charges, and so for proteins the average mass is measured. This may seem long-winded but fortunately the molecular mass of the sample can be calculated automatically, or at least semi-automatically, by the processing software associated with the mass spectrometer. This is of great help for multi-component mixture analysis where the m/z spectrum may well contain several overlapping series of multiply charged ions, with each component exhibiting completely different charge states.

Using electrospray or nanospray ionisation, a mass accuracy of within 0.01per cent of the molecular mass should be achievable, which in this case represents +/- 1.4 Da. In order to clarify electrospray/nanospray data, molecular mass profiles can be generated from the m/z spectra of high molecular mass, multiply charged samples. To achieve this, all the components are transposed onto a true molecular mass (or zero charge state) profile from which molecular masses can be read directly without any amendments or calculations.

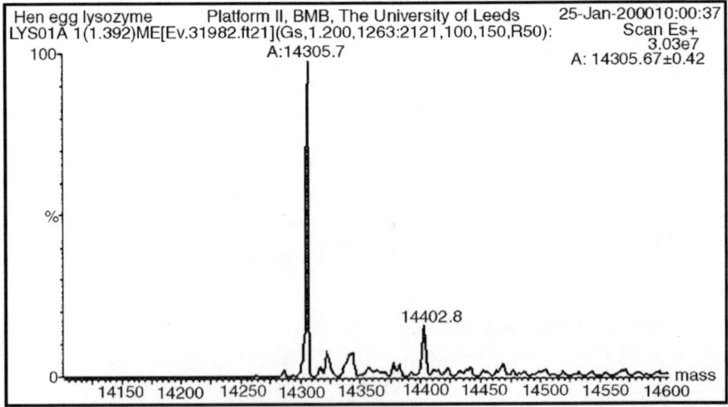

Fig. Molecular Mass Profile of Lysozyme Obtained by Maximum Entropy Processing of the m/z Spectrum

The m/z spectrum of lysozyme has been converted to a molecular mass profile using Maximum Entropy processing and the data are shown. The mass profile is dominated by a component of molecular mass 14,305.7 Da, with a series of minor peaks at higher mass, which is usually indicative of salt adducting *e.g.* Na (M+23), K (M+39), H_2SO_4 or H_3PO_4 (M+98). The molecular masses can be read easily and unambiguously, and a good idea of the purity of the protein is obtained on inspection of the molecular mass profile.

Proteins in their native state, or at least containing a significant amount of folding, tend to produce multiply charged ions covering a smaller range of charge states (say two or three). These charge states tend to have fewer charges than an unfolded protein would have, due to the inaccessibility of many of the protonation sites. In such cases, increasing the sampling cone voltage may provide sufficient energy for the protein to begin to unfold and create a wider charge state distribution centering on more highly charged ions in the lower m/z region of the spectrum.

The differences in m/z spectra due to the folded state of the protein are illustrated with the m/z spectra of the protein apo-pseudoazurin acquired under different solvent conditions. Analysis of the protein in 1:1 acetonitrile: 0.1per cent aqueous formic acid at pH2 gave a Gaussian-type distribution with multiply charged states ranging from n = 9 at m/z 1487.8 to n = 19 at m/z 705.3, centering on n = 15 (lower trace).

The molecular mass for this protein was 13,381 Da. Analysis of the protein in water gave fewer charge states, from n = 7 at m/z 1921.7 to n = 11 at m/z 1223.7, centering at n = 9 (upper trace). Not only has the charge state distribution changed, the molecular weight is now 13,444 Da which represents an increase of 63 Da and indicates that copper is remaining bound to the protein. Many types of protein complexes can be observed in this way, including protein-ligand, protein-peptide, protein-metal and protein-RNA macromolecules.

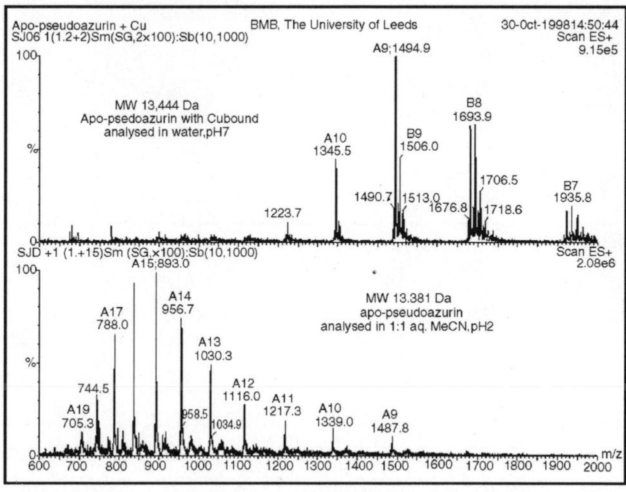

Positive ESI-MS m/z spectra of the protein apo-pseudoazurin analysed in water at pH7 (upper trace) and in 1:1 acetonitrile:0.1per cent aq. formic acid at pH2 (lower trace).

MATRIX ASSISTED LASER DESORPTION IONIZATION

Matrix Assisted Laser Desorption Ionisation (MALDI) deals well with thermolabile, non-volatile organic compounds especially those of high molecular mass and is used successfully in biochemical areas for the analysis of proteins, peptides, glycoproteins, oligosaccharides, and oligonucleotides. It is relatively straightforward to use and reasonably tolerant to buffers and other additives. The mass accuracy depends on the type and performance of the analyser of the mass spectrometer, but most modern instruments should be capable of measuring masses to within 0.01per cent of the molecular mass of the sample, at least up to ca. 40,000 Da.

MALDI is based on the bombardment of sample molecules with a laser light to bring about sample ionisation. The sample is pre-mixed with a highly absorbingmatrix compound for the most consistent and reliable results, and a low concentration of sample to matrix works best. The matrix transforms the laser energy intoexcitation energy for the sample, which leads to sputtering of analyte and matrix ions from the surface of the mixture. In this way energy transfer is efficient and also the analyte molecules are spared excessive direct energy that may otherwise cause decomposition. Most commercially available MALDI mass spectrometers now have a pulsed nitrogen laser of wavelength 337 nm.

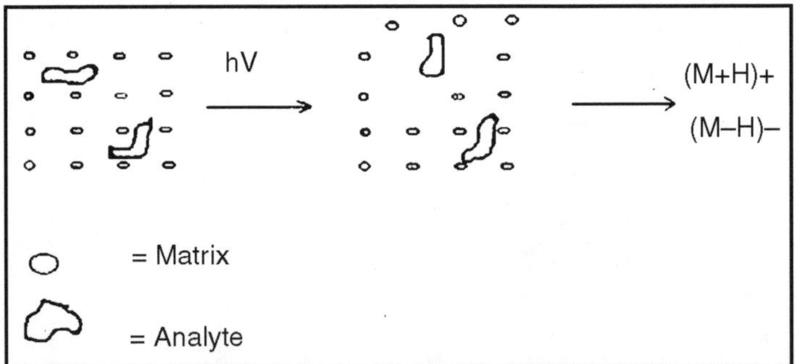

Fig. Matrix Assisted Laser Desorption Ionisation (MALDI)

The sample to be analysed is dissolved in an appropriate volatile solvent, usually with a trace of trifluoroacetic acid if positive ionisation is being used, at a concentration of ca. 10 pmol/L and an aliquot (1-2 L) of this removed and mixed with an equal volume of a solution containing a vast excess of a matrix.

A range of compounds is suitable for use as matrices: sinapinic acid is a common one for protein analysis while alpha-cyano-4-hydroxycinnamic acid is often used forpeptide analysis. An aliquot (1-2 L) of the final solution is applied to the sample target which is allowed to dry prior to insertion into the high vacuum of the mass spectrometer. The laser is fired, the energy arriving at the sample/matrix surface optimised, and data accumulated until a m/z spectrum of reasonable intensity has been amassed.

The time-of-flight analyser separates ions according to their mass(m)-to-charge(z) (m/z) ratios by measuring the time it takes for ions to travel through a field free region known as the flight, or drift, tube. The heavier ions are slower than the lighter ones.

The m/z scale of the mass spectrometer is calibrated with a known sample that can either be analysed independently (external calibration) or pre-mixed with the sample and matrix (internal calibration).

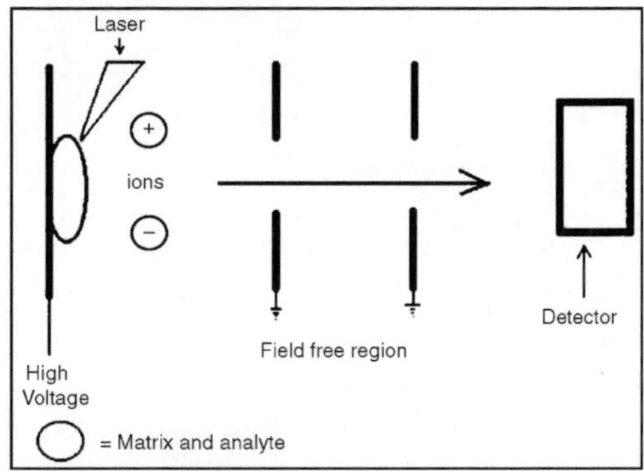

Fig. Simplified Schematic of MALDI-TOF Mass Spectrometry (linear mode).

MALDI is also a "soft" ionisation method and so results predominantly in the generation of singly charged molecular-related ions regardless of the molecular mass, hence the spectra are relatively easy to interpret.

Fragmentation of the sample ions does not usually occur. In positive ionisation mode the protonated molecular ions ($M+H^+$) are usually the dominant species, although they can be accompanied by salt adducts, a trace of the doubly charged molecular ion at approximately half the m/z value, and/or a trace of a dimeric species at approximately twice the m/z value.

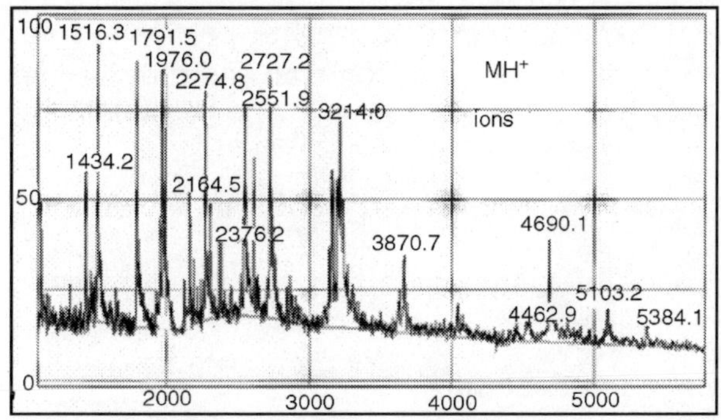

Fig. Positive Ionisation MALDI m/z Spectrum of a Peptide Mixture using Alpha-cyano-4-hydroxycinnamic acid as Matrix.

Positive ionisation is used in general for protein and peptide analyses. In negative ionisation mode the deprotonated molecular ions ($M-H^-$) are usually the most abundant species, accompanied by some salt adducts and possibly traces of dimeric or doubly charged materials. Negative ionisation can be used for the analysis of oligonucleotides and oligosaccharides.

POSITIVE OR NEGATIVE IONIZATION

If the sample has functional groups that readily accept a proton (H^+) then positive ion detection is used *e.g.* amines $R-NH_2 + H^+ = R-NH_3^+$ as in proteins or peptides. If the sample has functional groups that readily lose a proton then negative ion detection is used *e.g.* carboxylic acids $R-CO_2H = R-CO_2^-$ and alcohols R-OH = R-O- as in saccharides or oligonucleotides

Tandem mass spectrometry (MS-MS): Structural and sequence information from mass spectrometry.

TANDEM MASS SPECTROMETRY

Tandem mass spectrometry (MS-MS) is used to produce structural information about a compound by fragmenting specific sample ions inside the mass spectrometer and identifying the resulting fragment ions. This information can then be pieced together to generate structural information regarding the intact molecule. Tandem mass spectrometry also enables specific compounds to be detected in complex mixtures on account of their specific and characteristic fragmentation patterns. A tandem mass spectrometer is a mass spectrometer that has more than one analyser, in practice usually two. The two analysers are separated by a collision cell into which an inert gas (*e.g.* argon, xenon) is admitted to collide with the selected sample ions and bring about their fragmentation. The analysers can be of the same or of different types, the most common combinations being:

- *Quadrupole*: Quadrupole
- *Magnetic sector:* Quadrupole
- *Magnetic sector:* Magnetic sector
- *Quadrupole:* Time-of-flight.

Fragmentation experiments can also be performed on certain single analyser mass spectrometers such as ion trap and time-of-flight instruments, the latter type using a post-source decay experiment to effect the fragmentation of sample ions.

TANDEM MASS SPECTROMETRY ANALYSES

The basic modes of data acquisition for tandem mass spectrometry experiments are as follows:

Product or Daughter Ion Scanning

The first analyser is used to select user-specified sample ions arising from a particular component; usually the molecular-related (*i.e.* $(M+H)^+$ or $(M-H)^-$)

ions. These chosen ions pass into the collision cell, are bombarded by the gas molecules which cause fragment ions to be formed, and these fragment ions are analysed *i.e.* separated according to their mass to charge ratios, by the second analyser. All the fragment ions arise directly from the precursor ions specified in the experiment, and thus produce a fingerprint pattern specific to the compound under investigation. This type of experiment is particularly useful for providing structural information concerning small organic molecules and for generating peptide sequenceinformation.

Precursor or Parent Ion Scanning

The first analyser allows the transmission of all sample ions, whilst the second analyser is set to monitor specific fragment ions, which are generated by bombardment of the sample ions with the collision gas in the collision cell. This type of experiment is particularly useful for monitoring groups of compounds contained within a mixture which fragment to produce common fragment ions, *e.g.* glycosylated peptides in a tryptic digest mixture, aliphatic hydrocarbons in an oil sample, orglucuronide conjugates in urine.

Constant Neutral Loss Scanning

This involves both analysers scanning, or collecting data, across the whole m/z range, but the two are off-set so that the second analyser allows only those ions which differ by a certain number of mass units (equivalent to a neutral fragment) from the ions transmitted through the first analyser. *e.g.* This type of experiment could be used to monitor all of the carboxylic acids in a mixture. Carboxylic acids tend to fragment by losing a (neutral) molecule of carbon dioxide, CO_2, which is equivalent to a loss of 44 Da or atomic mass units. All ions pass through the first analyser into the collision cell. The ions detected from the collision cell are those from which 44 Da have been lost.

Selected/Multiple Reaction Monitoring

Both of the analysers are static in this case as user-selected specific ions are transmitted through the first analyser and user-selected specific fragments arising from these ions are measured by the second analyser. The compound under scrutiny must be known and have been well-characterised previously before this type of experiment is undertaken. This methodology is used to confirm unambiguously the presence of a compound in a matrix *e.g.* drug testing with blood or urine samples. It is not only a highly specific method but also has very high sensitivity.

PEPTIDE SEQUENCING BY TANDEM MASS SPECTROMETRY

The most common usage of MS-MS in biochemical areas is the product or daughter ion scanning experiment which is particularly successful for peptide andnucleotide sequencing.

PEPTIDE SEQUENCING: H_2N-CH(R')-CO-NH-CH(R")-CO_2H

Peptides fragment in a reasonably well-documented manner (P. Roepstorrf, J. Fohlmann, Biomed. Mass Spectrom., 1984, 11, 601; R. S. Johnson, K. Biemann,Biomed. Environ. Mass Spectrom., 1989, 18, 945). The protonated molecules fragment along the peptide backbone and also show some side-chain fragmentation with certain instruments (Four-Sector Tandem Mass Spectrometry of Peptides, A. E. Ashcroft, P. J. Derrick in "Mass Spectrometry of Peptides" ed. D. M. Desiderio, CRC Press, Florida, 1990).

There are three different types of bonds that can fragment along the amino acid backbone: the NH-CH, CH-CO, and CO-NH bonds. Each bond breakage gives rise to two species, one neutral and the other one charged, and only the charged species is monitored by the mass spectrometer. The charge can stay on either of the two fragments depending on the chemistry and relative proton affinity of the two species.

Hence there are six possible fragment ions for each amino acid residue and these are labelled as in the diagram, with the a, b, and c" ions having the charge retained on the N-terminal fragment, and the x, y", and z ions having the charge retained on the C-terminal fragment. The most common cleavage sites are at the CO-NH bonds which give rise to the b and/or the y" ions. The mass difference between two adjacent b ions, or y"; ions, is indicative of a particular amino acid residue.

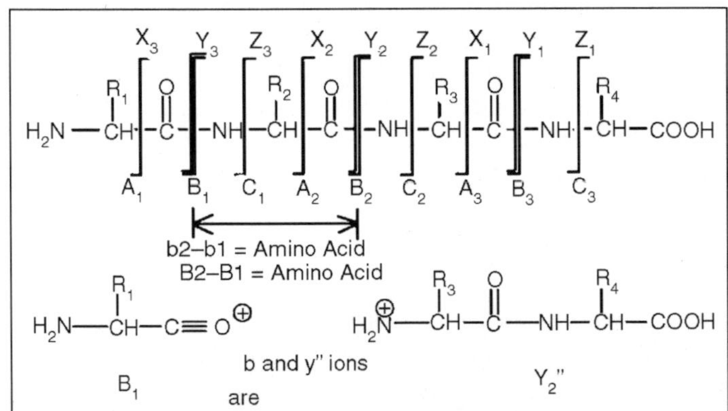

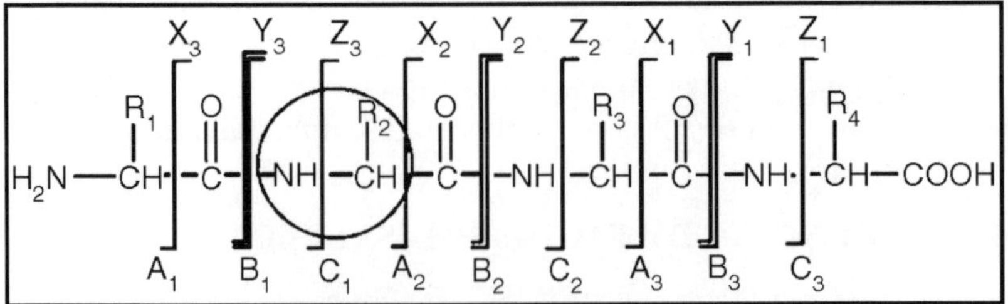

Fig. Peptide Sequencing by Tandem Mass Spectrometry - Backbone Cleavages

The extent of side-chain fragmentation detected depends on the type of analysers used in the mass spectrometer. A magnetic sector - magnetic sector instrument will give rise to high energy collisions resulting in many different types of side-chain cleavages. Quadrupole - quadrupole and quadrupole - time-of-flight mass spectrometers generate low energy fragmentations with fewer types of side-chain fragmentations.

Immonium ions (labelled “i”) appear in the very low m/z range of the MS-MS spectrum. Each amino acid residue leads to a diagnostic immonium ion, with the exception of the two pairs leucine (L) and iso-leucine (I), and lysine (K) and glutamine (Q), which produce immonium ions with the same m/z ratio, *i.e.* m/z 86 for I and L, m/z 101 for K and Q. The immonium ions are useful for detecting and confirming many of the amino acid residues in a peptide, although no information regarding the position of these amino acid residues in the peptide sequence can be ascertained from the immonium ions. An example of an MS/MS daughter or product ion spectrum is illustrated below.

The molecular mass of the peptide was measured using standard mass spectrometric techniques and found to be 680.4 Da, the dominant ions in the MS spectrum being the protonated molecular ions ($M+H^+$) at m/z 681.4.

These ions were selected for transmission through the first analyser, then fragmented in the collision cell and their fragments analysed by the second analyser to produce the following MS/MS spectrum.

The sequence (amino acid backbone) ions have been identified, and in this example the peptide fragmented predominantly at theCO-NH bonds and gave both b and y” ions. (Often either the b series or the y” series predominates, sometimes to the exclusion of the other). The b series ions have been labelled with blue vertical lines and the y” series ions have been labelled with red vertical lines.

The mass difference between adjacent members of a series can be calculated *e.g.* b3-b2 = 391.21 - 262.16 = 129.05 Da which is equivalent to a glutamine (E) amino acid residue; and similarly y4 - y3 = 567.37 - 420.27 = 147.10 Da which is equivalent to a phenylalanine (F) residue. In this way, using either the b series or the y” series, the amino acid sequence of the peptide can be determined and was found to be NFESGK (n.b. the y” series reads from right to left!). The immonium ions at m/z 102 merely confirm the presence of the glutamine (E) residue in the peptide.

A protein identification study would proceed as follows:

- The protein under investigation would be analysed by mass spectrometry to generate a molecular mass to within an accuracy of 0.01per cent.
- The protein would then be digested with a suitable enzyme. Trypsin is useful for mass spectrometric studies because each proteolytic fragment contains a basic arginine (R) or lysine (K) amino acid residue,

and thus is eminently suitable for positive ionisation mass spectrometric analysis. The digest mixture is analysed - without prior separation or clean-up - by mass spectrometry to produce a rather complex spectrum from which the molecular weights of all of the proteolytic fragments can be read. This spectrum, with its molecular weight information, is called a peptide map. (If the protein already exists on a database, then the peptide map is often sufficient to confirm the protein.)

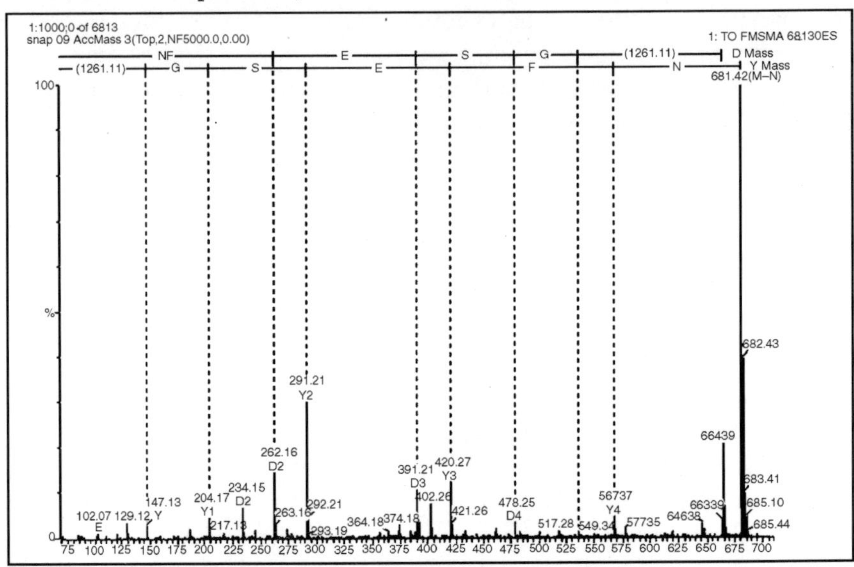

Fig. Peptide Sequencing by Tandem mass Spectrometry - an MS-MS Daughter or Product ion Spectrum.

For these experiments the mass spectrometer would be operated in the "MS" mode, whereby the sample is sprayed and ionised from the nanospray needle and the ions pass through the sampling cone, skimmer lenses, Rf hexapole focusing system, and the first (quadrupole) analyser. The quadrupole in this instance is not used as an analyser, merely as a lens to focus the ion beam into the second (time-of-flight) analyser which separates the ions according to their mass-to-charge ratio.

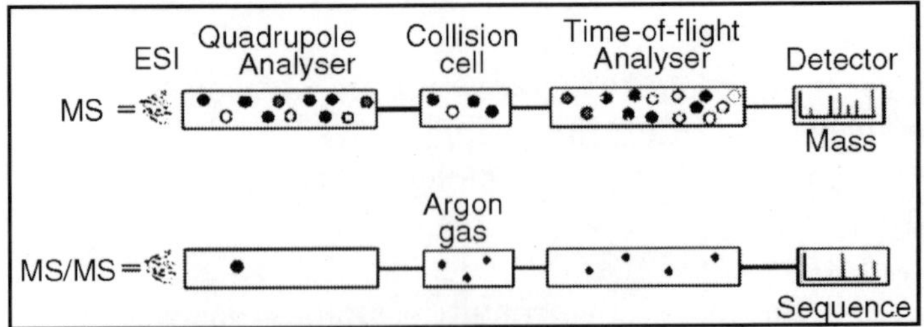

Fig. Q-TOF Mass Spectrometer Operating in MS (upper) and MS/MS mode (lower) modes.

- With the digest mixture still spraying into the mass spectrometer, the Q-Tof mass spectrometer is switched into "MS/MS" mode. The protonated molecular ions of each of the digest fragments can be independently selected and transmitted through the quadrupole analyser, which is now used as an analyser to transmit solely the ions of interest into the collision cell which lies inbetween the first and second analysers. An inert gas such as argon is introduced into the collision cell and the sample ions are bombarded by the collision gas molecules which cause them to fragment. The optimum collision cell conditions vary from peptide to peptide and must be optimised for each one. The fragment (or daughter or product) ions are then analysed by the second (time-of-flight) analyser. In this way an MS/MS spectrum is produced showing all the fragment ions that arise directly from the chosen parent orprecursor ions for a given peptide component. An MS/MS daughter (or fragment, or product) ion spectrum is produced for each of the components identified in the proteolytic digest. Varying amounts of sequence information can be gleaned from each fragmentation spectrum, and the spectra need to be interpreted carefully. Some of the processing can be automated, but in general the processing and interpretation of spectra will take longer than the data acquisition if accurate and reliable data are to be generated.

The amount of sequence information generated will vary from one peptide to another, Some peptide sequences will be confirmed totally, other may produce a partial sequence of, say, 4 or 5 amino acid residues. Often sequence "tag" of 4 or 5 residues is sufficient to search a protein database and confirm the identity of the protein.

PEPTIDE SEQUENCING IN SUMMARY

Peptides fragment along the amino acid backbone to give sequence information. Peptides ca. 2500 Da or less produce the most useful data. The amount of sequence information varies from one peptide to another. Some peptides can generate sufficient information for a full sequence to be determined; others may generate a partial sequence of 4 or 5 amino acids.

A protein digest can be analysed as an entire reaction mix, without any separation of the products, from which individual peptides are selected and analysed by the mass spectrometer to generate sequence information. About 4 L of solution is required for the analysis of the digest mixture, with a concentration based on the original protein of ca. 1-10 pmol/L. MS/MS sequencing is a sensitive technique consuming little sample. Sometimes the full protein sequence can be verified; some proteins generate sufficient information to cover only part of the sequence. 70 - 80per cent coverage is reasonable. Often a sequence "tag" of 4/5 amino acids from a single proteolytic peptide is sufficient to identify the protein from a database.

The final point in this summary means that mass spectrometers have been found to be extremely useful for proteomic studies, as illustrated below. The proteomics procedure usually involves excising individual spots from a 2-D gel and independently enzymatically digesting the protein(s) contained within each spot, before analysing the digest mixture by mass spectrometer in the manner outlined above. Electrospray ionisation or MALDI could be used at this step.

The initial MS spectrum determining the molecular masses of all of the components in the digest mixture can often provide sufficient information to search adatabase using just several of the molecular weights from this peptide map. If the database search is not fruitful, either because the protein has not been catalogued, is previously uncharacterised, or the data are not accurate or comprehensive enough to distinguish between several entries in the database, then further information is required.

This can be achieved by sample clean-up and then MS/MS studies to determine the amino acid sequences of the individual proteolytic peptides contained in the digest mixture, with which further database searching can be carried out.

OLIGONUCLEOTIDE SEQUENCING BY TANDEM MASS SPECTROMETRY

Oligonucleotide sequencing: P-S(B)-P-S(B)-P-S(B). Oligonucleotide sequencing can also be achieved by tandem mass spectrometry although it is not so well documented. However fragmentation patterns have been established and reported. The experimental principle is similar to that of peptide sequencing, in that individual species are mass measured in MS mode of instrument operation, and then their molecular-related ions selected by the first (quadrupole) analyser to be transmitted into the collision cell where they undergo fragmentation after bombardment with a collision gas. The fragments are analysed by the second (time-of-flight) analyser to produce an MS/MS product, or daughter, ion spectrum showing all the fragment ions that arise directly from the chosen parent or precursor ions.

Negative electrospray ionisation is often the preferred ionisation method. The optimisation of the fragmentation conditions varies from component to component and diligence must be taken to ensure the best conditions are employed. Data processing and interpretation is again of paramount importance for accurate, reliable results and hence sequence information.

PROTEIN MASS MAPPING

Now we are going to describe more in detail how using mass spectrometry is possible to map a protein or a peptide. This is a procedure where a protein or peptide is degraded under controlled conditions using a chemical reaction or specific enzymes. After purification by means of High performance Liquid Chromatography (HPLC), protein fragments are analysed using mass spectrometry, using Fast Atom Bombardment (FAB) or Matrix-Assisted Laser-Desorption Ionization (MALDI), last technique is currently more often used. There are several databases available where masses of proteolytic peptides expected from enzymatic degradation of proteins of known sequence can be found; these values can match with the fragments of analysed unknown proteins in order to determine their sequence. Historically, nanomole amounts have been requires for sequencing by mass spectrometry, however, as instrumentation and methods improve, more and more problems can be solved with sample amounts in the 100 pmol range.

SEQUENCE DETERMINATIONS

Next figure describe the concept of mass mapping of peptide fragments resulting from controlled degradation of protein. In this case, trypsin is used, cleaving the peptide bond on C-terminal side of R or K. The mass of the expected peptide fragments can be calculated; mass-spectral peaks observed for the expected peptide fragments confirm the sequence of the original peptide.

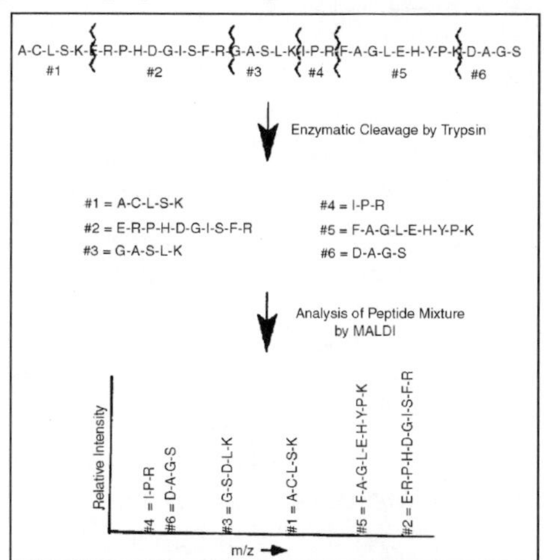

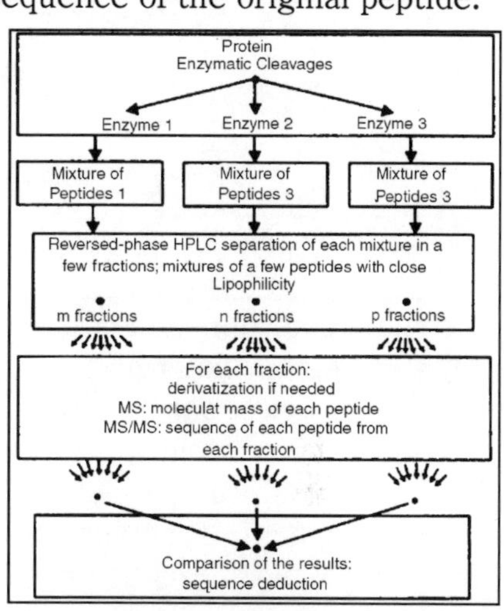

In general, the strategy followed in sequencing proteins using mass spectrometry can be summarized in the next diagram:

PROTEIN IDENTIFICATION

Protein identification requires total or partial determination of their sequences by the method of Edman degradation. In some particular cases protein identification can be also based on their recognition by specific antibodies. Edman degradation limits this method to the isolated polypeptides that are not blocked on the N-terminal side. Moreover, this technique requieres a long analysis time and a large amount of sample. Without any doubt, mass spectrometry is now the most efficient way to identify proteins. The strategy used is depicted in the figure. This method allows peptides to be obtained from a two-dimensional gel electrophoresis with certainty, quickly and at high sensitivity. This method is based on comparison of the data obtained from mass spectrometry with those predicted for all proteins contained in a database. The efficiency of the method results from the development of mass spectrometry into a rapid and sensitive method to analyse peptides and proteins and also from the availability of larger and larger databases.

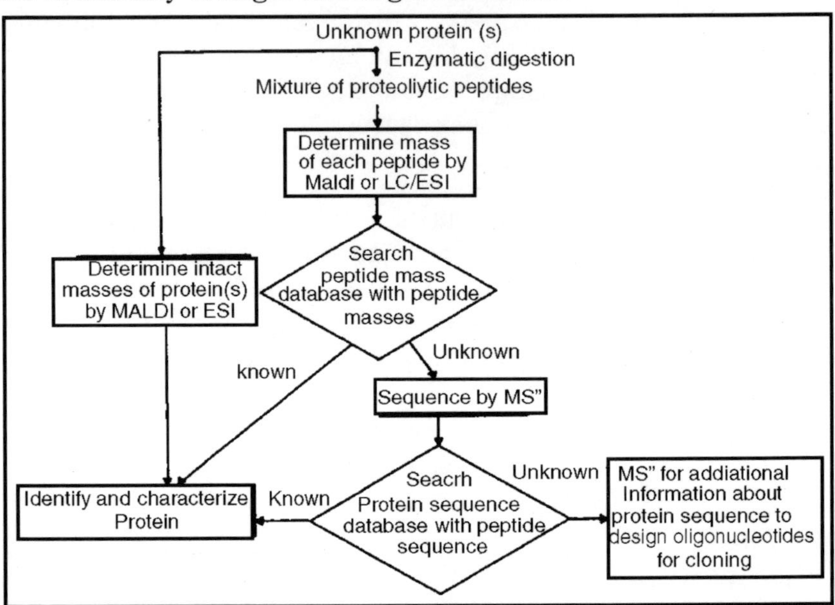

Accurate determination of the molecular weight of a protein is useful for its identification and the determination of its purity. Owing to the possibility of post-translational modifications that are not contained in the database, the correct mass often is not sufficient for identification of a protein but it does facilitate the search. On the other hand, the peptide mixture obtained by cleavage of a protein by enzymes or specific reactants is characteristic of a protein, because the postranslational modifications only affect a small number of peptides obtained.

PROTEIN CLASSIFICATION

Protein classification is motivated by the notion of "descriptive biology". When faced with tremendous amounts of highly complex data, such as with the set of all proteins, one way to understand the data is by classification: the act of associating or grouping proteins into classes using certain criteria. One such criterion is protein sequence identity, where sequential similarity led to the development of phylogenetic trees and multiple sequence analyses. The same is done in protein structure classification, where the effort is to identify groups of similar proteins, with the hope that this will yield information about their biochemical function and biological purpose.

Proteins are classified by simultaneously applying a number of criteria, including sequence homology (evolutionary relatedness), function, folding motifs, structural features, and so on. The resulting hierarchies and clusters of protein structures provide a notion of the distance between two proteins and their structures. A couple of popular classification schemes are linked. Note that a fair amount of manual annotation and classification was necessary to build these systems.

PROTEIN ALIGNMENT

The core computational problem of protein classification, using sequence or structure, is the problem of comparing two proteins. For structural classification, one method for comparison is *structural alignment*, which identifies an ideal superimposition between two protein structures, in order to compare them.

SSAP, Dali, Foldminer, Lock, and Geometric Hashing are algorithms which have been designed in part to align whole protein structures.

Despite differences in algorithmic approach, all of these algorithms essentially evolved from the need to assign the best possible correlation between points in one structure and points in another.

The problem of finding the optimal alignment is polynomial in the number of atoms in biological data, where we are assured that atoms cannot fall within a certain distance to each other (Van der Waals forces enforce this), but without this constraint the problem is exponential.

Protein alignment has been used for the classification and comparison of proteins in many existing algorithms.

These include:

- Dali is a structural comparison algorithm based on pairwise distance matrices. Dali uses patterns of residue contacts. The alignments are found using a randomized search.
- FoldMiner and LOCK 2. FoldMiner finds protein structures similar to an input structure by performing alignment the query structures secondary structure elements with proteins in its database using the LOCK 2 algorithm. LOCK 2 uses a combination of geometric hashing and dynamic programming to optimize the alignments of secondary structure elements of different proteins. Once a set of alignments to similar structures are found, motifs consisting of similar secondary structure arrangements are constructed and used to refine the similarity search.
- Sequential Structure Alignment Programme (SSAP) Given two protein structures, SSAP returns a structural alignment.

CLASSIFICATION

Once alignment algorithms have been implemented, it is possible to explore different classifications of proteins. Naturally, it would be intuitive to classify proteins solely according to their structure, but much richer data is available as well. Current classifications of proteins integrate sequence and structure information in order to maximize their utility.

These include the following:

- SCOP (Structural Classification of Protein) is a database of all proteins whose structures have been determined, organized by family (evolutionary relationship), superfamily (structural and functional similarity), and fold (similar secondary structure, with similar arrangement and topological connections). SCOP was constructed largely by manual inspection and annotation.
- CATH Protein Structure Classification is another database of protein structures, organized by Class (secondary structure content), Architecture (orientation of secondary structures), Topology (overall shape and connectivity), and Homologous Superfamily (evolutionary relationship inferred based on sequence and structure similarity). CATH uses SSAP (the Sequential Structural Alignment Programme, a secondary structure element-based method) for structural comparison.

The biological purpose of designing Global Stuructural Alignment algorithms was the identification, classification, and ultimately prediction, of protein function, under the hypothesis that protein structure dictates protein function. Simultaneously, it was realised that small changes to proteins could lead to massive changes in function, or nothing at all. This suggested that global alignment and global structure comparison (as well as global sequence alignment and global sequence comparison) should not be the only tools used for function prediction.

In particular, it was realised that active sites, clusterings of amino acids on the surface of proteins and a tiny minority of the entire protein, were often strongly related to protein function. In a continuation of the effort to predict protein function through structural comparison, algorithms were developed to compare functionally relevant substructures of proteins. We refer to these algorithms collectively as local structure alignment algorithms.

LOCAL MATCHING: GEOMETRIC HASHING, POSE CLUSTERING AND MATCH AUGMENTATION

Algorithms for local structure alignment address the similar computational problem of selecting a correspondence between a*motif*, a tiny substructure of a protein, often between 3 and 20 amino acids, and a *target*, a full protein structure. Once a correspondence has been established, the "distance" of the motif to the identified part of the target is measured using lRMSD.

Some algorithms for local structure alignment are based on pattern matching algorithms. Pattern matching algorithms seek target substructures called matches which have maximal geometric similarity to the motif. An excellent example of this type of algorithm is Geometric Hashing, a very flexible framework for geometric pattern matching under noisy constraints. Geometric Hashing, has been adapted to alignment by atom position, by backbone C-alpha, multiple structural alignment, and alignment of hinge-bending and flexible protein models.

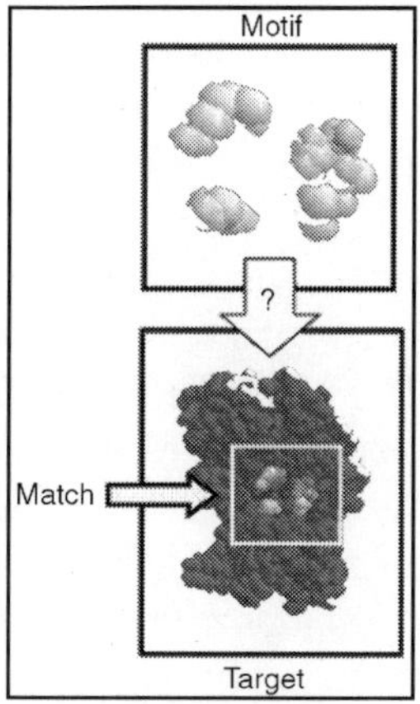

Motifs

A motif S is a set of m points $s_1..., s_m$ in three dimensions, whose coordinates are taken from backbone and side-chain atoms. Each *motif point* s_i in the motif has an associated *rank* $p(s_i)$, a measure of the functional significance of the motif point. Each s_i also has a set of alternate amino acid *labels* $l(s_i)$ in {GLY, ALA...}, which represent residues this amino acid has mutated to during evolution. Labels permit our motifs to simultaneously represent many homologous active sites with slight mutations, not just a single active site. In this paper, we obtain labels and ranks using Evolutionary Trace (ET).

Other motifs have been designed with other approaches. Motifs have been composed of points on the Connolly surface representing electrostatic potentials, of hinge-bending sets of points in space, of sets of "pseudo-centers" representing protein-ligand interactions, or of points taken from atom coordinates with evolutionary data,to name a few. Depending on how motif points are defined, they have different labels associated with them and these labels need to be taken into account when comparing motifs.

Protein Function Prediction

Local structure comparison algorithms mainly target the biological problem of Protein Function Prediction. Ideally, a function prediction pipeline should address the following subproblems:

- The design of effective motifs
- The efficient identification of matches
- The effective filtering of matches

Suppose for a moment that we have hand-designed motifs.

Identification of Matches

Many such algorithms exist, but differ fundamentally in that they are optimized for comparing different types of motifs. There are algorithms for comparing graph-based motifs, algorithms for finding catalytic sites, and the seminal Geometric Hashing framework which can search for many types of motifs, including motifs based on atom position, points on Connolly face centers catalytic triads and flexible protein models. *Match Augmentation* (MA) is described below.

MA compares a motif S to a target T, a protein structure encoded as $|T|$ target points: $T=\{t_1...t_{|T|}\}$, where each ti is taken from coordinates, and labeled $I(t_i)$ for the amino acid to which ti belongs. A match M is a bijection correlating all motif points in S to a subest of T of the form $M = \{(s_{a1},t_{b1}), (s_{a2},t_{b2}) ... (s_{a|s|},t_{|s|})\}$. Referring to the Euclidean distance between points a and b as $||a-b||$, an acceptable match requires:

Criterion 1 i, s_{ai} and t_{bi} are biologically compatible: $I(t_{bi})\in I(s_{ai})$.

Criterion 2 LRMSD alignment, via rigid transformation A of S, causes $\forall i, ||A(s_{ai})-t_{bi}||<\varepsilon$, our threshold for geometric similarity.

MA takes as input a motif S and a target T. MA outputs the match with smallest LRMSD among all matches that fulfill the criteria. Partial matches correlating subsets of S to T are rejected. By establishing a threshold for acceptable geometric similarity, the second criterion causes MA to return match LRMSDs bounded above by ε. We find that ε =7Å permits the identification of structurally distant matches when no matches with lower LRMSD exist, while still efficiently identifying matches with high structural similarity.

Match Augmentation

Rank information prioritizes motif data and MA was designed in a prioritized fashion, where correspondences with higher ranked points are identified first. MA is composed of two parts: *Seed Matching* and *Augmentation*. The purpose of Seed Matching is to identify a match for the *seed* $S' = \{s_1,s_2,s_3\}$, the three highest ranked motif points. The k lowest lRMSD *seed matches* are passed to Augmentation to be iteratively expanded into matches for the remaining motif points, in descending rank order. Augmentation outputs the match with smallest lRMSD.

Seed Matching

Seed Matching identifies all sets of 3 target points $T' = \{t_A,t_B,t_C\}$ which fulfill our matching criteria with the highest ranked 3 motif points, $S'= \{s_1,s_2,s_3\}$. In this stage, we represent the target as a geometric graph with coloured edges. There are exactly three unordered pairs of points in S', and we name them red, blue and green. In the target, if any pair of target points t_i,t_j fulfills our first two criteria with either red, blue or green, we draw a corresponding red blue or green edge between t_i,t_j in the target. Once we have processed all pairs of target points, we find all three-coloured triangles in T. These are the Seed Matches, a set of three-point correlations to S' that we sort by lRMSD and pass to Augmentation.

Augmentation

Augmentation is an application of depth first search that begins with the list of seed matches. Assuming that there are more than four motif points, we must find correspondences for the unmatched motif points within the target. Interpret the list of seed matches as a stack of partially complete matches. Pop off the first match, and considering the lRMSD alignment of this match, plot the position p of the next unmatched motif point s_i relative to the aligned orientation of the motif. In the spherical region V around p, identify all target points t_i, compatible with s_i, inside V. Now compute the lRMSD alignment of all correlated points, include the new correlation (s_i, t_i). If the new alignment satisfies our first two criteria and there are no more unmatched motif points, put this match into a heap which maintains the match with smallest lRMSD. If there are more unmatched motif points, put this partial match back onto the stack. Continue to test correlations in this manner, until V contains no more target points that satisfy our criteria. Then, return to the stack, and begin again by popping off the first match on the stack, repeating this process until the stack is empty.

Filtering Matches

Structural similarity is important to functional annotation only if a strong correlation exists between identifiably significant structural similarity and functional similarity. However, the existence of a match alone does not guarantee functional similarity. lRMSD can be a differentiating factor. If matches of homologous proteins represent statistically significant structural similarity over what is expected by random chance, we could differentiate on lRMSD, as long as we can evaluate the statistical significance of the lRMSD of a match.

BLAST first calculated the statistical significance of sequence matches with a combinatorial model of the space of similar sequences. Determining the statistical significance of structural matches has also been attempted. Modeling was applied for the PINTS database to estimate the probability of a structural match given a particular LRMSD.

An artificial distribution was parameterized by motif size and amino acid composition in order to fit a given data set, and the p-value is calculated relative to that distribution. Another approach was taken in the algorithm JESS, using comparative analysis to generate a significance score relative to a specific population of known motifs. Both methods have some disadvantages.

The artificial models of PINTS are not parameterized by the geometry of motifs, and, all else equal, produce identical distributions for motifs of different geometry. JESS, on the other hand, is dependent on a set of known motifs; should this set change, all significance scores would have to be revised.

Local structural alignment methods operate on the assumption that local structural and chemical similarity implies functional similarity. A statistical model has been developed that can be used to identify the degree of similarity sufficient to follow this implication. Given a match m with lRMSD r between motif S and target T, exactly one of two hypotheses must hold:

- H_0: S and T are structurally dissimilar
- H_A: S and T are structurally similar

The proposed statistical model implements this measurement by computing a *motif profile*. Motif profiles are frequency distributions of match lRMSDs between S and the entire Protein Data Bank (PDB), which is essentially a large set of functionally unrelated proteins. A motif profile is essentially a histogram, where the vertical axis measures the number of matches at each specific lRMSD, which is measured on the horizontal axis. Motif profiles provide very complete information about matches typical of H_0. If we suspect that a match m has lRMSD r indicative of functional similarity, we can use the motif profile to determine the probability p of observing another match m' with smaller lRMSD by computing the volume under the curve to the left of r, relative to the entire volume.

The probability p, often referred to as the p-value, is the measure of statistical significance. With a standard of statistical significance alpha, if p is less than alpha, then we say that the probability of observing a match m' with lRMSD r' less than r is so low that we reject the null hypothesis in favour of the alternative hypothesis. This process means that if a match m with lRMSD r has a p-value exactly equal to alpha, then this lRMSD is the highest lRMSD for which our statistical model predicts that m identifies structural and chemical similarity sufficient to imply functional similarity. Matches with this property are considered to be statistically significant.

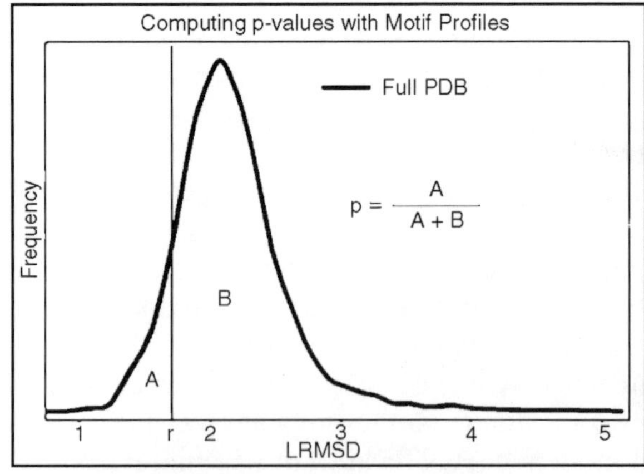

Fig. The Use of Motif Profiles.

Designing Effective Motifs

Given a motif representing a specific biochemical function, the task of any algorithm seeking to predict protein functions is to identify other proteins with similar biological functions. This is immediately affected by how well the motif represents the biological function - protein structures are flexible, dynamic objects, and any computational representation of these objects is likely to be inaccurate in some manner. In particular, since it is the computational representation that is compared, the fidelity of representation is essential for the effectiveness of the structural comparison approach.

An effective motif must simultaneously fulfill two criteria:

- The motif must be sensitive
- The motif must be specific

Motifs must maintain geometric and chemical similarity, in respect to the characteristics compared by the comparison algorithm, to functional homologs. This ensures that algorithms searching for the motif identify proteins with similar function.

Sensitivity is measured as the proportion of acceptable matches to functional homologs relative to the total number of functional homologs. Specific motifs must maintain geometric and chemical dissimilarity, in respect to the characteristics compared by the comparison algorithm, to functionally unrelated proteins.

This ensures that algorithms searching for the motif accidentally identify less matches to functionally unrelated proteins. Specificity is measured as the proportion of rejected matches to functionally unrelated proteins, relative to all functionally unrelated proteins. The ideally effective motif is 100per cent sensitive and 100per cent specific.

Under most conditions, effective motifs have been designed by hand. However, a few recently studies exist which examine the relationship between elements of the motif and the sensitivity and specificity of the motif. These studies resulted in the design of MultiBind, an algorithm which identifies conserved binding patterns among functionally homologous active sites, in order to generate motifs which represent only conserved binding patterns. Another study of motif design produced Geometric Sieving, an algorithm for maximizing the Geometric Uniqueness of motifs from functionally unrelated proteins.

Putting together effective motif design, an efficient matching algorithm, and a statistical scoring of the results can lead to an automated functional annotation pipeline for proteins.

SIMPLE PROTEINS

- *Albumins*: Blood (serumbumin); milk (lactalbumin); egg white (ovolbumin); lentils (legumelin); kidney beans (phaseolin); wheat (leucosin). Globular protein; soluble in water and dilute salt solution;

precipitated by saturation with ammonium sulfate solution; coagulated by heat; found in plant and animal tissues.

- *Globulins*: Blood (serum globulins); muscle (myosin); potato (tuberin); Brazil nuts (excelsin); hemp (edestin); lentils (legumin). Globular protein; sparingly soluble in water; soluble in neutral solutions; precipitated by dilute ammonium sulfate and coagulated by heat; distributed in both plant and animal tissues.
- *Glutelins*: Wheat (glutenin); rice (oryzenin). Insoluble in water and dilute salt solutions; soluble in dilute acids; found in grains and cereals.
- *Prolamines*: Wheat and rye (gliadin); corn (zein); rye (secaline); barley (hordein). Insoluble in water and absolute alcohol; soluble in 70per cent alcohol; high in amide nitrogen and proline; occurs in grain seeds.
- *Protamines*: Sturgeon (sturine); mackerel (scombrine); salmon (salmine); herring (clapeine). Soluble in water; not coagulated by heat; strongly basic; high in arginine; associate with DNA; occurs in sperm cells.
- *Histones*: Thymus gland; pancreas; nucleoproteins (nucleohistone). Soluble in water, salt solutions, and dilute acids; insoluble in ammonium hydroxide; yields large amounts of lysine and arginine; combined with nucleic acids within cells.
- *Scleroproteins*: Connective tissues and hard tissues. Fibrous protein; insoluble in all solvents and resistant to digestion.
  - *Collagen*: connective tissues, bones, cartilage, and gelatin. Resistant to digestive enzymes but altered to digest gelatin by boiling water, acid, or alkali; high in hydroxylrpline.
  - *Elastin*: Ligaments, tendons, and arteries. Similar to collagen but cannot be converted to gelatin.
  - *Keratin*: Hair, nails, hooves, horns, and feathers. Partially resistant to digestive enzymes; contains large amounts of sulfur, as cystine.

CONJUGATED PROTEINS

- *Nucleoproteins*: Cytoplasm of cells (ribonucleoprotein); nucleas of chromosomes (deoxyribonucleoprotein) viruses, and bacteriophages. Contains nucleic acids, nitrogen, and phosphorus. Present in chromosomes and in all living forms as a combination of protein with either RNA or DNA.
- *Mucoprotein*: Saliva (mucin); egg white (ovomucoid). Proteins combined with amino sugars, sugar acids, and sulfates.
- *Glycoprotein*: Bone (osseomucoid); tendons (tendomucoid); carilage (chondromucoid). Containing more than 4per cent hexosamine, mucoproteins; if less than 4per cent, then glycoproteins.
- *Phosphoproteins*: Milk (casein); egg yolk (ovovitellin). Phosphoric acid joined in ester linkage to protein.

- *Chromoproteins*: Hemoglobin; myoglobin; flavoproteins; respiratory pigments; cytochromes. Protein compounds with such nonprotein pigments as heme; coloured proteins.
- *Lipoproteins*: Serum lipoprotein; brain, nerve tissues, milk, and eggs. Water-soluble protein conjugated with lipids; found dispersed widely in all cells and all living forms.
- *Metallo proteins*: Ferritin; carbonic anhydrase; ceruloplasmin. Proteins combined with metallic atoms that are not parts of a nonprotein prosthetic group.

DERIVED PROTEINS

- *Proteans*: Edestan (from elastin) and myosan (from myosin). Results from short action of acids or enzymes; insolvent in water.
- *Proteases*: Intermediate products of protein digestion. Soluble in water; uncoagulated by heat; and precipitated by saturated ammonium sulfate; result from partial digestion of protein by pepsin or trypsin.
- *Peptones*: Intermediate products of protein digestion. Same properties as proteases except that they cannot be salted out; of smaller molecular weight that proteases.
- *Peptides*: Intermediate products of protein digestion. Two or more amino acids joined by a peptide linkage; hydrolyzed to individual amino acids.

5

Pharmacokinetic

A young child given an im injection might ask "How will that 'ouch' get from there to my sore throat"? The answer to this question is the basis of pharmacokinetics. That is, how drugs move around the body and how quickly this movement occurs. During this semester many of the processes which control the absorption, distribution, metabolism, and excretion of drugs will be discussed.

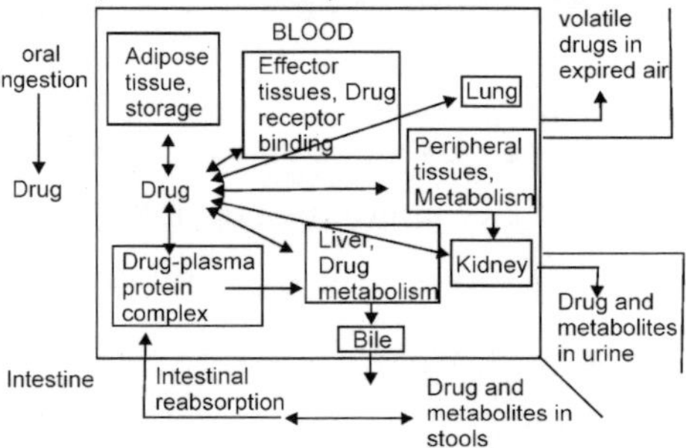

Fig. Complex picture of drug interactions in the body. This Figure gives an idea of the complexity of drug disposition. Shown in this Figure are many of the steps to getting drug from one site in the body to another. Many of these processes are enzyme induced. However the overall picture often is much simpler. Many of these processes maybe fast or not significant for any given drug.

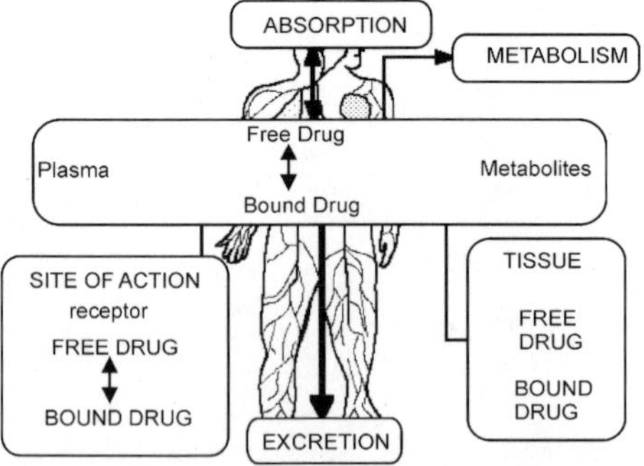

Fig. Figure of processes involved in drug transport. Here the major processes are represented in a less physiological fashion. It is with this approach that we will look at much of the course material this semester. The headings Absorption, Distribution, Metabolism, and Excretion are important.

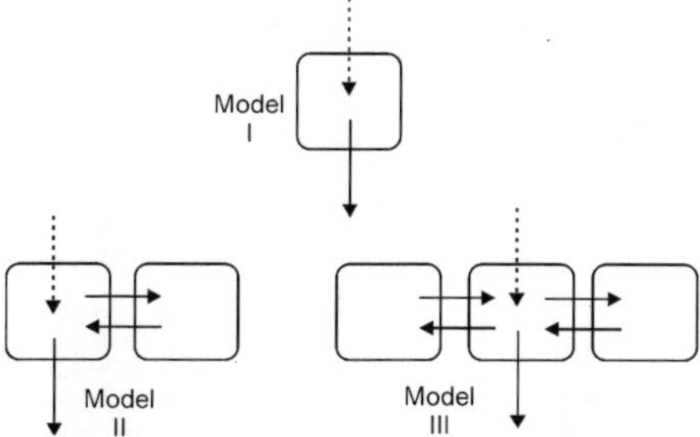

Fig. Figure of one, two, and three compartment pharmacokinetic models. Fortunately many of the processes involved in drug movement around the body are not saturated at normal therapeutic dose levels. The pharmacokinetic - mathematical models that can be used to describe plasma concentration as a function of time can then be much simplified. The body may even be represented as a single compartment or container for some drugs. For other drugs a two or three compartment model is found to be necessary.

One Compartment Model

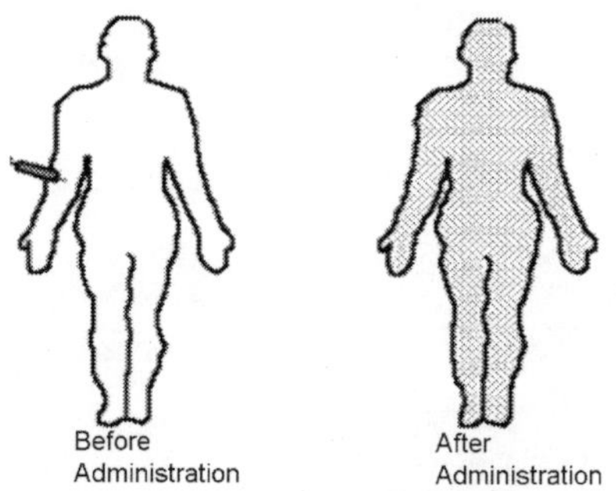

Fig. Figure of body before and after a rapid I.V. bolus injection, considering the body to behave as a single compartment. In order to simplify the mathematics it is often possible to assume that a drug given by rapid intravenous injection, a bolus, is rapidly mixed. This Figure represents the uniformly mixed drug very shortly after administration.

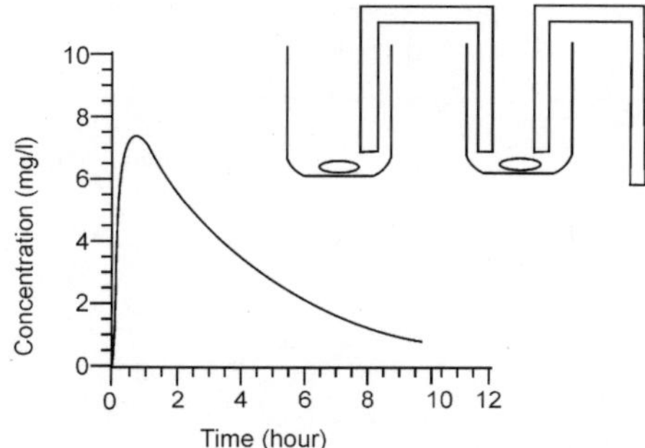

Fig. Figure of oral curve and beakers. We can picture oral administration as water flowing from one bucket (representing the GI tract) into a second beaker (representing the body). At first drug flows into the 'body' beaker and the level rises, as drug concentration rises, then after peaking the levels start to fall as elimination overtakes absorption. We have a few experiments in lab where the body is represented as a beaker. In the lab experiment a dye concentration represents drug concentration in the body.

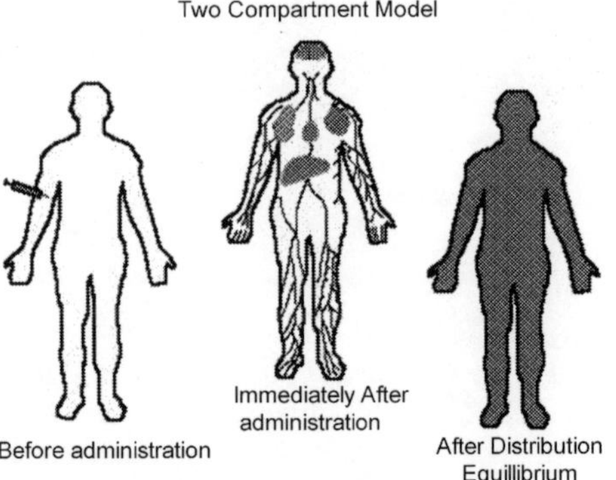

Fig. Figure of an intravenous bolus injection with a two compartment model. Often a one compartment model is not sufficient to represent the pharmacokinetics of a drug. A two compartment model often has wider application. Here we consider the body is a central compartment with rapid mixing and a peripheral compartment with slower distribution. The central compartment is uniformly mixed very shortly after drug administration, whereas it takes some time for the peripheral compartment to reach a pseudo equilibrium.

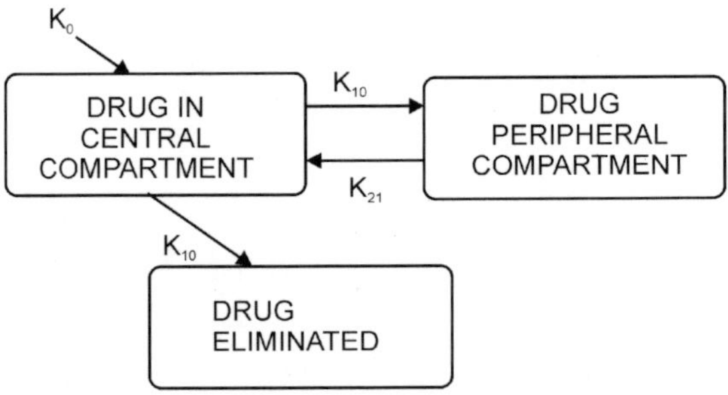

Fig. A diagram of a two compartment model showing the parameters to be measured. The processes of distribution and excretion can be represented by the rate constants k12, k21, and k10. The rate constant k0 representing an infusion or absorption process. The drug appears to be dissolved in the body volume. This volume is the 'apparent' volume of distribution.

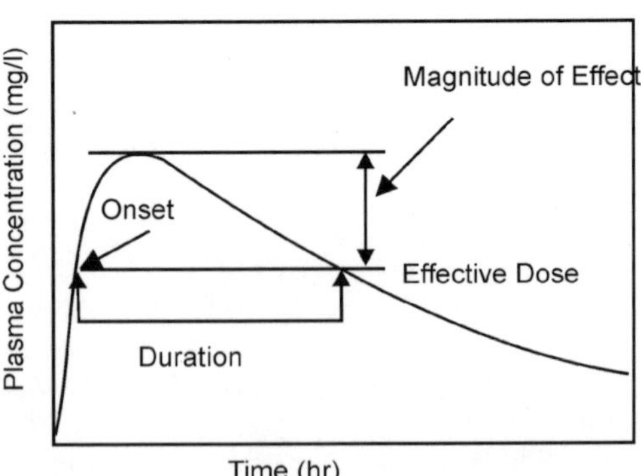

Fig. Figure showing effect as a function of time. From a graph such as this we can see the relationship between drug concentration and drug effect. If a drug has to reach an effective concentration at a receptor site this will be reflected as a required blood concentration.

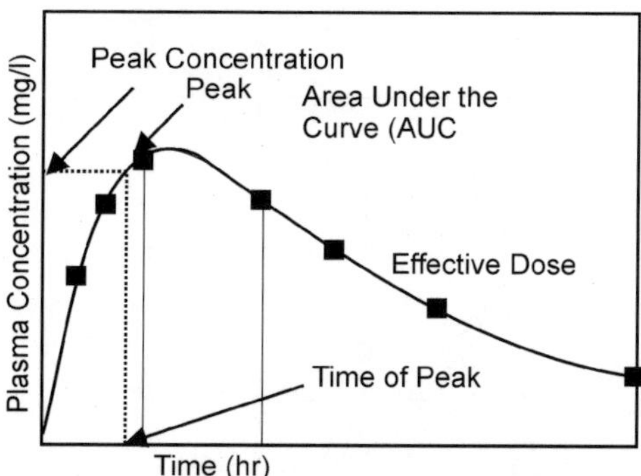

Fig. Figure of biopharmaceutic parameters over a blood time curve. This Figure shows some of the biopharmaceutic parameters which can be used to measure drug product performance. Later in the semester we will use the trapezoidal method of calculating AUC.

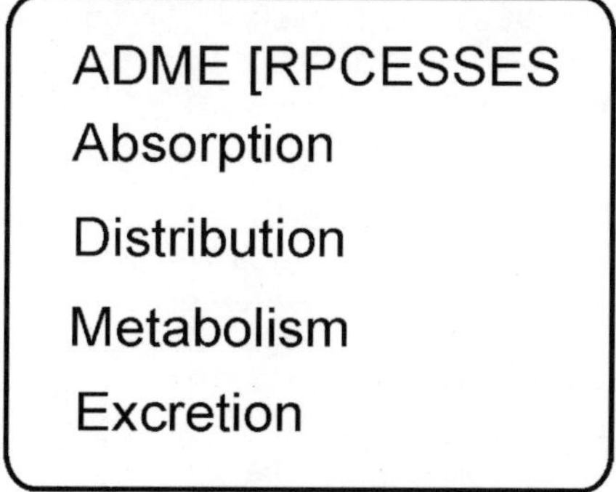

Fig. Figure listing the four pharmacokinetic processes. We will briefly consider each of these processes in turn. A (bsorption) D(istribution) M(etabolism) E(xcretion).

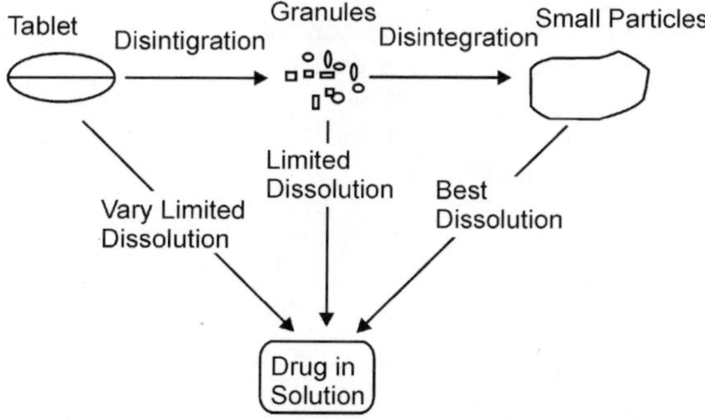

Fig. Figure showing the processes involved in the dissolution of a tablet before absorption. A drug cannot be absorbed across the intestinal wall as a solid. It must first dissolve in the fluid of the G-I tract. Tablets are carefully formulated, designed, to stay together in the bottle during transport but break up quickly once they are in an aqueous environment. This can be an easy or difficult job depending on the drug and the dose required. There are therefore dissolution tests specified to ensure that tablet formulations work.

Also it may be appropriate to conduct experiments with human volunteers to ensure that the tablet does release the drug as it should.

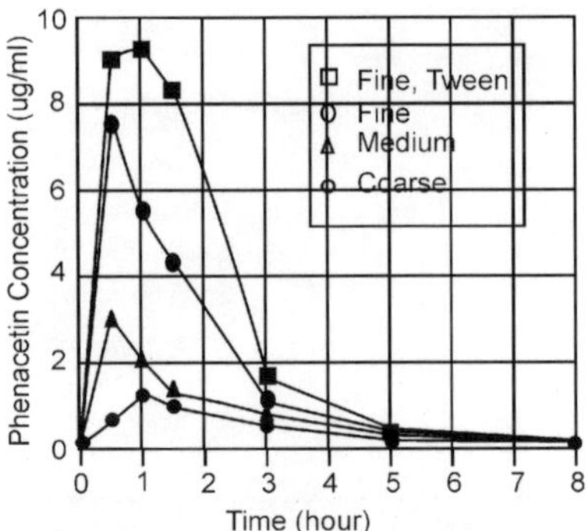

Fig. Figure showing plasma phenactin versus time curve after various suspensions. The effect of particle size on drug absorption is shown in this Figure. Generally speaking the smaller the particle size the quicker the absorption. By increasing the particle surface area it is possible to increase the dissolution rate. However very small particle can clump together. Therefore a wetting agent such as Tween 80 can have a beneficial effect on the overall absorption. The intestinal fluids usually contain some materials which can act as wetting agents, however drug dissolution testing *in vitro* may neglect this effect.

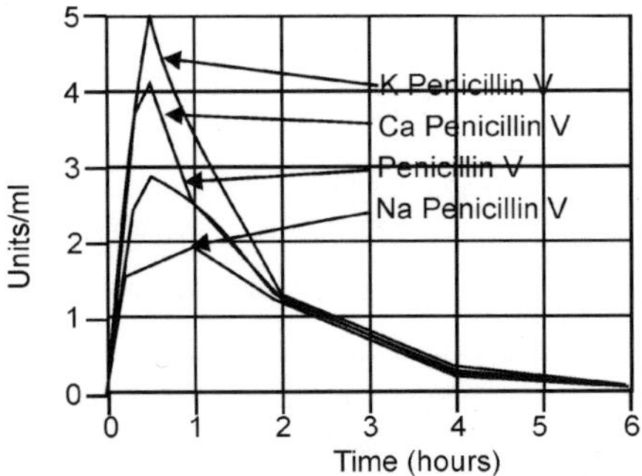

Fig. 1.14: Figure showing plasma penicillin concentration versus time curve after oral administration of various salts. The rate at which a drug dissolves is dependent on the solubility of the drug. A common occurrence is that different salts will have quite different solubility characteristics, and again somewhat different to the free acid (or base) form. In the case of penicillin V it appears that only drug which is dissolved quickly can be absorbed.

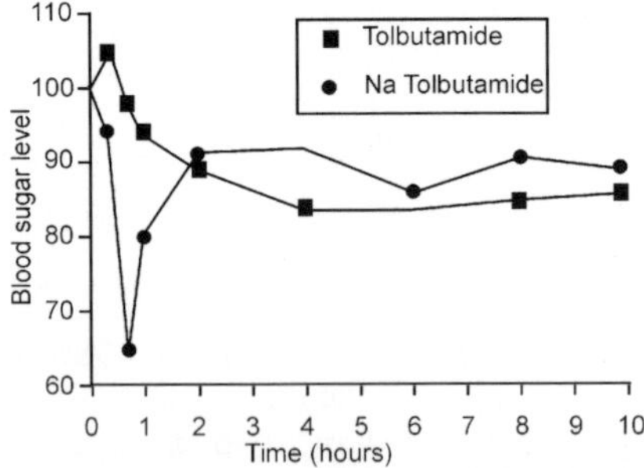

Fig. Figure showing blood sugar levels after tolbutamide acid and salt (redrawn from Wagner, J.G. 1961 Biopharmaceutics: absorption aspects, *J. Pharm. Sci.* Rapid dissolution and absorption is not always the objective. Sometimes a slower release is required. In the case of tolbutamide, used to lower blood sugar concentrations, a more sustained release is better causing a more gradual reduction in blood sugar.

The effect of dissolution rate on the absorption and biological Response of tolbutamide (1.0g) and sodium tolbutamide (1.0g equivalent) when formulated in compressed tablets.

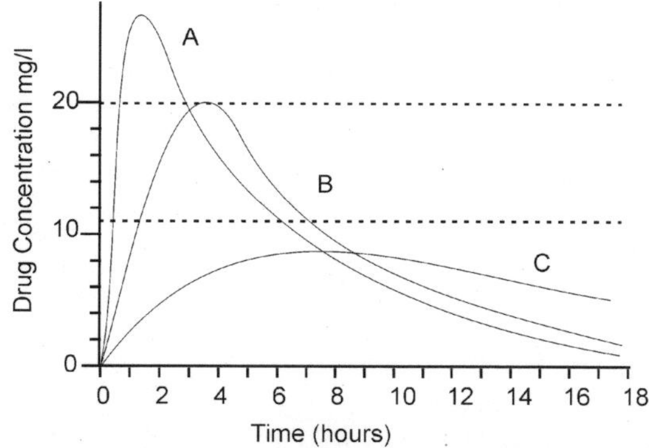

Fig. Figure showing plasma concentration time curves for three theoretical formulations with different ka values. The plasma concentrations achieved can be controlled by the rate of drug absorption. As shown product I would be toxic. A smaller dose, or a slower formulation should be considered. Formulation II appears to be effective in the dose and formulation used. The dosage form III appears to be too slow and thereby ineffective. If it is a drug requiring a sustained effect this formulation may be more useful at a higher dose or after repeated doses.

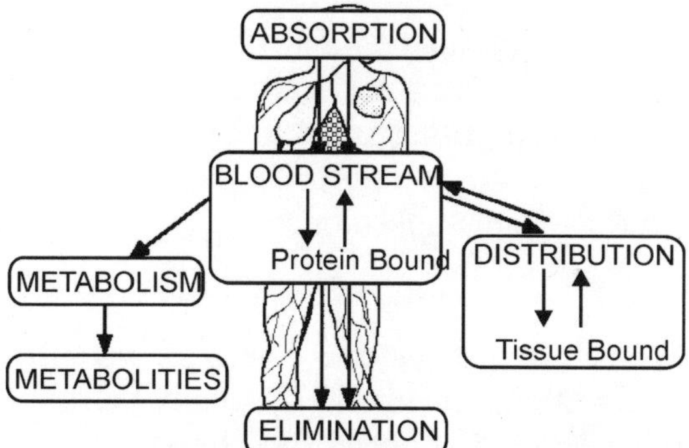

Fig. Figure showing the four processes schematically. Leading to the next process elimination.

ONE COMPARTMENT I.V. BOLUS

Definition: Pharmacokinetics is the study of drug and/or metabolite kinetics in the body. It deals with a mathematical description of the rates of drug movement into, within and exit from the body. It also includes the study of drug metabolism or biotransformation rates. The body is a very complex system and a drug undergoes many steps as it is being absorbed, distributed through the body, metabolized or excreted (ADME).

The drug also interacts with receptors and causes therapeutic and/or toxic responses. Although the details of drug kinetics are complicated it is fortunate that we can often approximate drug kinetic processes using "simple" mathematical models.

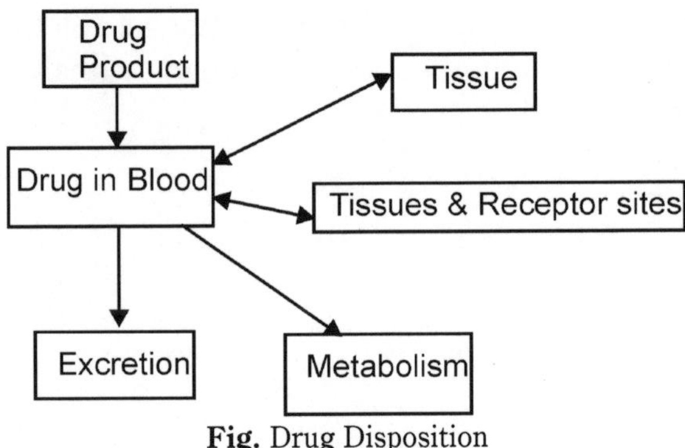

Fig. Drug Disposition

A. ASSUMPTIONS

We will start the course with a one compartment - linear model. Also, we will first consider drug kinetics after a rapid intravenous injection, an IV bolus injection. According to this model we will consider the body to behave as a single well- mixed container. To use this model mathematically we need to make a number of assumptions.

1. One Compartment

The drug in the blood is in rapid equilibrium with drug in the extravascular tissues. The drug concentration may not be equal in each tissue or fluid however we will assume that they are proportional to the concentration of drug in the blood at all times. This is not an exact representation however it is useful for a number of drugs to a reasonable approximation.

2. Rapid Mixing

We also need to assume that the drug is mixed instantaneously in blood or plasma. The actual time taken for mixing is usually very short, within a few of minutes, and in comparison with normal sampling times it is insignificant. We usually don't sample fast enough to see drug mixing in the blood.

3. Linear Model

We will assume that drug elimination follows first order kinetics. First order kinetics means that the rate of change of drug concentration by any process is directly proportional to the drug concentration remaining to undertake that process. Remember first order kinetics is an assumption of a linear model not a one compartment model. If we have a linear if we double the dose, the concentration will double at each time point.

B. FIRST-ORDER KINETICS

To illustrate first order kinetics we might consider what would happen if we were to give a drug by iv bolus injection, collect blood samples at various times and measure the plasma concentrations of the drug. We might see a steady decrease in concentration as the drug is eliminated, as shown in Figure given below.

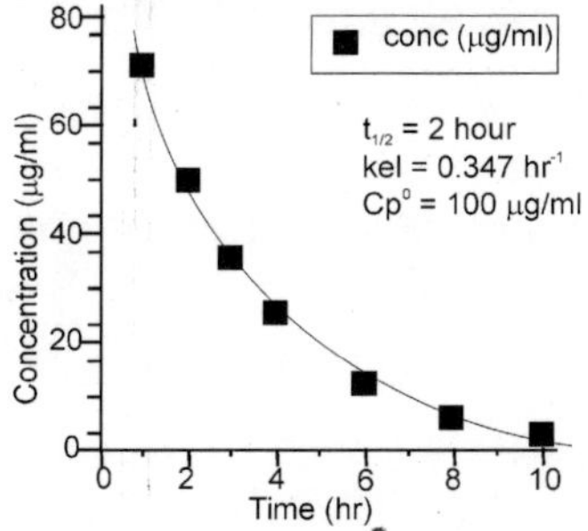

Fig. Linear Plot of Concentration versus Time

1. Rate versus Cp

If we measure the slope of this curve at a number of times we are actually measuring the rate of change of concentration at each time point $\frac{\Delta Cp}{\Delta t}$ represented by the straight line tangents in Figure given below.

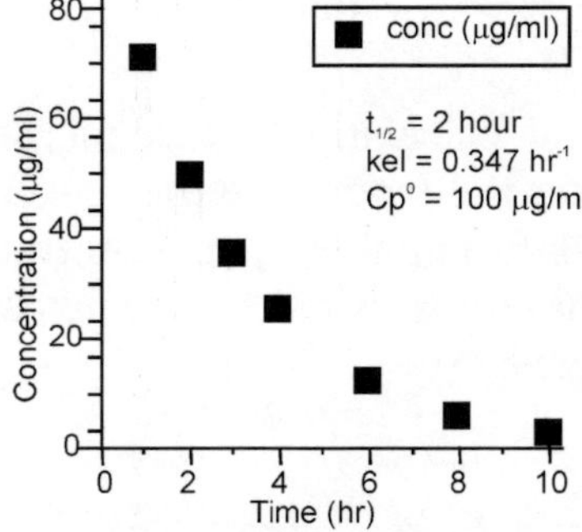

Fig. Same as Figure given above with Tangents shown.

Now if we plot this rate of change versus the plasma concentration, for each data point, we will get a straight line when first order kinetics are obeyed. This is shown in Figure given below.

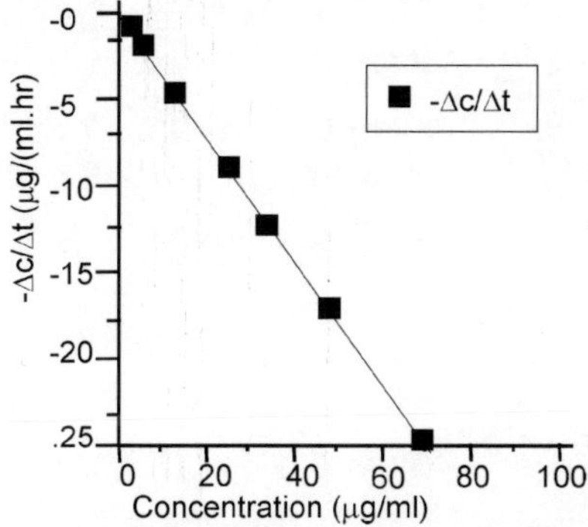

Fig. Plot of $\Delta Cp/\Delta t$ versus Cp for first order plot.

This behaviour can be expressed mathematically as:-

Rate of Change of C_P versus time $= \dfrac{\Delta Cp}{\Delta t} = kel \bullet Cp$

Change in $Cp = \Delta Cp$

Change in time $= \Delta t$

Proportionality constatn called the elimination rate constant, $kel = kel \bullet Cp$ Equation-1

C. PLASMA DATA

1. Scheme or Diagram

The one compartment pharmacokinetic model can be represented schematically as:-

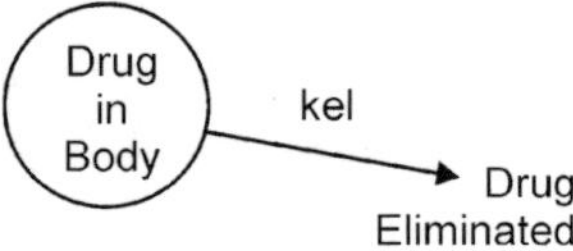

Fig. Scheme for a One Compartment Model, Intravenous Bolus Administration

2. Differential Equation

Going back to the slope calculations, if we measure the slope over small intervals we are calculating the tangent to the line. We can now say that the rate of elimination is the differential of the concentration with respect to time as Δt - - - > 0 then $\Delta Cp/\Delta t$ - - - > dCp/dt which gives:-

$$\frac{dCp}{\Delta t} = kel \bullet Cp$$

Equation -2. Rate of Change of Drug Concentration - First Order, IV Bolus

Equation -2 is a differential equation for the one-compartment model after IV bolus administration. With the calculus term dCp/dt we are going from the gross or large time interval term $\Delta Cp/\Delta t$ to the continuously varying dCp/dt term.

3. Elimination Rate Constant, kel

We should now distinguish between the elimination rate and the elimination rate constant. The rate (tangent or slope, dCp/dt) changes as the concentration changes, however, for a linear model the rate constant (kel) is constant, it does not change.

4. Integrated Equation

We could use the equation

$$\frac{dCp}{dt} = kel \bullet Cp$$

to calculate kel. Plotting - dCp/dt versus Cp would give kel as the slope of the straight line. Howver, in practice, it is difficult to measure *dCp/dt* (the tangent to the line drawn through the *Cp* versus time plot) accurately and so this equation is not often used directly.

The problem is the differential term. Mathematically, we get rid of this term by integrating the equation. We can go through this one because it is easy and also to see what is involved in the process, but for other differential equations we'll just use the answer.

Starting with

$$\frac{dCp}{dt} = kel \bullet Cp$$

(Equation-2 from earlier)

Rearranging gives

$$\frac{dCp}{Cp} = -kel \bullet dt$$

Equation -3. Differential Equation Rearranged

Integrating both sides gives

$$\int_{Cp(0)}^{Cp(t)} \frac{dCp}{Cp} = -kel \bullet \int_{t=0}^{t=t} dt$$

Equation -4. Integration of the Rearranged Equation

This gives (by looking the answer in Maths tables)

$$[InCp]_{Cp(0)}^{Cp(t)} = -kel \bullet = [t]_0^t$$

Equation -5. Rearrange the Integrated Equation

Note that the integral of 1/x is ln(x), when ln represents log to the base e. This leads to the utility of the log to base e which is used extensively in the area of pharmacokinetics.

Expanding Equation -5 gives

$$\ln Cp^t - \ln Cp^0 = - kel * t + kel * 0$$

Equation -6. Natural log of Cp versus Time

Or

$\ln Cp^t = \ln Cp^0$ - kelt

Equation -7. Integrated Equation for ln *Cp* versus Time

Note the use of natural log to base e

Rearranging gives

$$in[\frac{Cp(t)}{Cp(0)}] = -kel \bullet t$$

Equation -8. Rearranging the Integrated Equation

Taking the antilog (base e) of both sides gives

$$Cp^t = Cp^0 \bullet e^{-kel \bullet t}$$

Equation -9. Another form of the integrated equation

This is a single exponential equation. The fall in plasma concentration is therefore called monoexponential decay

Looking back at the ln (base e) equation; we can convert that into log (base 10), common logs, by dividing by 2.303 giving

$$\log Cp^t = \log Cp^0 - \frac{kel \bullet t}{2.303}$$

Equation -10. Log base 10 *Cp* versus Time

This is another form of the integrated equation

Both of these integrated (logarithmic) forms represent a straight line equation, that is of the form: $y = a - m * t$ with a = intercept and m = slope.

Plotting ln (*Cp*) versus t should give a straight line with a slope of - kel and an intercept of ln Cp^0.

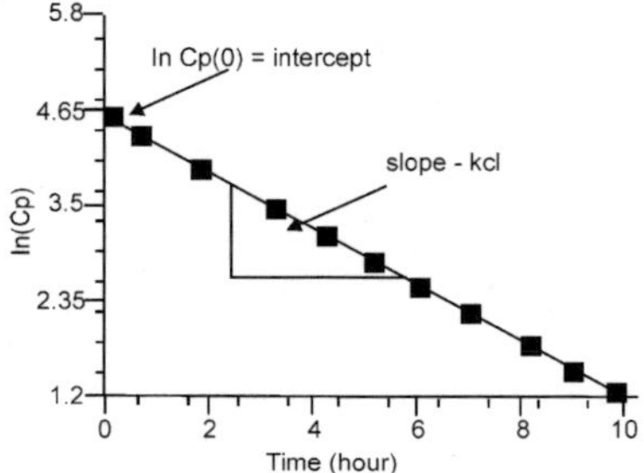

Fig. Linear plot of *Cp* versus time, showing intercept and slope.

Notice, no Units for ln (*Cp*) but units of hour for time (X axis).

Units: Slope has units of time^{-1} thus kel has units of time^{-1} *e.g.* min^{-1}, hr^{-1}.

Now we can measure kel by determining *Cp* versus time and plotting ln *Cp* versus time.

On Semi-log Graph Paper

This plot allows us to calculate kel given *Cp* at various times.

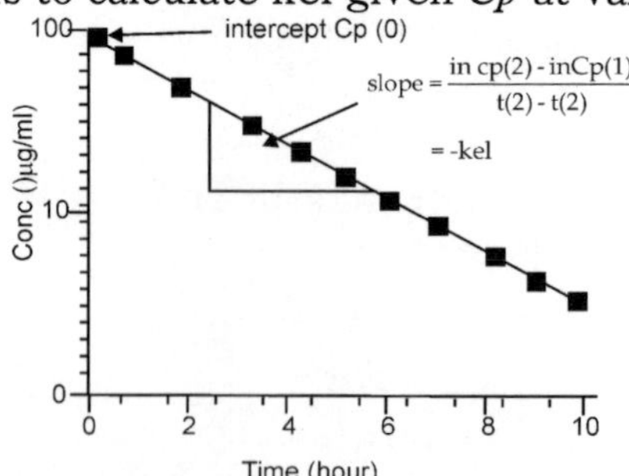

Fig. Semi-log plot of *Cp* versus time, showing slope and intercept.

Plasma Concentration versus Time Plots

- Semi-log

Table. Example Values for Elimination Rate Constant and Half-life for Elimination.

	kel, hr^{-1}	$t_{1/2}$, *hr*
Acetaminophen	0.28	2.5
Diazepam	0.021	33
Digoxin	0.017	40
Gentamicin	0.35	2.1
Lidocaine	0.43	1.6
Theophylline	0.063	11

5. Apparent Volume of Distribution, V

We can also use the equations above to calculate the plasma concentration at any time when we know kel and Cp^0. However, usually we don't know Cp^0 ahead of time, but we do know the dose. A dose in mass units, maybe in mg. To calculate Cp^0 we need to know the volume that the drug is distributed into. That is, the apparent volume of the mixing container, the body. This apparent volume of distribution is not a physiological volume. It won't be lower than blood or plasma volume but it can be much larger than body volume for some drugs. It is a mathematical 'fudge' factor relating the amount of drug in the body and the concentration of drug in the measured compartment, usually plasma.

$$\text{Definition: } V = \frac{amount}{concentration\ measured\ in\ plasma}$$

Equation -11. Definition for Apparent Volume of Distribution

$$V = \frac{x}{Cp}$$

Equation -12. Relationship between Amount and Concentration

Immediately after the intravenous dose is administered the amount of drug in the body is the dose. Thus:-

$$V = \frac{DOSE}{Cp^0}$$

Equation -13. Volume calculated from Cp^0

Or

$$Cp^0 = \frac{DOSE}{V}$$

Equation -14. Initial Concentration

Table. Example Values for Apparent Volume of Distribution[2].

Drug	V (l/kg)	V (l, 70 kg)
Sulfisoxazole	0.16	11.2
Phenytoin	0.63	44.1
Phenobarbital	0.55	38.5
Diazepam	2.4	168
Digoxin	7	490

The last figure, for digoxin, is much larger than body volume. Drug must be extensively distributed into tissue, leaving low concentrations in the plasma, thus the body as a whole appears to have a large volume, of distribution. Remember, this is not a physiological volume.

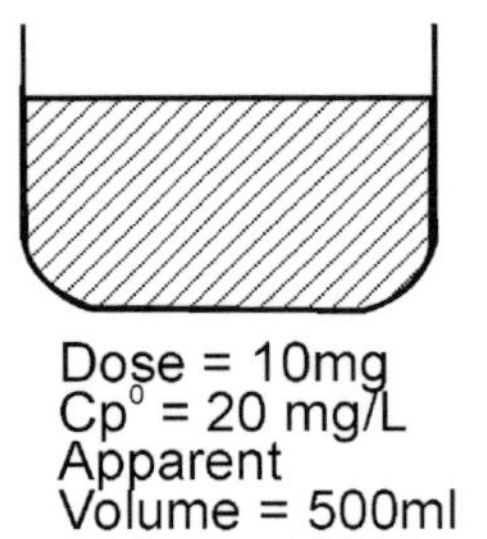

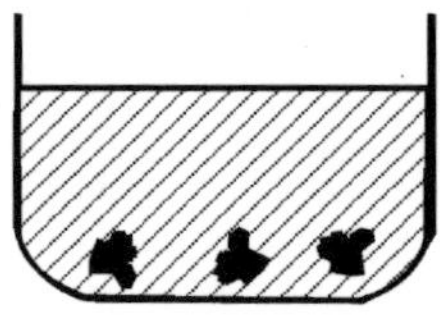

Fig. Apparent Volume of Distribution.

In summary these equations apply:

$$Cp = \frac{DOSE}{V} \bullet e^{-kel-t}$$

Equation -15. Concentration as a Function of Time since

$$Cp^0 = \frac{DOSE}{V}$$

(Equation -14, from above)

Example Calculations:

1. After a dose of 500 mg, $V = 30$ litre, $kel = 0.2\ hr^{-1}$

The following plasma concentrations can be calculated

$$Cp = Cp0 * e- kel * t$$

$$Cp = \frac{DOSE}{y} \bullet e^{-kel \bullet t}$$

Thus:

$Cp^0 = 500/30 = 16.7$ mg/litre $Cp^{2\ \text{hours}} = 11.2$ mg/litre

$Cp^{4\ \text{hours}} = 7.5$ mg/litre

Table. Enter Values into Each Field.

IV Bolus Dose:	500	
Apparent Volume of Distribution:	30	Cannot be zero
Elimination Rate Constant:	0.2	
Time since IV Dose:	2	
The answer Cp^t is:		

Example Calculations:

2. We can also calculate the pharmacokinetic parameters kel and V if we know the dose given and the plasma concentrations at two (or more) times after an I.V. bolus administration. This time we could use the equation:

$\ln Cp = \ln Cp^0$ - kel*t

If $Cp^{2\text{ hours}} = 4.5$ mg/litre and $Cp^{6\text{ hours}} = 3.7$ mg/litre after a 400 mg I.V. bolus dose then:

$$slope = -kel = \frac{in\,3.7 - in\,4.5}{6-2}$$

$$= \frac{1.308 - 1.504}{4} = -\frac{0.196}{4} = -\,0.0489\,hr^{-1}$$

thus $kel = 0.0489\,hr^{-1}$

Now $\ln Cp^{2\text{ hr}} = \ln Cp^0 - kel * t$

$\ln 4.5 = \ln Cp^0 - 0.0489 \times 2$

$\ln Cp^0 = 1.504 + 0.098 = 1.602$

$$Cp^0 = 4.96 = \frac{DOSE}{V}$$

$$V = \frac{DOSE}{Cp^0} = \frac{400}{4.96} = 80.6 liter$$

Example Calculations:

3. Given kel (= $0.17\,hr^{-1}$) and $V = (25\,L)$ for a given drug we can calculate the dose required, by rapid IV bolus, to achieve a plasma concentration of 2.4 *ug/ml* (= 2.4 *mg/L*) at 6 hours.

Thus $Cp^6 = Cp^0 * e^{-kel.t}$

$$Cp^0 = \frac{DOSE}{V} = e^{-kel-t}$$

Example Calculations:

4. After an I.V. bolus dose of 500 mg the data collected in Table were collected.

Table. Concentration versus Time Data.

Time (hr)	1	2	3	4	6	8	10
Cp (mcg/ml)	72	51	33	20	14	9	4

Calculate kel and V.

Plot the data on semi-log graph paper and determine Cp^1, Cp^2, $t1$ and t^2.

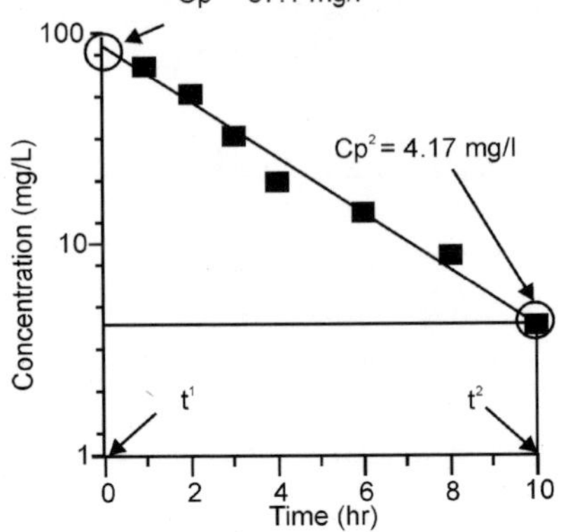

Fig. Plot of *Cp* Versus Time on Semi-log Graph Paper After an I.V. Bolus Dose of 500 mg.

$$kel = \frac{In\,Cp_1 - In\,Cp_2}{t_2 - t_2}$$

$$= \frac{In\,87.1 - In\,4.17}{10.0}$$

$$= 3.04/10 = 0.304\ hr^{-1}$$

$$V = \frac{Dose}{Cp^0} = \frac{500}{87.1} = 5.74L$$

6. Area under the Plasma Concentration Time Curve, AUC

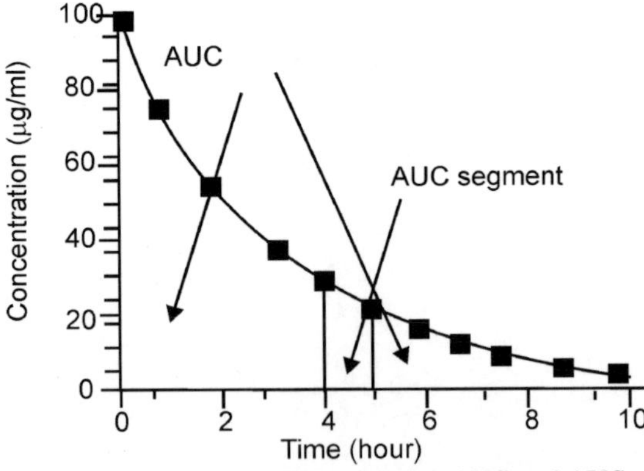

Fig. Linear Plot of Cp versus Time showing AUC and AUC segment.

We can continue by looking at two more parameters. These are the area under the plasma concentration time curve (*AUC*) and the half-life of elimination. First *AUC*. The *AUC* value is very useful for calculating the relative efficiency of different drug products (We'll talk about this later). It will also give us another method of calculating the apparent volume of distribution, not just from Cp^0.

The *AUC* is calculated by adding these segments together. Each very narrow segment has an area = $Cp*dt$. Thus the total area has the area, *AUC*.

$$AUC = \int_{t=0}^{t=0} Cp^t \bullet dt$$

Equation -16. AUC for a Very Narrow Segment

calculus uses very narrow segments

Since

$$Cp^t = Cp^o \bullet e^{-kel \bullet t} = \frac{DOSE}{V} \bullet e^{-kel \bullet t}$$

then

$$AUC = \frac{DOSE}{V} \bullet \int_{t=0}^{t=\bullet} e^{-kel \bullet t} \bullet dt$$

$$= \frac{DOSE}{V} \bullet \left[\frac{e^{-kel \bullet t}}{-kel}\right]_{t=0}^{t=\infty}$$

at $t = 0$, $e^{-kel*t} = 1$

at $t = \infty$, $e^{-kel*t} = 0$

Therefore

$$AUC = \frac{DOSE}{V} \bullet \left[0 - \frac{1}{-kel}\right]$$

or

$$AUC = \frac{DOSE}{V \bullet kel} = \frac{Cp^0}{kel}$$

Equation -17. *AUC* Calculated from Concentration and kel

Analytical integration (exact solution, given exact values for V and kel)

[Note: From $t = 0 -> t =$ [[infinity]], $AUC = Cp^0/kel$ and for $t = t ->$ t= [[infinity]], $AUC = Cp^t/kel$]

or

$$V = \frac{DOSE}{AUC \bullet kel}$$

Equation -18. Volume of Distribution Calculated from Dose, *AUC* and kel

We could use equation 20 to calculate the *AUC* value if we knew *DOSE*, kel, and V; but usually we don't and have to calculate *AUC* directly from the *Cp* versus time data.

We need then a different approach, which is called the trapezoidal rule. Numerical (approximate) solution

a) Trapezoidal rule

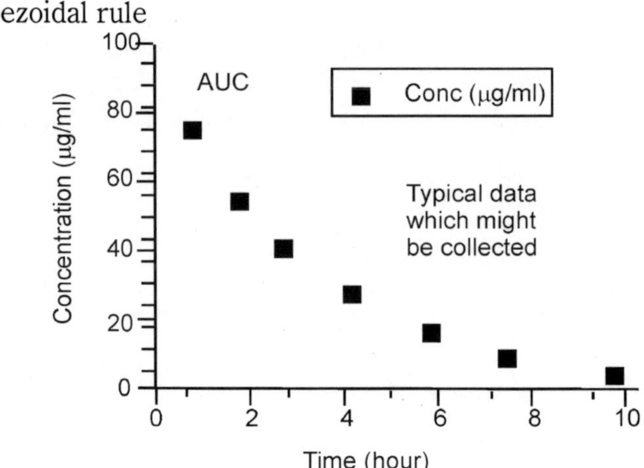

Fig. Linear Plot of *Cp* versus Time showing Typical Data Points

We can calculate the *AUC* of each segment if we consider the segments to be trapezoids. [Four sided figures with two parallel sides].

The area of each segment is then given by the average concentration x segment width.

There fore

$$\text{AUC}^{2\text{-}3} = \frac{Cp^2 + Cp^3}{2} \bullet (t^3 - t^2)$$

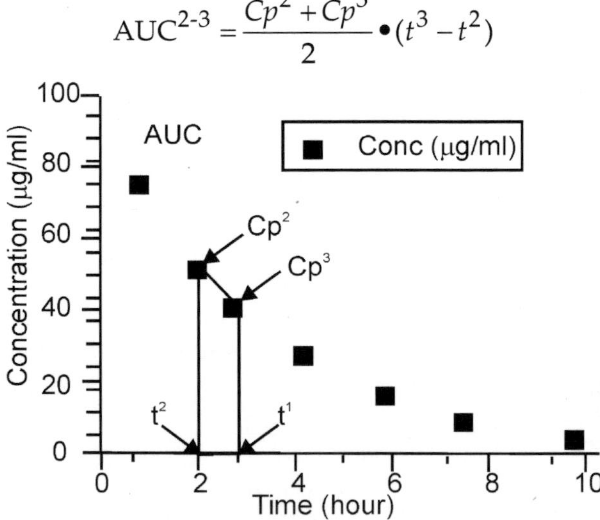

Fig. Linear Plot of *Cp* versus Time showing One Trapezoid

The area from the first to last data point can then be calculated by adding the areas together.

$$AUC^{1\text{-}n} = \Sigma \left\{ \frac{Cp^1 + Cp^2}{2} \bullet (t^2 - t^1) \right\}$$

$$+\left\{\frac{Cp^3 + Cp^2}{2} \bullet (t^3 - t^2)\right\} + \ldots$$

Note: Summation of data point information (non-calculus).
This gives:

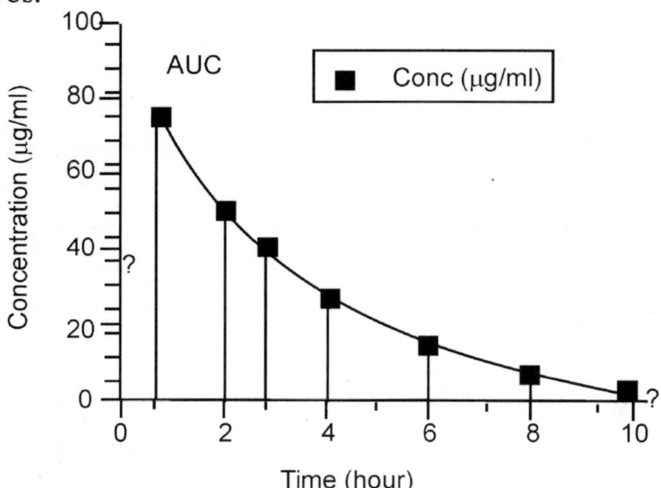

Fig. Linear plot of *Cp* versus time showing areas from data 1 to data n

We now have two more areas to consider. The first and the last.

First if we give a rapid I.V. bolus the zero plasma concentration Cp^0 can be determined by extrapolation.

Thus

$$AUC^{0\text{-}1} = \left\{\frac{Cp^0 + Cp^1}{2} \times t^1\right\}$$

The final segment can be calculated if we go back to the mathematical equation.

$$AUC^{t(last)^{-\infty}} = \int_{t=t(last)}^{t=\infty} Cp \bullet dt$$

$\frac{Cp^{last}}{kel}$ can be derived

Therefore the total AUC can be calculated as,-

$$AUC^{0-\infty} = AUC^{0-t(last)} + AUC^{t(last)-\infty}$$

$$= \Sigma\left\{\frac{Cp^0 + Cp^1}{2} \bullet t^1\right\} + \left\{\frac{Cp^1 + Cp^2}{2} \bullet (t^2 - t^1)\right\} + \;..+ \frac{cp^{last}}{kel}$$

Table. Calculation of AUC.

Time (hr)	Concentration (μg.hr/ml)	Δ AUC	AUC (μg/ml)
0	100		
1	71	85.5	85.5
2	50	60.5	146.0
3	35	42.5	188.5
4	25	30.0	218.5
6	12	37.0	255.5
8	6.2	18.2	273.7
10	3.1	9.3	283.0
Total		8.9	291.9

7. Half-life

Another important property of first order kinetics is the half-life of elimination, $t^{1/2}$.

The half-life is the time taken for the plasma concentration to fall to half its original value. Thus if *Cp* = concentration at the start and *Cp*/2 is the concentration one half-life later then:-

$$In\frac{Cp}{2} = In\,Cp - kel \bullet t_{1/2}$$

$$In\left[\frac{Cp}{2} \bullet \frac{1}{Cp}\right] = -\,kel \bullet t_{1/2}$$

$$\text{In } 2 = kel * t1/2$$

or

$$t_{1/2} = \frac{0.693}{kel}$$

OR

$$kel = \frac{0.693}{t_{1/2}}$$

Note: Independent of concentration, a property of first order processes

These equations can be used as an approximate method of calculating kel. If we look at a plot of *Cp* versus time on semi-log graph paper.

The steps to take

- Draw a line through the points (this tends to average the data)
- Pick any *Cp* and t^1
- Determine *Cp*/2 and t^2

- Calculate $t_{1/2}$ as $(t^2 - t^1)$

Then kel = $0.693/t^{1/2}$

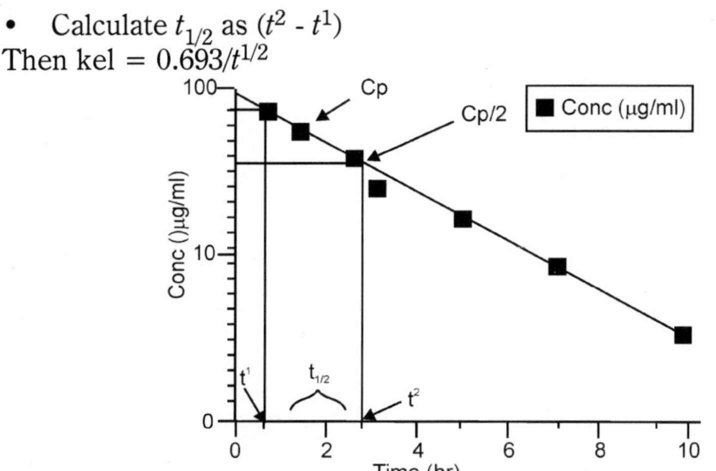

Fig. Semi-log Plot of *Cp* versus Time with Some Data and a Line

Also Consider Determining Cp/4 or Cp/8 for two Half-lives or Three Half-lives, Respectively

The line smooths out the bumps. There may be bad data points, so by putting in a line you 'sort of' average the data. The half-life is the same whether going from 40 to 20 or from 10 to 5 *mg/L*. This is a property of the first order process.

Note:

Go from:

Cp - > *Cp*/2 in 1 half-life *per cent* 50.0 per cent lost 50.0 per cent
Cp - > *Cp*/4 in 2 half-lives *i.e.* 25.0 per cent lost 75.0 per cent
Cp - > *Cp*/8 in 3 half-lives *i.e.* 12.5 per cent lost 87.5 per cent
Cp - > *Cp*/16 in 4 half-lives *i.e.* 6.25 per cent lost 93.75 per cent
Cp - > *Cp*/32 in 5 half-lives *i.e.* 3.125 per cent lost 96.875 per cent
Cp - > *Cp*/64 in 6 half-lives *i.e.* 1.563 per cent lost 98.438 per cent
Cp - > *Cp*/128 in 7 half-lives *i.e.* 0.781 per cent lost 99.219 per cent

Thus over 95 per cent lost or eliminated in 5 half-lives. Typically considered the completion (my definition unless told otherwise) of the process, although in theory it takes an infinite time. Others may wish to wait 7 half-lives where over 99per cent of the process is complete.

Analysis of Urine Data

So far we have looked at most of the information we can get from plasma data following a rapid intravenous dose of a drug using a one compartment model. There is another part of the model which can be sampled. Sometimes it is not possible to collect blood or plasma samples but we may be able to measure the amount of drug excreted into urine.

- We may not want to take repeated blood samples from certain patient populations, for example pediatrics

- The apparent volume of distribution maybe so large that plasma concentrations are too small to measure.

If we collect data for amount of drug excreted into urine it may be possible to determine the elimination rate constant or half-life and other pharmacokinetic parameters.

Excretion Unchanged - No Metabolism

First we'll consider the case in which the drug is excreted totally as the unchanged drug into urine.

Scheme or Diagram

The scheme is then:-

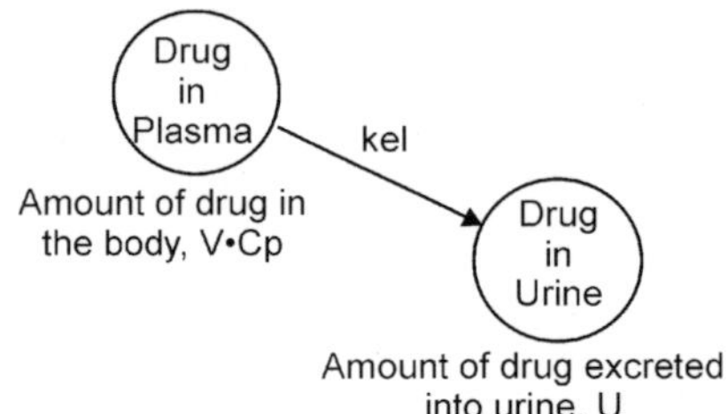

Fig. Scheme for drug excreted into urine, one compartment

Differential Equation

Since the rate of elimination from plasma is the same as the rate of appearance of drug into urine.

$$\frac{dU}{dt} = -\frac{V \bullet dcp}{dt} = +kel \bullet Cp \bullet V$$

Equation V-1. Differential Equation for Cumulative amount Excreted

Since according to this model, the drug is either in the body or has been eliminated into urine.

$$\text{Dose} = \text{Amount in body} + \text{Amount excreted} = V * Cp + U$$

Plot Types

Cumulative Amount Excreted Versus Time

The U versus time is a mirror image of the amount of drug in the body $V*Cp$ versus time. As we lose drug from the body, it will appear in urine. We can derive an equation for U versus time by integrating the differential equation.

(Equation -a)

$$\frac{dU}{dt} = kel \bullet Cp \bullet V$$

Differential Equation

Since

$$Cp = Cp^0 * e^{-kel * t} \text{ and } V * Cp^0 = DOSE$$

$$dU = DOSE * kel * e^{-kel * t} * dt$$

then

$$U = DOSE\,[1 - e^{-kel * t}]$$

Equation -b. Integration Equation for U

Cumulative amount excreted into urine at time = t

At $t = 0$; $e^{-kel * t} = 1$

then $U^0 =$ ***DOSE*** [1 - 1] = 0

At $t = \infty$; $e^{-kel * t} = 0$

then $U = {}^{\infty}$ *DOSE* [1 - 0] = *DOSE*

The cumulative amount excreted into urine is one way of representing this data. It is fairly qualitative and it is difficult to get quantitative results directly. There are other ways of looking at this data which can give you more information.

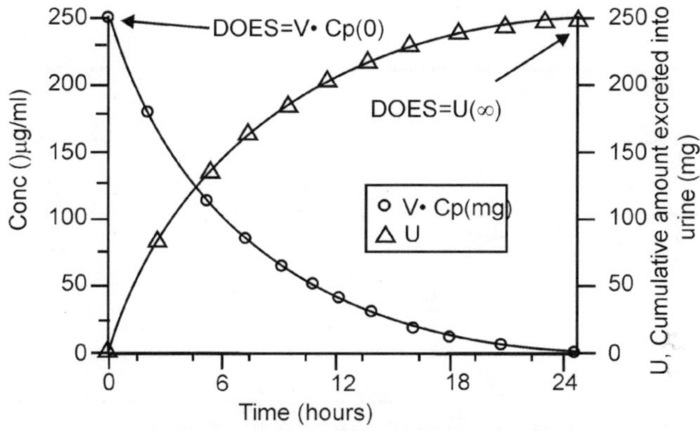

Fig. Plot of *Cp* versus Time and *U* versus Time

Rate of excretion (R/E)

A second method is the rate of excretion versus time plot. Going back to the differential equation.

$$\frac{dU}{dt} = kel \bullet V \bullet Cp = DOSE \bullet Kel \bullet e^{-kel \bullet t}$$

Equation -c. Rate of Change of U versus Time

Taking the logarithms of both sides gives:-

$$In\frac{dU}{dt} = In\,(DOSE \bullet kel) - kel \bullet t$$

Thus by plotting ln (dU/dt) versus time you should get a straight line with a slope of - *kel*.

It may look like a strange way of plotting the data, but actually it's quite convenient to use because urine data results are collected as an amount of drug excreted during a time interval. The amount excreted is the product of the volume of urine voided and concentration of drug in the sample. Again, this is a rate measurement. Since we estimate d*U*/d*t* as $\Delta U/\Delta t$, an average rate of excretion over the collection interval, the t value used with this plot is the time at the midpoint of the collection interval.

Example Ampicillin almost 100per cent (actually closer to 90per cent) excreted unchanged into urine.

Table. Example Data Analysis of Drug in Urine Data.

Time Interval (mg)	Amount Excreted Excreted	Cumulative Amount (hr) (mg)	Midpoint Time (mg/hr)	Rate of Excretion	A.R.E. (mg)(hr)
0 - 0.5	103	103	0.25	206	397
0.5 -1	82	185	0.75	164	315
1 - 2	117	302	1.5	117	198
2 - 4	119	421	3	59.5	79
4 - 8	67	488	6	16.8	12
8 - 12	10	498	10	2.5	2
12 - 24	2	500	18	0.17	-
24 -	-	500			

After giving an IV dose of 500 mg, urine is collected and assayed for drug content. Data collected is time interval versus amount (mg) excreted during the time interval. The cumulative amount excreted is readily calculated.

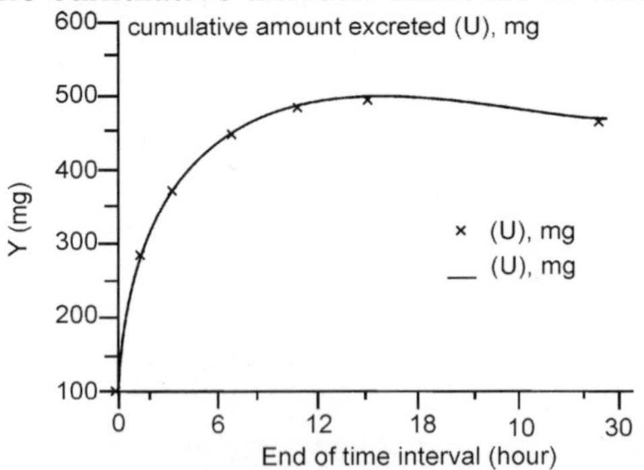

Fig. Plot of Cumulative Amount Excreted versus Time.

The plot shows U rapidly increasing at first then leveling off to U^{∞}. U^{∞} = DOSE for this set of data. Notice that $U^{\infty}/2$ (250 mg) is excreted in about $1_{1/2}$ hours. Otherwise it is a fairly qualitative representation of the data.

We can then calculate the rate of excretion during each time interval. Then the time point is the midpoint time. If we plot $\Delta U/\Delta t$ versus $t_{mid\ point}$ on semi-log graph paper we have the blue squares on the graph paper. As you can see this gives a straight line plot.

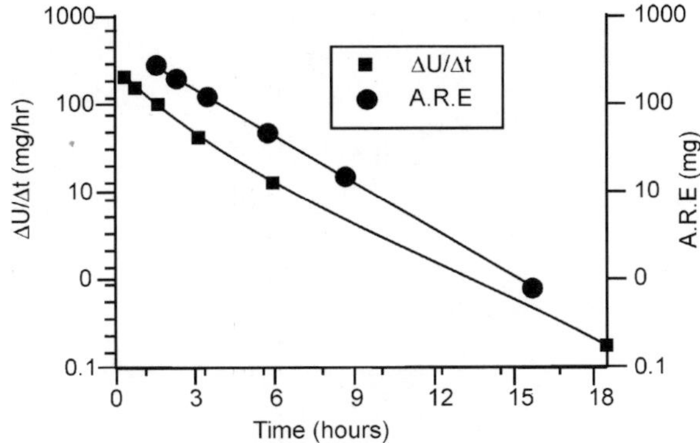

Fig. Plot of Rate of Excretion and A.R.E. versus Time

From the equation before we have:-

Intercept = ln (DOSE * kel)

Slope = - kel

$$-\frac{\text{In}228 - \text{In}10}{0-7.1}$$

$$\frac{5.429 - 2.303}{7.1} = -0.440^{\text{hr}^{-1}}$$

$$\text{kel} = 0.440 \text{ hr}^{-1} \ (t_{1/2} = 1.58 \text{ hr})$$

Consequently with this plot we can estimate kel and $t_{1/2}$. A disadvantage of this type of plot is that the error present in "real" data can obscure the straight line and lead to results which lack precision. Also it can be difficult to collect frequent, accurately timed urine samples. This is especially true when the elimination half-life is small.

Amount Remaining to be Excreted (A.R.E.)

There is a third method of plotting the data which is commonly used. That is the amount remaining to be excreted (A.R.E.) plot.

The equation describing this plot can be derived from the differential equation.

$$\frac{dU}{dt} = \text{kel} \bullet V \bullet Cp$$

(Equation -a)

Since,

$$\text{DOSE} = \text{Amount in body} + \text{Amount eliminated}$$

Thus,

$$\text{DOSE} = V * Cp + U = U^{\infty}$$

U^{∞}, total amount excreted

Then

$$U^{\infty} - U = V.Cp$$

$$\frac{dU}{dt} = kel \bullet \left(U^{\infty} - U\right)$$

Integrating gives:

$$\ln (U^{\infty} - U) = \ln U^{\infty} - kel * t$$

Alternate Derivation:

$$U = U^{\infty} \bullet \left[1 - e^{-kel \bullet t}\right]$$

$$U = U^{\infty} - U^{\infty} \bullet e^{-kel \bullet t}$$

$$U^{\infty} - U = U^{\infty} * e^{-kel * t}$$

$$\ln (U^{\infty} - U) = \ln U^{\infty} - kel * t$$

Thus by plotting ln (U^{∞} - U) versus time we should get a straight line with a slope of - kel. The term (U^{∞} - U) is called the amount remaining to be excreted (A.R.E.). If we subtract U from U^{∞} at each time point we are calculating A.R.E. or (U^{∞} - U). These results are shown as red circles on the semi- log graph paper.

$$\text{Slope} = \frac{\text{In}\,500 - \text{In}\,12.2}{0 - 8}$$

$$= -\frac{6.215 - 2.501}{8} = -0.464\,\text{hr}^{-1}$$

$$kel = 0.464\ \text{hr}^{-1}$$

One disadvantage of this approach is that the errors are cumulative, with collection interval, and the total error is incorporated into the U^{∞} values and therefore into each A.R.E. value. Another problem is that total (all) urine collections are necessary. One missed sample means errors in all the results calculated.

Metabolism and Excretion

So far we have considered elimination by excretion into urine only. Usually drugs are eliminated by excretion and metabolism, with possibly more than one metabolite involved.

Scheme or diagram

Schematically this can be represented as:-

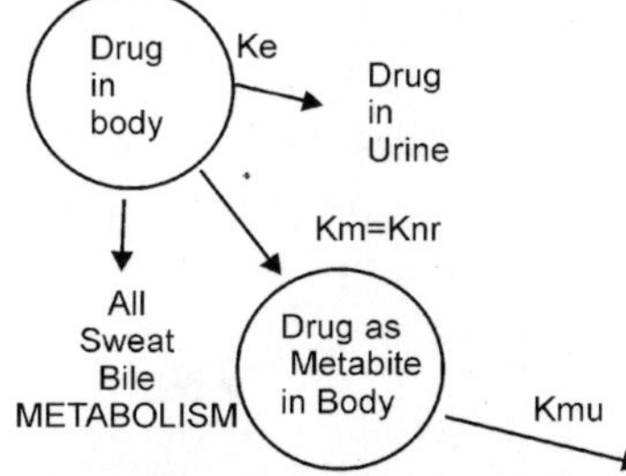

Fig. Schematic for drug eliminated by excretion and metabolism

ke is the excretion rate constant and km is the metabolism rate constant. Here we have two parallel pathways for elimination (with others as a shadow). We can write the differential equations for the three components shown in this Figure. There could be more pathways. It may be appropriate to specify excretion by exhalation, in sweat, or as is commonly the case, more than one metabolite.

Differential Equation

For V*Cp, amount of drug in the body

$$\frac{V \bullet dCp}{dt} = -ke \bullet V \bullet Cp - km \bullet V \bullet Cp$$

$$= -(ke + km) * V * Cp$$

Equation -d. Rate of Change of V x dCp
with terms for excretion and metabolism
and since we call ke + km = kel

$$\frac{V \bullet dCp}{dt} = -kel \bullet V \bullet Cp$$

Equation -e. Rate of Change of V x Cp

This is the same as before with one elimination pathway. The integrated equation will also be exactly the same as before:-

$$V * Cp = DOSE * e^{-kel * t}$$

For U, the amount excreted into urine

$$\frac{dU}{dt} = kel \bullet V \bullet Cp$$

Equation -f. Rate of Change of U versus Time
Notice we have ke here in place of kel
Then substituting for Cp we get

$$\frac{dU}{dt} = ke \bullet DOSE \bullet e^{-kel \bullet t}$$

Equation -g. Rate of Change of U versus Time
after integrating we get

$$U = \frac{ke \bullet DOSE}{kel} \bullet \left[1 - e^{-kel \bullet t}\right]$$

Equation -h. Integration Equation for U versus Time
Again, note: ke is in the numerator of Equation -h and not kel
For M, the amount of drug which has been metabolized the equations are:-

$$\frac{dM}{dt} = km \bullet V \bullet Cp$$

Equation -i. Rate of Change of M versus Time

and

$$M = \frac{ke \bullet DOSE}{kel} \bullet \left[1 - e^{-kel \bullet t}\right]$$

Equation -j. Integration Equation for M versus Time
At

$$t^{\infty} = ; e^{-kel * t} \longrightarrow 0$$

Then

$$U^{\infty} = \frac{ke \bullet DOSE}{kel}$$

Equation -k. Equation for U versus Time
and

$$M^{\infty} = \frac{km \bullet DOSE}{kel}$$

Equation -l Equation for M^{∞} versus Time
Note

$$U^{\infty} + M^{\infty} = DOSE$$

This provides two new parameters, the fraction excreted unchanged in urine, fe, and the fraction metabolized, fm

$$fe = \frac{U^{\infty}}{DOSE} = \frac{ke}{kel}$$

Equation -m. Fraction Excreted as Unchanged Drug

$$fm = \frac{M^{\infty}}{DOSE} = \frac{km}{kel}$$

Equation -m. Fraction Excreted as Metabolite
The plots we did before for U, dU/dt, and A.R.E. have the same significance as before.

Plot Types

Cumulative amount excreted versus time

$$U = \frac{ke \bullet DOSE}{kel} \bullet \left[1 - e^{-kel \bullet t}\right]$$

(Equation -h)

250 200 150 100 50 0
U (fe = 0.75) (mg)
DOSE
U (fe=0.75)
0 6 12 10 30
Time (hour)

Fig. Linear Plot of U versus Time showing Approach to U^{∞} not equal to DOSE.

Rate of Excretion (R/E)

$$\text{In}\left[\frac{dU}{dt}\right] = \text{in}(ke \bullet DOSE) - kel \bullet t$$

Equation. Natural log of Rate of Excretion versus Time
Note: ke * DOSE not kel * DOSE

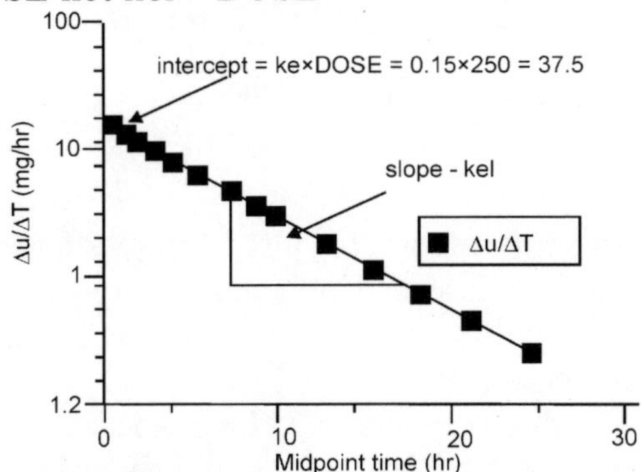

Fig. Semi-log Plot of DU/Dt versus $\text{Time}_{midpoint}$ Showing Slope = - kel with fe = 0.75, kel = 0.2 hr^{-1}; ke = 0.15 hr^{-1}

Amount Remaining to be Excreted (A.R.E.)

$$U = \frac{ke \bullet DOSE}{Kel} \bullet \left[1 - e^{-kel \bullet t}\right]$$

(Equation -h)

$$= U^{\infty} - U^{\infty} * e^{-kel * t}$$

$$(U^{\infty} - U) = U^{\infty} * e^{-kel * t}$$

then

$$\ln (U^{\infty} - U) = \ln U^{\infty} - kel * t$$

$$U^{\infty} = \frac{ke \bullet DOSE}{Kel} = fe \bullet DOSE$$

Note ke
Thus,

$$(U^{\infty} - U) = \ln(fe \bullet Dose) - kel \bullet t$$

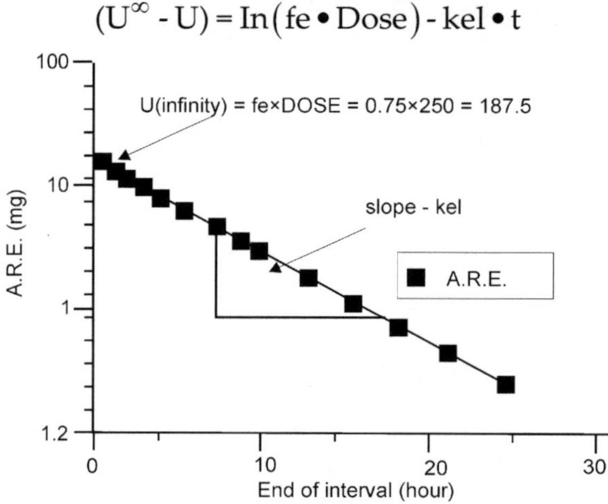

Fig. Semi-Log Plot of A.R.E. versus Time

Fraction Excreted or Metabolized, fe or fm

Renal Function

We can now use this information to start to understand dosage adjustments for patients with poor kidney function. These patients will have reduced ability to excrete some drugs. That is the ke value for a drug will be lower in these patients than in normal patients.

Depending on the value of fe this may have a large effect on kel or it may be insignificant. Fortunately there are a number of clinical tests for renal function which can be used.

One common one is creatinine clearance. Creatinine is formed in the body and is excreted almost entirely by filtration in the kidney. The normal creatinine clearance value is similar to the glomerular filtration rate of 120 to 130 ml/min. We can measure the CLCr prior to drug treatment and adjust the dosage accordingly.

For example. Vancomycin fe = 0.95 (Dose 500 mg; V = 33L; Cp^0 = 15 mg/L)

The normal kel = 0.116 hr^{-1} ($t_{1/2}$ = 6 hr)

$$fe = \frac{ke}{kel}$$

Equation -p. Fraction Excreted into Urine

thus

$$ke = fe * kel = 0.95 * 0.116 = 0.110 \ hr^{-1}$$

$$km = fm * kel = 0.05 * 0.116 = 0.006 \ hr^{-1}$$

Now consider a patient with a creatinine clearance of 12 to 13 ml/min. About 1/10 th of the normal kidney function. ke should then be about 1/10 of normal in this patient.

therefore

$$ke^{patient} = 0.011 \ hr^{-1}$$

Now

$$kel^{patient} = ke^{patient} + km$$

probably unchanged

$$= 0.011 + 0.006 \ hr^{-1} = 0.017 \ hr^{-1} \ (t_{1/2} = 41 \ hour)$$

Thus the half-life changes from 6 hours to 41 hours in a patient with impaired renal function. Therefore it takes seven times longer for the body to get rid of half the dose. If repeated doses were given based on a normal half-life the levels in this patient would rapidly reach toxic concentrations.

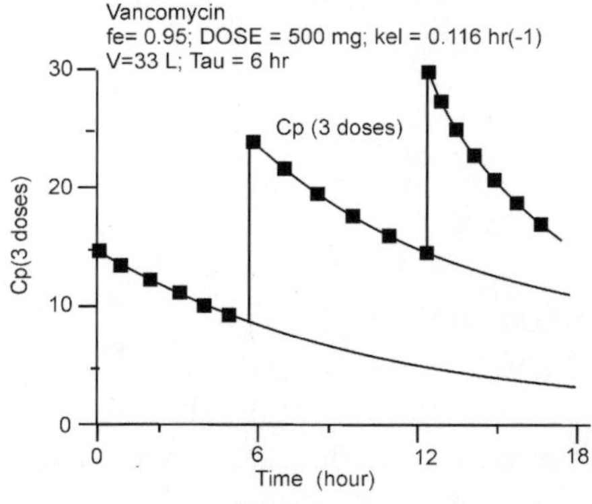

Fig. Plot of Cp versus Time after Multiple Doses in Normal Patient.

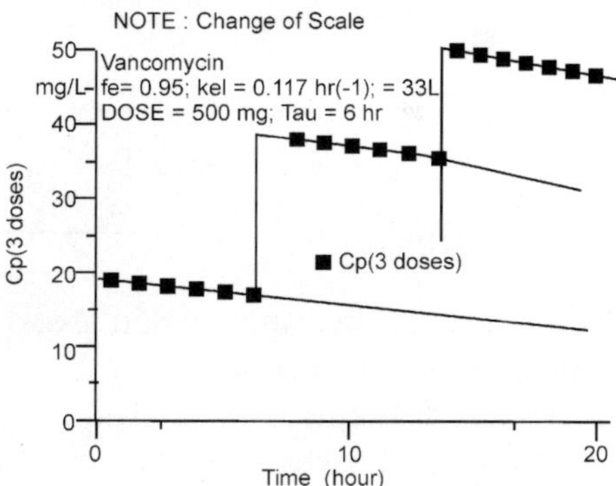

Fig. Plot of Cp versus Time after Multiple Doses.

For another drug such as erythromycin, fe = 0.15 (Dose = 250 mg) the normal kel = 0.58 hr^{-1} ($t_{1/2}$ = 1.2 hr)

$$ke^{normal} = 0.58 \times 0.15 = 0.087 \ hr^{-1}$$

$$km = 0.58 \times 0.85 = 0.493 \text{ hr}^{-1}$$

if the patient ke is reduced by tenth.

$$ke^{patient} = 0.009 \text{ hr}^{-1}$$

$$kel^{patient} = 0.009 + 0.493 = 0.502 \text{ hr}^{-1} \ (t_{1/2} = 1.4 \text{ hr})$$

Thus the half-life changes from 1.2 hour to 1.4 hours.

Clearance, CL

At this point we can define another pharmacokinetic parameter, clearance. Clearance can be defined as the volume of plasma which is completely cleared of drug per unit time. The symbol is CL and the units are ml/min, L/hr, *i.e.* volume per time. Another way of looking at Clearance is to consider the drug being eliminated from the body ONLY via the kidneys. [If we were to also assume that all of the drug that reaches the kidneys is removed from the plasma then we have a situation where the clearance of the drug is equal to the plasma flow rate to the kidneys. All of the plasma reaching the kidneys would be cleared of drug.]

The amount cleared by the body per unit time is dU/dt, the rate of elimination (also the rate of excretion in this example). To calculate the volume which contains that amount we can divide by Cp. That is the volume = amount/ concentration. Thus:-

$$CL = \frac{dU}{dt} \bullet \frac{1}{Cp}$$

Equation -q. Clearance as the Ratio between Rate of Excretion and Cp

Since

$$\frac{dU}{dt} = kel \bullet V \bullet Cp$$

$$CL = \frac{kel \bullet V \bullet Cp}{Cp} = kel \bullet V$$

Equation -r. Clearance calculated from kel and V

As we have defined the term here it is the total body clearance. We have considered that the drug is cleared totally by excretion in urine. Below we will see that the total body clearance can be divided into a clearance due to renal excretion and that due to metabolism.

Clearance is a useful term when talking of drug elimination since it can be related to the efficiency of the organs of elimination and blood flow to the organ of elimination. It is useful in investigating mechanisms of elimination and renal or hepatic function in cases of reduced clearance of test substances. Also the units of clearance, volume/time (*e.g.* ml/min) are easier to visualize, compared with elimination rate constant (units 1/time, *e.g.* 1/hr).

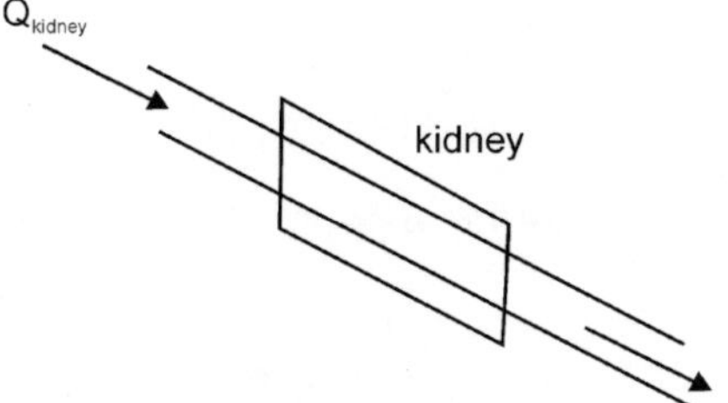

Renal Clearance = Q_{kidney}
if Drug removed totally form blood flowing into kidney
Fig. Representation of Renal Clearance.

Total body clearance, CL, can be separated into clearance due to renal elimination, CLr and clearance due to metabolism, CLm.

$$CLr = ke * V \text{ (renal clearance)}$$

and

$$CLm = km * V \text{ (metabolic clearance)}$$

Note

$$CL = CLr + CLm$$

Another method of calculating CL can be derived
Integrating

$$\frac{dU}{dt} = ke \bullet V \bullet Cp = CL_r \bullet Cp$$

gives

$$U^{\infty} = CL_r \bullet \int_0^{\infty} Cp \bullet dt = CL_r \bullet AUC$$

thus

$$CL_r = \frac{U^{\infty}}{AUC}$$

Equation -s. Renal Clearance calculated from U^{∞} and AUC also

$$CL_m = \frac{M^{\infty}}{AUC}$$

Equation -t. Metabolic Clearance calculated from M^{∞} and AUC
and

$$CL = \frac{DOSE}{AUC}$$

Equation -u. Clearance calculated from Dose and AUC

This equation uses the DATA only (without fitting a line through the data or modeling the data) using the trapezoidal rule. Thus this is a model independent method.

From Equation -q

$$\frac{dU}{dt} = CL \bullet Cp$$

thus a plot of dU/dt versus Cp will give a straight line through the origin with a slope equal to the clearance, CL.

Intravenous Infusion

Commonly in a hospital setting a patient will receive a drug by intravenous infusion. The inconvenience of administering the drug over a long time is not a real problem with bedridden patients. Some may already be receiving intravenous fluids.

If a drug is chemically stable and is compatible with the intravenous fluid it may be added to the fluid and thereby be given by slow infusion. Some drugs cannot be given by rapid intravenous injection. Therefore they may be given by slower IV infusion over 15 or 30 minutes.

Continuous Infusion

Scheme or Diagram

Giving the drug by infusion will alter the kinetics of the drug. Schematically:

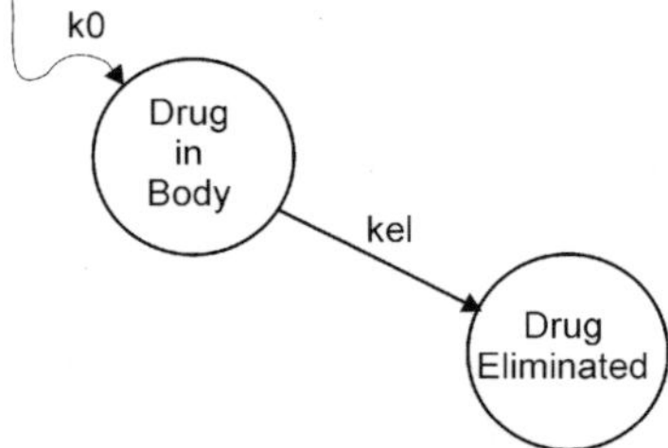

Fig. Scheme for one compartment Intravenous Infusion

Here we have added an infusion rate constant, k0 to the Figure presented earlier. This is a zero order process so the units of k0 would be amount per time; for example 25 mg/min.

Differential and Integrated Equation

The differential equation for V*Cp is then:

$$\frac{V \bullet dCp}{dt} = k0 - V \bullet kel \bullet Cp$$

input positive from infusion

Output negative by elimination

Equation I-1. Differential Equation During an IV Infusion.

This is the differential equation during the infusion period and it can be integrated to give:

$$Cp = \frac{K0}{V \bullet kel}\left[1 - e^{-kel \bullet t}\right]$$

Equation I-2. Integrated Equation for Cp versus Time

Table. Javascript Calculators using Equation I-2.

Calculate Cp Given k0, kel and V at time t		**Calculate k0 required to give Cp at time t**	
Enter your own values into each field		Enter your own values into each field	
Desired Cp (mass/volume)	100		
kel (first order reciprocal time)	10	kel (first order reciprocal time)	k0 (zero order mass/time)
V (volume)	0.15	V (vo lume)	0.15
t (time)	10	t (time)	10
Cp (mass/volume) is:	1	k0 (mass/time) is:	1

You may notice that Equation I-2 for Cp is quite similar to Equation -h we had before for the cumulative amount of drug excreted into urine. As you might expect the plot of Cp would be similar in shape.

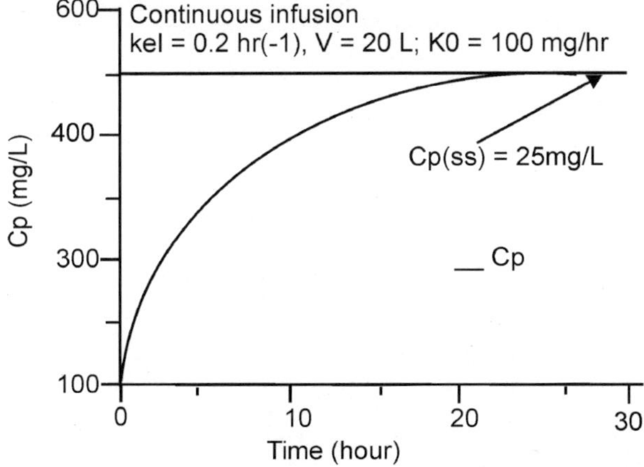

Fig. Linear Plot of Cp versus Time During a Continuous Infusion.

Plasma Concentration versus Time Plots

- Linear
- Semi-log

If we continue the infusion indefinitely then we will approach a steady state plasma concentration when the rate of infusion will be equal to the rate of elimination.

This is because the rate of infusion will be constant whereas the rate of elimination will increase as the plasma concentration increases. At steady state the two rates become equal. We can determine the steady state concentration from the differential equation by setting the rate of change of Cp, *i.e.* dCp/dt = 0.

Then

$$\frac{V \bullet dCp}{dt} = 0 = k0 - kel \bullet V \bullet Cp^{ss}$$

therefore

$$Cp^{ss} = \frac{K0}{kel \bullet V} = \frac{K0}{Cl}$$

Equation I-3. Steady State Concentration after Continuous Infusion

This could also be calculated from the integrated equation by setting $e^{-kel * t} = 0$ at t =.

We can now calculate the infusion rate necessary to produce some desired steady state plasma level. For Example:

A desired steady state plasma level of theophylline maybe 15 mg/L. The average half-life of theophylline is about 4 hr and the apparent volume of distribution is about 25 litre. What infusion rate is necessary? First

$$kel = 0.693/4 = 0.17 \ hr^{-1}$$

then

$$k0 = kel * V * Cp = 0.17 * 25 * 15 = 63.8 \ mg/hr$$

We would probably use an infusion of 60 mg/hr which would produce a Cp^{ss} value given:

$$Cp^{ss} = \frac{K0}{kel \bullet V}$$

$$= \frac{60}{0.17 \bullet 25} = 14.1 mg/L$$

Time to Reach Steady State

Another important factor is the time to reach the steady state concentration. For instance, the time to reach half the steady state can be derived:

Since

$$Cp^{ss} = \frac{K0}{kel \bullet V}$$

(see Equation I-3)

and

$$Cp = \frac{Cp^{ss}}{2} = Cp^{ss} \bullet \left[1 - e^{-kel \bullet t_{HALF}}\right]$$

then

$$Cp = \frac{Cp^{ss}}{2} = Cp^{ss} \bullet \left[1 - e^{-kel \bullet t_{HALF}}\right]$$

$$\frac{1}{2} - 1 = e^{-kel \bullet t_{HALF}}$$

or

$$e^{kel * t_{HALF}} = 2$$

taking the antilog of both sides

$$kel * t_{HALF} = \ln 2 = 0.693$$

Thus

$$t_{HALF} = 0.693/kel = t_{1/2} \text{ for elimination}$$

Thus the approach to Cp^{ss} is exponential in nature and is controlled by the elimination process NOT the infusion process. NOTE however that the value of Cp^{ss} IS controlled by k0.

Halfway	**to steady state**	**in**	**one**	**half-life**
75per cent	"	"	2	"
87.5per cent	"	"	3	"
94per cent	"	"	4	"

For theophylline with a $t_{1/2}$ equal to 4 hours the time to reach 94per cent of steady state will be 16 hours. We could calculate how long it might take to reach a therapeutic concentration. For theophylline this might be 10 mg/L

Thus

$$Cp = \frac{k0}{v \bullet kel}\left[1 - e^{-kel \bullet t}\right]$$

(see Equation I-2)

Using the values from before

k0 = 60 mg/hr; kel = 0.17 hr^{-1}; V = 25 L; and Crequired = 10 mg/L

$$10 = \frac{60}{0.17 \bullet 25} \bullet \left[1 - e^{-0.17 \bullet t}\right]$$

$$0.708 = 1 - e^{-0.17 * t}$$

thus

$$0.292 = e^{-0.17 * t}$$

therefore

$$-0.17 * t = -1.231 \text{ or } t = 7.24 \text{ hr}$$

Thus if we started an infusion to achieve a steady state plasma concentration of approximately 15 mg/L (actually 14.1 mg/L) it would take 7.25 hours to reach a therapeutic level.

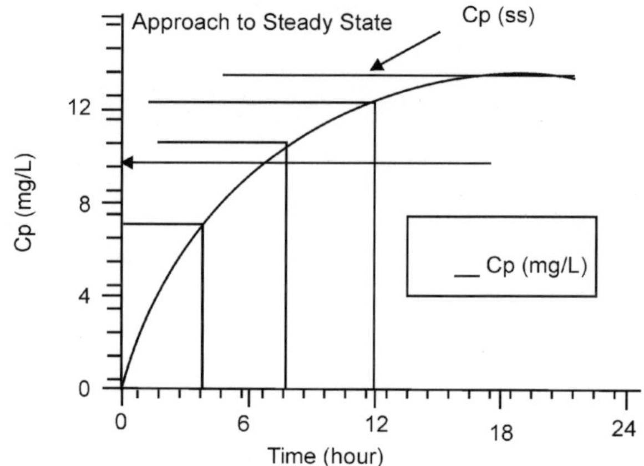

Fig. Plot of Cp versus Time showing Approach to Steady State

Combined Infusion and Bolus Administration

One reason we give a drug by IV infusion of course is because we need a quick therapeutic response.

One way to achieve a therapeutic concentration more quickly is to give a loading dose by rapid intravenous injection and then start the slower maintenance infusion. For Drugs which can be given as a bolus:-

For example, theophylline again.

To achieve Cp^{ss} = 14.1 mg/L; k0 = 60 mg/hr; V = 25 L; kel = 0.17 hr^{-1}.

A loading dose can be calculated from

$$Cp^0 = \frac{DOSE}{V}$$

(Equation I-4)

thus

$$DOSE = V * Cp^0 = 25 \text{ x } 14.1 = 353 \text{ mg}$$

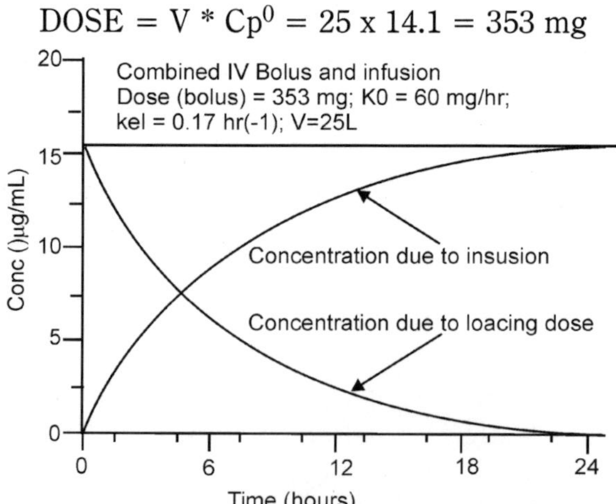

Fig. Linear Plot of Cp versus Time Showing Bolus, Infusion, and ombined Curves

Combined Slow and Fast Infusion

Alternately we can give a loading dose by rapid infusion and then give a slower maintenance infusion once the plateau concentration is achieved.

For example. Using the previous data

For theophylline, kel = 0.17 hr^{-1}; V = 25 L; with a required Cp = 14.1 mg/L

If we wish to give a loading infusion over 30 minutes we need to give the infusion at a rate which will produce Cp = 14.1 mg/L at 30 minutes. Therefore:-

$$Cp^{30\ min} = 14.1\ mg/L$$

$$Cp = \frac{k0}{v \bullet kel}\left[1 - e^{-kel \bullet t}\right]$$

(Equation I-2 above)

$$14.1 = \frac{k0}{0.17 \times 25} \bullet \left[1 - e^{-0.17 \times 0.5}\right]$$

thus

$$k0 = 735\ mg/hr$$

Therefore we need to give a dose of 367 mg over 30 minutes to achieve a plasma concentration of 14.1 mg/L at 30 minutes.

It is important to realise what the steady state plasma concentration would be if we didn't turn this fast infusion off.

$$Cp = \frac{k0}{v \bullet kel} = \frac{735}{0.17 \times 25} = 173 mg/L$$

which would be quite toxic.

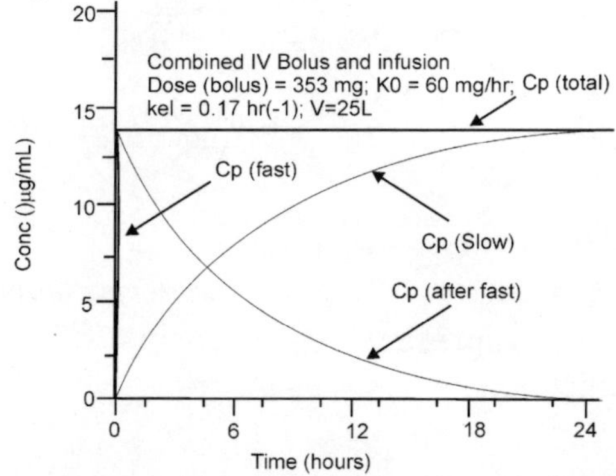

Fig. Linear Plot of Cp versus Time showing Combined and Separate Curves for Both Infusions

Consequently we would need to ensure that at 30 minutes the rapid infusion rate was slowed from 735 mg/hr to 60 mg/hr. One way to do this is to only provide 367 mg (or 360 mg) in the infusion syringe at first.

The dosing regimen (or controlled sequence of drug administration) to achieve the desired plasma concentration is:-

- A loading dose by IV infusion of 367 mg/30 minutes followed by
- A maintenance IV infusion of 60 mg/hr

Post infusion

Before moving on to discussing various routes of drug administration, we can look at the equation for plasma concentration after an infusion is stopped.

Remember that the equation for plasma concentration versus time during an IV infusion is:-

$$Cp = \frac{k0}{v \bullet kel} = \left[1 - e^{-kel \bullet 1}\right]$$

(Equation I-2 from earlier)

If the infusion is continued indefinitely then the plasma concentration approaches a steady state plasma concentration.

$$Cp^{ss} = \frac{K0}{kel \bullet V}$$

(Equation I-3 from earlier)

If however the infusion is stopped the plasma concentration can be expected to fall.

Scheme or Diagram

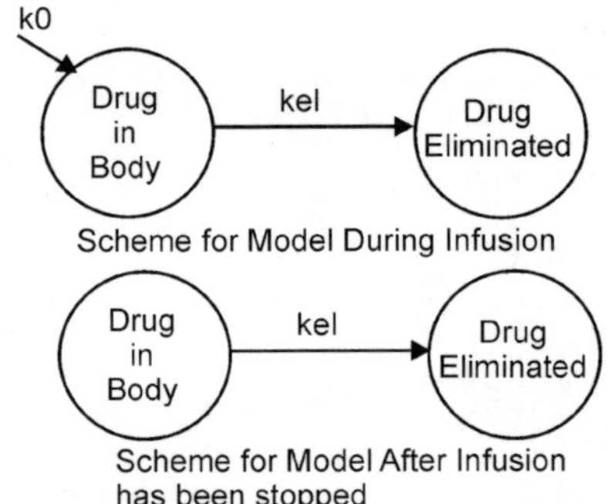

Fig. During and After an IV Infusion - One Compartment Model

The scheme shown to represent 'after the infusion is stopped' is the same as that for the bolus injection.

Equations

The equation for Cp versus time is shown above. At the end of the infusion period when t = T the plasma concentration can be calculated as:-

$$Cp^{T} = \frac{k0}{kel \bullet V} \bullet \left[1 - e^{-kel \bullet T}\right]$$

Equation I-5. Concentration at the End of an IV Infusion

Once the infusion is stopped all we have is a first order elimination.

Then

$$Cp^t = Cp^T \bullet e^{-kel \bullet (t-T)}$$

Equation I-6. Concentration after an IV Infusion has Stopped

where t is time counted from the start of the infusion. Then t - T is the time since the end of the infusion. Then

$$Cp^t = \frac{k0}{kel \bullet V} \bullet \left[1 - e^{-kel \bullet T}\right] \bullet e^{-kel \bullet (t-T)}$$

Equation I-7. Concentration during and after an IV Infusion

for

$$t > T$$

If t is less than or equal to T then set T = t. Then the term $e^{-kel * (t-T)}$ becomes = 1 and is not needed.

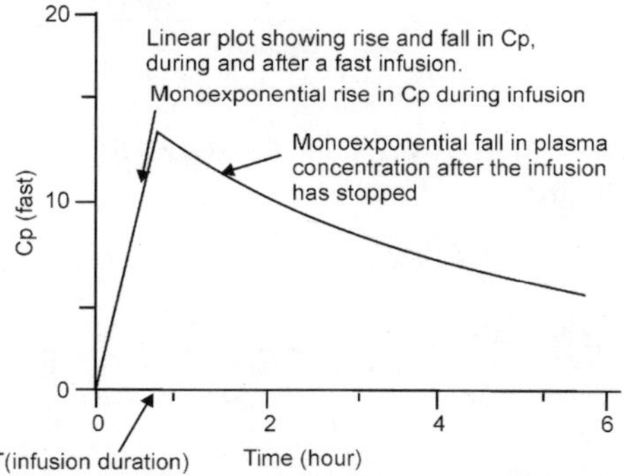

Fig. Linear Plot of Cp versus Time for Interrupted Infusion. Showing Monoexponential Rise and Fall

If we use the previous example data, thus V = 25 L; kel = 0.17 hr^{-1}; T = 0.5 hour; and k0 = 735 mg/hr, what would be the plasma concentration be at 4.5 hours (t = 4.5 hours).

That is if we stop the loading infusion and don't start the maintenance infusion.

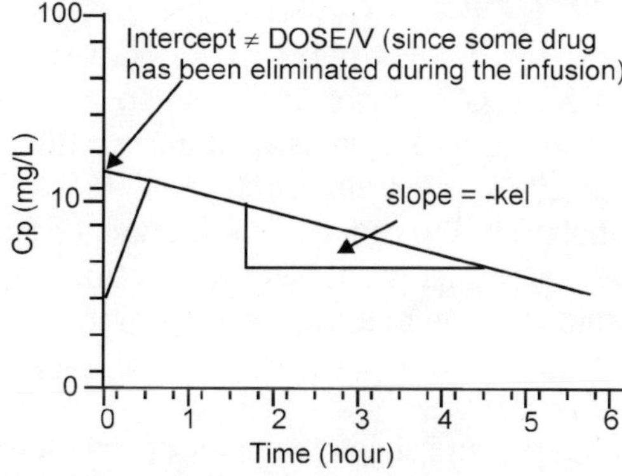

Fig. Semi-log Plot of Cp versus Time. NOTE: Intercept is not Cp^0

Example Calculation: Following a two-hour infusion of 100 mg/hr plasma was collected and analysed for drug concentration. Calculate kel and V.

Time (hr)	3	5	9	12	18	24
Cp (mg/L)	12	9	8	5	3.9	1.7

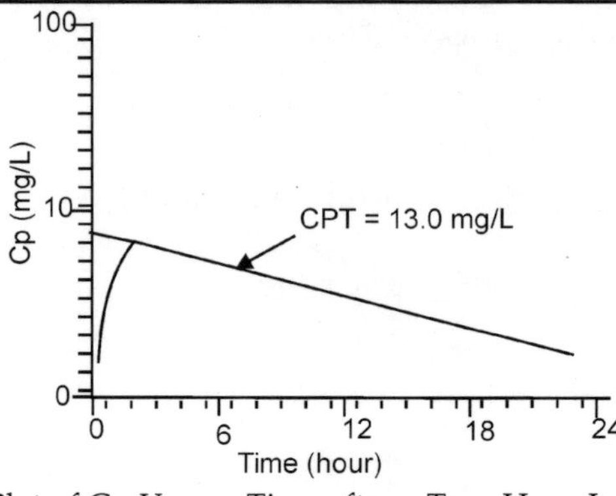

Fig. Plot of Cp Versus Time after a Two-Hour Infusion

The red line drawn through the data points and back to the Y-axis represents the best-fit line.

$$Cp^T = 13.0\, mg/L$$

$$\text{kel} = \frac{\text{In}\,\text{Cp}^1 - \text{In}\,\text{Cp}^2}{t^2 - t^1} = \frac{\text{In}\,13 - \text{In}\,1.9}{24 - 2} = 0.087\,\text{hr}^{-1}$$

$$\text{Cp}^T = \frac{k0}{\text{kel} \bullet V} \bullet \left[1 - e^{\text{kel}\bullet T}\right]$$

$$13 = \frac{100}{0.087 \bullet V} \bullet \left[1 - e^{-0087\bullet 2}\right]$$

$$V = 88.4 \bullet [1 - 0.840] = 14.1\,L$$

Routes of Drug Administration

An alternate method of classifying these routes of administration is ENTERAL and PARENTERAL. Enteral means to do with the GI tract and includes oral, buccal, and rectal. Parenteral means not through the alimentary canal and commonly refers to injections such as IV, IM, and SC; but could also include topical and inhalation. We can also distinguish IV from the rest, as with all others at least one membrane must be crossed, thus an absorption process is involved in the administration and the pharmacokinetics.

Oral

Only some advantages and disadvantages of oral administration will be presented in this Chapter.

Advantages:

- *Convenient:* Portable, no pain, easy to take.
- *Cheap:* No need to sterilize (but must be hygienic of course), compact, multi-dose bottles, automated machines produce tablets in large quantities.
- *Variety*: fast release tablets, capsules, enteric coated, layered tablets, slow release, suspensions, mixtures

Disadvantages:

Sometimes inefficient - high dose or low solubility drugs may suffer poor availability, only part of the dose may be absorbed. Griseofulvin was reformulated about 1970 to include the drug as a micronized powder. The recommended dose at that time was decreased by a factor of two because of the improved bioavailability.

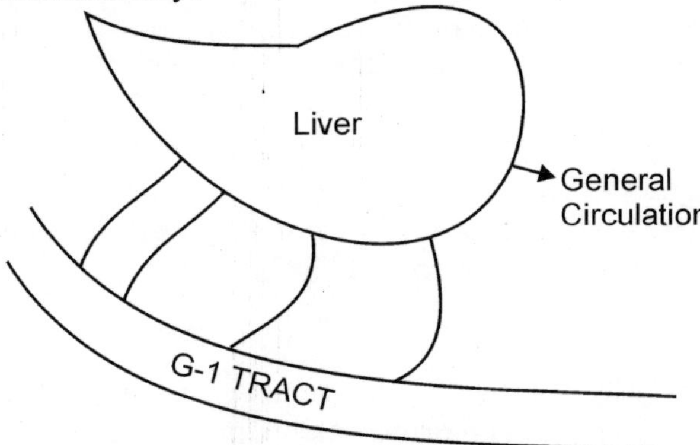

Fig. First Pass Effect

- *First-pass effect:* Drugs absorbed orally are transported to the general circulation via the liver. Thus drugs which are extensively metabolized will be metabolized in the liver during absorption.
  e.g. the propranolol oral dose is somewhat higher than the IV, the same is true for morphine. Both these drugs and many others are extensively metabolized in the liver.
- *Food:* Food and G-I motility can effect drug absorption. Often patient instructions include a direction to take with food or take on an empty stomach. Absorption is slower with food for tetracyclines and penicillins, etc. However, for propranolol bioavailability is higher after food, and for griseofulvin absorption is higher after a fatty meal.
- *Local effect*: Antibiotics may kill normal gut flora and allow overgrowth of fungal varieties. Thus, antifungal agent may be included with an antibiotic.
- Unconscious patient: Patient must be able to swallow solid dosage forms. Liquids may be given by tube.

Buccal/Sublingual

Some drugs are taken as smaller tablets which are held in the mouth or under the tongue. These are buccal or sublingual dosage forms. Buccal tablets are often harder tablets [4 hour disintegration time], designed to dissolve slowly. Nitroglycerin, as a softer sublingual tablet [2 min disintegration time], may be used for the rapid relief of angina. This ROA is also used for some steroids such as testosterone and oxytocin. Nicotine containing chewing gum may be used for cigarette smoking replacement.

Advantages:

- *First pass*: The liver is by-passed thus there is no loss of drug by first pass effect for buccal administration. Bioavailability is higher.
- *Rapid absorption*: Because of the good blood supply to the area absorption is usually quite rapid.
- *Drug stability*: pH in mouth relatively neutral (cf. stomach - acidic). Thus a drug may be more stable.

Disadvantages:

Holding the dose in the mouth is inconvenient. If any is swallowed that portion must be treated as an oral dose and subject to first pass metabolism. Small doses only can be accommodated easily.

Rectal

Most commonly by suppository or enema. Some drugs given by this route include aspirin, theophylline, chlorpromazine and some barbiturates

Advantages:

- *By-pass liver*: Some of the veins draining the rectum lead directly to the general circulation, thus by-passing the liver. Reduced first-pass effect.
- *Useful*: This route may be most useful for patients unable to take drugs orally or with younger children.

Disadvantages:

Erratic absorption - Absorption is often incomplete and erratic. However for some drugs it is quite useful. There is research being conducted to look at methods of improving the extent and variability of rectal administration. Not well accepted.

Intravenous

Drugs may be given into a peripheral vein over 1 to 2 minutes or longer by infusion. Rapid injections are used to treat epileptic seizures, acute asthma, or cardiac arrhythmias

Advantages:

- *Rapid*: A quick response is possible
- *Total dose*: The whole dose is delivered to the blood stream. Large doses can be given by extending the time of infusion. Veins relatively insensitive - to irritation by irritant drugs at higher concentration in dosage forms.

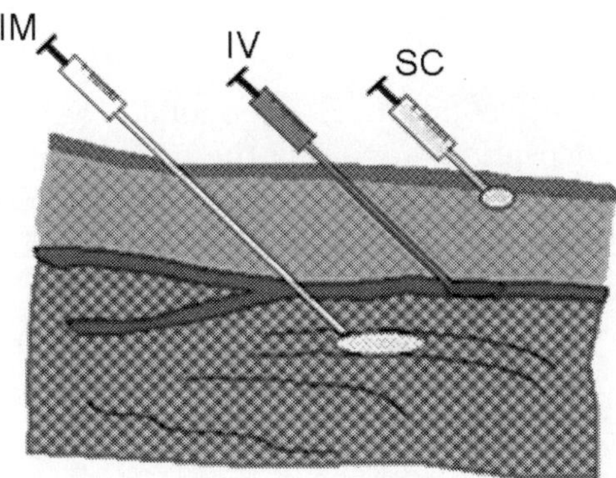

Fig. Showing IV, IM, and SC Injection

Disadvantages:

- *Suitable vein*: It may be difficult to find a suitable vein.
- *Maybe toxic*: Because of the rapid response, toxicity can be a problem with rapid drug administrations, could then give as an infusion, monitoring for toxicity.
- *Requires trained personnel*: Trained personnel are required to give intravenous injections.
- *Expensive*: Sterility, pyrogen testing and larger volume of solvent means greater cost for preparation, transport and storage.

Subcutaneous

This involves administration of the drug dose just under the skin.

Advantages:

- Can be given by patient, *e.g.* in the case of insulin
- Absorption slow but usually complete. Improved by massage or heat. Vasoconstrictor may be added to reduce the absorption of a local anesthetic agent, thereby prolonging its effect at the site of interest.

Disadvantages:

- Can be painful
- Irritant drugs can cause local tissue damage
- Maximum of 2 ml injection thus often small doses limit use.

Intramuscular

Advantages:

- Larger volume, than sc, can be given by IM
- A depot or sustained release effect is possible with IM injections, *e.g.* procaine penicillin

Disadvantages:

- Trained personnel required for injections. The site of injection will influence the absorption, generally the deltoid muscle is the best site
- Absorption is sometimes erratic, especially for poorly soluble drugs, *e.g.* diazepam, phenytoin. The solvent maybe absorbed faster than the drug causing precipitation of the drug at the site of injection.

Inhalation

- *Local effect*: Bronchodilators
- *Systemic effect*: General anesthesia
- Rapid absorption, byPassing the liver

Absorption of gases is relatively efficient, however solids and liquids are excluded if larger than 20 micron and even then only 10 per cent of the dose may be absorbed. Cromolyn is taken as a powder with 50 per cent of the particles within the range of 2 to 6 micron. Larger than 20 micron and the particles impact in the mouth and throat. Smaller than 0.5 micron and they aren't retained.

Topical

- *Local effect*: Eye drops, antiseptic, sunscreen, callous removal, etc.
- *Systemic effect*: *e.g.*, nitroglycerin ointment.

Absorption through the skin, especially via cuts and abrasions but also intact, can be quite marked. This can be a real problem in handling toxic materials in the laboratory or pharmacy.

Other ROA's

Other routes of administration include: intra-nasal, some systemic absorption has been demonstrated for propranolol and some low dose hormones; intra-arterial for cancer chemotherapy to maximize drug concentrations at the tumor site; and intrathecal directly into the cerebrospinal fluid.

Bibliograhy

Alimuddin Khan: *Basics of Thermodynamics*, Anmol Publication, Delhi, 2008.

B.K. Venkanna and B.V. Swati: *Basic Thermodynamics*, PHI Learning, Delhi, 2001.

Donald T. Haynie: *Biological Thermodynamics*, Cambridge University Press, New York, 2003.

G P Garg and M Prakash: *Pharmacokinetics*, Discovery Publishing House, Delhi, 2011.

G. Victor Rajamanickam and U. Subasini: *Pharmacokinetics and Biopharmaceutics*, New Academic Publication, Delhi, 2009.

Gayathri V. Patil and Harpal Singh: *Biopharmaceutics and Pharmacokinetics*, Shree Publication, Delhi, 2009.

Hirschel: *Basics of Aerothermodynamics*, Springer, New York, 2003.

Horsley: *Engineering Thermodynamics*, Springer, New York, 1999.

John G. Wagner: *Pharmacokinetics for the Pharmaceutical Scientist*, Technomic Publication, Delhi, 2008.

Jolles: *Proteomics in Functional Genomics: Protein Structure Analysis*, Springer, New York, 2005.

K K Jain: *Encyclopaedia of Chemical Thermodynamics, Vol. I to III*, Discovery Publishing House, Delhi, 2008.

Kamp: *Protein Structure Analysis: Preparation, Characterization and Microsequencing*, Springer, New York, 1999.

Mahendra R. Awode: *Chemical Thermodynamics (A Treatise on the Application of Thermodynamics of Chemical and Biochemical Systems)*, Dattsons, 2002.

Milo D. Koretsky: *Engineering and chemical Thermodynamics*, Wiley, Delhi, 2001.

Milo Gibaldi: *Biopharmaceutics and Clinical Pharmacokinetics*, Pharma Med Press, Delhi, 2008.

P. Chattopadhyay: *Engineering Thermodynamics*, Oxford University Press, Delhi, 2011.

Praveen Tyagi: *Chemical Thermodynamics*, Discovery Publishing House, Delhi, 2006.

R.K. Singal, Mridul Singal and Rishi Singal: *Engineering Thermodynamics*, I.K. International Publication, Delhi, 2009.

Rahul Gupta: *Engineering Thermodynamics*, Asian Books, Delhi, 2005.

Rajeev K. Prithiani: *Algorithms and Techniques for the Recognition of Various Protein Structures*, Vista International, Delhi, 2010.

Ronald D. Schoenwald: *Pharmacokinetic Principles of Dosing Adjustments : Understanding the Basics*, CRC Press, Delhi, 2011.

S.K. Das Gupta: *Chemical Thermodynamics*, Alp Books, Delhi, 2010.

Safaraz Niazi: *Textbook of Biopharmaceutics and Clinical Pharmacokinetics*, PharmaMed Press, Delhi, 2011.

Schulz: *Principles of Protein Structure*, Springer, New York, 2003.

Stephen H. Curry: *Drug Disposition and Pharmacokinetics With a Consideration of Pharmacological and Clinical Relationships*, PharmaMed Press, Delhi, 2008.

Suresh Bandari, Vijay Kumar Nagabandi and Raju Jukanti: *Experimental Approaches to Biopharmaceutics and Pharmacokinetics*, PharmaMed Press, Delhi, 2013.

Udai Veer: *Encyclopaedia of Thermodynamics (2 Vols-Set)*, Anmol Publication, Delhi, 2006.

V. Venkateswarlu: *Biopharmaceutics and Pharmacokinetics*, PharmaMed Press, Delhi, 2010.

Index

L

M

N

O

P

R

S

T

U

V